Understanding Laboratory Investigations

A text for nurses and health care professionals

Chris Higgins MSc FIBMS DMLM

Blackwell
Science

© 2000 by
Blackwell Science Ltd
Editorial Offices:
Osney Mead, Oxford OX2 0EL
25 John Street, London WC1N 2BL
23 Ainslie Place, Edinburgh EH3 6AJ
350 Main Street, Malden
  MA 02148 5018, USA
54 University Street, Carlton
  Victoria 3053, Australia
10, rue Casimir Delavigne
  75006 Paris, France

Other Editorial Offices:

Blackwell Wissenschafts-Verlag GmbH
Kurfürstendamm 57
10707 Berlin, Germany

Blackwell Science KK
MG Kodenmacho Building
7–10 Kodenmacho Nihombashi
Chuo-ku, Tokyo 104, Japan

The right of the Author to be identified as
the Author of this Work has been asserted
in accordance with the Copyright, Designs
and Patents Act 1988

First published 2000
Set in 10/12½ pt Century Book
by DP Photosetting, Aylesbury, Bucks
Printed and bound in Great Britain at
the Alden Press, Oxford and Northampton

The Blackwell Science logo is a
trade mark of Blackwell Science Ltd,
registered at the United Kingdom
Trade Marks Registry

DISTRIBUTORS

Marston Book Services Ltd
PO Box 269
Abingdon
Oxon OX14 4YN
(*Orders:* Tel: 01235 465500
         Fax: 01235 465555)

USA
Blackwell Science, Inc.
Commerce Place
350 Main Street
Malden, MA 02148 5018
(*Orders:* Tel: 800 759 6102
               781 388 8250
         Fax: 781 388 8255)

Canada
Login Brothers Book Company
324 Saulteaux Crescent
Winnipeg, Manitoba R3J 3T2
(*Orders:* Tel: 204 837 2987
         Fax: 204 837 3116)

Australia
Blackwell Science Pty Ltd
54 University Street
Carlton, Victoria 3053
(*Orders:* Tel: 03 9347-0300
         Fax: 03 9347-5001)

A catalogue record for this title
is available from the British Library

ISBN 0–632–04245–1

Library of Congress
Cataloging-in-Publication Data
is available

For further information on
Blackwell Science, visit our website:
www.blackwell-science.com

For Mary, Tom and Jon

Contents

Preface

The purpose of this book is to help nurses to understand better how the work of clinical laboratories contributes to patient care. It answers the following questions:

- Why is this test being ordered on my patient?
- What sort of sample is required?
- How is that sample obtained? And most importantly:
- What is the significance of the test result for my patient?

Answers to these questions must be based on an understanding of basic science. Care has been taken to introduce this science, which includes some basic biochemistry, physiology and anatomy, in a way which is accessible to all those with an interest in how the body works. Much will be familiar to nurses.

The format of the book is simple. After two introductory chapters (one of which emphasises the role of nursing staff in the process of laboratory testing), each chapter is devoted to consideration of a single test or group of related tests. Each of these chapters begins with some relevant biochemistry, physiology or anatomy to put the substance being measured (i.e. the test) in some physiological context. A consideration of the sample requirements for the test follows, and finally interpretation of the test results. Wherever possible patient pathology, symptoms and test results are related. A mock case history is included at the end of each chapter to illustrate the practical clinical use of the test being discussed and give a human face to the science.

It is not possible in a book of this size to discuss all of the tests performed in clinical laboratories in this degree of detail, so it has been necessary to be selective. The tests discussed are the most commonly requested, and those which nurses are most likely to encounter. Taken together the tests discussed in this book account for around 70–80% of the total workload of clinical laboratories in the average district general hospital.

Although the primary audience for this book is nursing staff, it should be of interest to other health care workers and also students of biomedical sciences interested in pursuing a career in laboratory medicine.

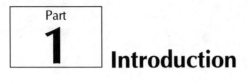

Part 1

Introduction

Chapter 1

Introduction to Clinical Laboratories

Patients may be subjected to many investigative procedures. These range in complexity from ward- or clinic-based measurements familiar to all nurses such as determining body temperature, pulse and blood pressure, through monitoring of heart function by electrocardiographic (ECG) machines, to highly sophisticated body imaging techniques such as X-ray and computed tomography (CT) scan. All of these require the presence of the patient; they are performed on the patient, if not by nurses, at least often in their presence.

In contrast, all the investigations described in this book are performed on samples removed from the patient. The remoteness of the patient from the site of laboratory testing helps to engender the understandable, though misguided, perception that laboratory testing has little to do with nursing care and therefore need not concern nurses. In fact there are several reasons why it is important for nursing staff to understand the work of clinical laboratories.

Nurses are in a unique position to satisfy the need that many patients express for information about the tests to which they are subjected (Fig. 1.1). This need may be to allay fears and anxieties for those who have never undergone such a test before, or it may simply reflect a right to know. Most laboratory tests are only minimally invasive but can only be done with a patient's informed consent. Of course, many patients will express no interest, but some have many questions which must be addressed.

Nurses often have responsibility for the collection and timely, safe transport of specimens. It is vital that anyone collecting samples is aware of the importance of good practice during this pretesting phase. There are some blood and urine tests (e.g. blood glucose testing and urine dipstick testing) which are performed in a ward or clinic setting by nurses. The pitfalls, limitations and clinical significance of such testing have to be appreciated by those performing these investigations. The development of technology has allowed the introduction of chemical analysers into intensive care units. This trend to 'near patient testing' is likely to continue, with more nurses becoming involved in the analytical process.

Nurses are frequently involved in the documentation of laboratory results. It is important that they are familiar with the terminology and format of laboratory reports and are able to identify abnormal results, particularly those which warrant immediate clinical intervention. Traditionally the clinical interpretation of test results has been the responsibility of doctors, but the developing role of the clinical nurse specialist may well necessitate more nurses becoming involved in this process. In any case nursing staff need to know what impact laboratory test results have for the formulation of nursing care plans.

Finally there are those nurses whose professional role involves unusually close co-operation with laboratory workers. These include haematology nurse specialists, infection control nurses and diabetic nurse specialists.

All the tests described in this book are performed in clinical pathology laboratories.

The final part of this introductory chapter serves to describe in outline the work of the five sub-disciplines of clinical pathology and the range of patient types and samples tested (Table 1.1).

The clinical chemistry laboratory

Clinical chemistry (also known as chemical pathology, clinical biochemistry) is concerned with the diagnosis and monitoring of disease by measuring the concentration of chemicals, principally in blood and in urine. Occasionally, chemical analysis of faeces and other body fluids, for example cerebrospinal and pleural fluid, is useful. Blood is a chemically complex fluid containing many inorganic ions, proteins, hormones, enzymes, carbohydrates and lipids, along with two dissolved gases, oxygen and carbon dioxide. In health the blood concentration of each substance is maintained within limits which reflect normal whole body and cellular metabolism. However, disease is often associated with one or more disturbances in this delicate balance of blood chemistry; it is this general principle which underlies the importance of chemical testing of blood in the diagnostic process. The range of pathologies in which chemical testing of blood and urine has proven diagnostically useful is diverse and includes disease of the kidney, liver, heart, lungs and endocrine system. Some cancer cells release chemical substances into blood. Measurement of these so-called tumour markers allows a

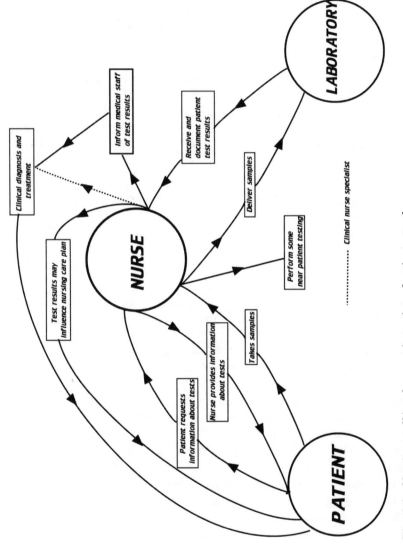

Fig. 1.1 Nursing staff involvement in testing of patient samples.

Table 1.1 Range of samples useful for laboratory investigation.

	Sample type

Chemical analysis	Usually blood or urine
	Less commonly:
	  Faeces
	  Cerebrospinal fluid (CSF): the fluid which surrounds the brain and spinal cord
	  Pleural fluid: the abnormal accumulation of fluid in the pleural cavity of the lungs
	  Ascitic fluid: abnormal fluid which accumulates in the peritoneal cavity

Haematological analysis	Usually blood only Occasionally bone marrow biopsy also useful

Microbiological analysis	Urine, blood, faeces, sputum. Swabs from almost any accessible site including nose, throat, eye, ear, wounds, vagina, etc.
	Less commonly:
	  Cerebrospinal fluid
	  Pleural fluid
	  Skin scrapings
	  Nails
	  Vomit

Histopathological examination	Tissue specimens only
Cytopathological	Cells recovered by scraping the surface of tissues (e.g. cervix) or aspirating abnormal fluids (e.g. cysts) Also urine and sputum are useful
Immunological analysis	Usually blood only

limited role for the clinical chemistry laboratory in the diagnosis and monitoring of malignant disease. Nutritional deficiencies can be identified by chemical analysis of blood.

In addition to its diagnostic role, clinical chemistry is also involved in the monitoring of treatment. This role is most evident among patients receiving intravenous fluid replacement therapy or parenteral nutrition, who require regular monitoring of some aspects of blood chemistry. The blood concentration of some drugs must be monitored to ensure maximum therapeutic effect and minimum toxicity.

Most chemical testing of blood and urine is performed on highly sophisticated, automated machinery. A typical modern clinical chemistry analyser can process around 200–400 samples an hour with the option to perform up to 20 or more tests on each sample. Results of the most commonly requested tests are usually available within 24 hours of receipt of the specimen. Some more specialised tests are performed only once a week. All laboratories offer an urgent 24-hour-a-day service for a limited range of tests; results of such urgently requested tests are usually available within an hour. Intensive care patients often require frequent and urgent monitoring of some aspects of blood chemistry. In these circumstances limited blood testing is performed by nursing staff using dedicated analysers sited within intensive care units.

The haematology laboratory

Haematology is concerned principally with the investigation and monitoring of diseases which affect the number, size and appearance of the cellular or formed elements of blood. These are red blood cells (erythrocytes), white blood cells (leucocytes) and platelets. The full blood count (FBC) is the most frequently requested laboratory test, reflecting the range of common and less-common disorders which affect both the numbers and appearance of these cells. It is in fact not one but a battery of tests.

The modern haematology analyser is able to process FBC tests at the rate of 100 samples per hour. The detailed information about the blood cells which these analysers provide has dramatically reduced the number of specimens which need to be examined under the microscope, but the microscope remains an essential tool to the haematologist for examination of bone marrow biopsy specimens and in some circumstances blood. Apart from the cells in blood, haematology is also concerned with measurement of the concentration of some of the proteins present in blood which are involved in the process of blood coagulation.

Disorders of the blood in which haematology testing is important include haematological malignancy (e.g. the leukaemias, Hodgkin's disease, myeloma), anaemia, and diseases such as haemophilia in which disturbances of blood coagulation result in an increased tendency to bleed. Some haematology tests including the FBC are useful in the diagnosis or clinical management of some common, non-haematological diseases. For example, infectious disease is usually associated with an increase in the number of white blood cells. Anaemia is often a feature of many chronic inflammatory disorders such as rheumatoid arthritis or may result from diseases of nutritional deficiency.

Many patients at risk of heart and blood vessel disease are given tablets which tend to prevent the blood from clotting. This anticoagulation therapy must be monitored by regular blood testing to prevent excessive bleeding, a potentially dangerous side effect of such therapy.

Most haematology test results are routinely available within 12–24 hours. However, if the need is clinically justified, results of some haematology tests can be made available within an hour or so, at any time of the day or night.

The clinical microbiology laboratory

Clinical microbiology is concerned with the diagnosis of disease caused by infective agents, mostly bacteria, but also viruses, fungi and parasitic worms. Most of the work involves the isolation and identification of bacteria from many sorts of sample, including urine, sputum, faeces, blood, cerebrospinal fluid and swabs taken from a variety of infected sites. Bacteria can sometimes be seen by examining these specimens under the microscope, but more precise identification can only be made after culture (growth of bacteria on nutrient-enriched media). One of the problems encountered by the microbiologist dealing with clinical specimens is that many sorts of bacteria are normally present in many sites around the body; indeed in some cases they are essential for normal health. The microbiologist must isolate those that are pathogenic (i.e. cause disease) from those that may normally be present, and from any bacterial contaminant introduced during sample collection. Some body fluids are normally sterile; these include blood, cerebrospinal fluid, and fluid aspirated from joints and the pleural cavity. Bacteria isolated from these sites are always pathogenic. Having isolated and identified the species or strain of pathogenic bacterium, the next step is to test the sensitivity of the organism to a range of antibiotics. This information helps in deciding which antibiotic therapy is likely to be most effective in eradicating the infection.

Blood testing plays a limited but important and evolving role in detecting infections caused by organisms which are difficult to isolate by culture. During any infection the immune system produces antibodies directed at specific antigens present on the surface of the invading organism. A rising amount of the antibody in blood provides evidence of current infection. The specific antigens present on the surface of organisms also provide a means of identifying infective agents. Testing blood for the presence of viral antigens is an important means of diagnosing viral infections such as those which cause hepatitis and AIDS.

Microbiological investigation may take from several days to several weeks to complete; this delay is governed largely by the speed of bacterial growth in culture. Initial microscopical examination can be made immediately on receipt of the specimen and results can usually be made available on the day the sample is received in an interim report.

Microbiology laboratories operate a 24-hour service for the rare cases when urgent culture and microscopical examination of samples are necessary. These include suspected cases of immediate life-threatening infections of blood (septicaemia) and the central nervous system (meningitis).

Quite apart from its diagnostic role, hospital microbiology laboratories play an important role with infection control nurses in the monitoring and prevention of nosocomial infectious disease, that is, infectious disease acquired by patients whilst in hospital – a growing problem.

The blood transfusion laboratory

Blood transfusion is concerned with the provision of a safe supply of blood and blood products. In contrast to other pathology departments, blood transfusion has a limited diagnostic function. In some senses its function more resembles a pharmacy in that its main purpose is to supply therapeutic products. With the possible exception of very severe blood loss involving more than half the total blood volume, the transfusion of whole blood is rarely necessary. The most frequently needed blood product is red cells, to correct anaemia and to replace blood lost during surgery or as a result of trauma. Much less commonly, the white cells of blood, platelets and the proteins present in plasma are therapeutically useful.

The National Blood Service (NBS) is responsible for the collection and supply of safe, donated blood to hospital blood transfusion laboratories. Here each donated unit of blood must be tested for compatibility with the patient's blood before it can be transfused. The transfusion of incompatible blood can have very serious health consequences and is potentially fatal. Advances in compatibility testing have ensured that compatible blood can be made available for transfusion usually well within an hour of a patient's blood sample arriving in the laboratory; this service is available 24 hours a day.

Blood transfusion departments also have an important specific diagnostic role for some forms of haemolytic anaemia, in which the body produces antibodies against its own red cells. One important aspect of this work is haemolytic disease of the newborn, a potentially fatal condition in which the red cells of the developing foetus are destroyed by antibodies present in the mother's blood. All pregnant women are tested for the presence of such antibodies.

The histopathology laboratory

Histopathology (also known as morbid anatomy or cellular pathology) is the oldest of all the five disciplines and is concerned with the diagnosis of disease by microscopical examination of tissue samples (biopsies). The rationale for this approach is that disease processes, e.g. malignancy, inflammation, infection, etc., are characterised by specific changes at the tissue and cellular level which are evident when viewed under the microscope. There are many ways of recovering tissue samples from the body. Tissues from the gastrointestinal tract, lungs and urinary tract are commonly sampled at the time of endoscopic examination. An endoscope is an instrument used to visually examine internal organs directly by fibre optics. The instrument includes small forceps which can be used to remove small pieces of tissue during the examination. Tissue may be taken during surgery by incision or excision biopsy. Incision biopsy is the removal of a sample cut from an area of diseased tissue, whereas excision biopsy involves removal of the whole area of diseased tissue.

Before transport to the laboratory, biopsy specimens must be 'fixed' in a chemical fixative, usually formalin, to preserve structure. This process can take from a few hours to a whole day depending on the size of the specimen. In the laboratory, 'fixed' specimens are impregnated with paraffin wax, allowed to harden and then cut into very thin sections just 3–5 μm thick. These wafer-thin sections are then mounted on glass microscope slides and stained with chemicals before examination under the microscope. The whole process from reception of specimen to issue of a histopathological report can take from one to three or four days depending on the size of the biopsy sample. Sometimes it is important to make a diagnosis very quickly, and in these circumstances a frozen section is performed. Tissue is 'fixed' immediately by freezing. This process allows sections to be cut almost immediately the sample is removed from the patient. The sections are stained and examined under the microscope. This rapid technique allows a diagnosis of, for example, breast cancer to be made in a half an hour or so whilst the patient remains anaesthetised on the operating table. Armed with a laboratory report, the surgeon can proceed immediately to surgical treatment if a malignancy is discovered.

Microscopical examination of tissue removed from the patient is probably most widely used in the diagnosis and staging of malignant disease in organs throughout the body. It is also used in the differential diagnosis of non-malignant disease of the liver, kidney, lungs and gastrointestinal tract. It has a role in the diagnosis of disorders of the connective tissue and skin. More recently it has been used in the early diagnosis of tissue rejection among patients who have received transplanted organs.

Clearly all histopathological tests are invasive, often requiring surgical intervention to recover samples. Both financial and patient safety consideration ensure that, unlike other laboratory investigations, histopathological investigations are usually reserved for those patients in whom there is a strong suspicion of serious disease.

Finally post-mortem examinations, that is, the examination of bodies and tissues removed from bodies to determine the exact cause of death, are conducted in the histopathology department.

Cytopathology

This is a sub-discipline of histopathology. It involves recovery of individual cells for microscopical examination rather than tissue samples. Sample recovery is less invasive than that required for histopathological investigation. Typically cells are scraped from the surface of organs such as the cervix of the uterus, and the mucosal surface of the duodenum, stomach and lungs. Cells can also be recovered by aspiration using a fine needle and syringe, from the pleural and peritoneal cavities, or from solid tumours, for example in the breast. The cells are spread on to a glass microscope slide, fixed and stained and then examined under the microscope. Cytopathology is almost exclusively concerned with diagnosis of pre-malignant and malignant disease. The cervical smear test, used to screen women for cervical cancer, accounts for a large proportion of the workload of the cytopathology laboratory.

The immunology laboratory

Immunology is concerned principally with blood testing for the diagnosis of autoimmune diseases, in which the body's normally protective immune system produces an immune response against itself. One consequence is the production of antibodies against normal tissue. These are called autoantibodies. The detection in blood of organ-specific autoantibodies is helpful in the diagnosis of many diseases with an autoimmune component including some thyroid disorders, pernicious anaemia, and some forms of kidney and liver disease. More rarely, tissues may be microscopically examined for the presence of the complex formed when an autoantibody reacts with its complementary antigen. For example, the autoimmune disease systemic lupus erythematosus (SLE), which affects many organ systems, can be diagnosed by microscopical examination of a skin biopsy for the presence of such complexes.

Laboratory staffing

Clinical laboratories are staffed by biomedical science graduates called medical laboratory scientific officers (MLSOs), alternative title biomedical scientists (BMSs) who are responsible for the analysis of samples. They are helped in this task by medical laboratory assistants (MLAs). Cytoscreeners are a specially trained group whose work is confined largely to the examination of cervical smears. Each pathology department is headed by a medically qualified doctor of consultant status who has specialised in one area of laboratory medicine. In some laboratories this role is filled by non-medically qualified clinical scientists. They provide a consultancy for clinicians on all aspects of laboratory medicine. Thus they might advise both on the most appropriate laboratory investigation in particular cases, and on the clinical significance of test results. Haematology consultants also have clinical responsibility for patients suffering haematological disease (e.g. leukaemia). Consultants attached to clinical chemistry departments are often responsible for the medical care of patients suffering diabetes and other metabolic and endocrine disorders, whilst a microbiology consultant is responsible, with the control of infection nurse, for the formulation and implementation of the hospital's control of infection policy. Histopathological diagnoses are made by a consultant histopathologist who also performs all post-mortem examinations.

Around 85 million pathology test requests are processed annually by around 400 NHS clinical pathology departments in England and Wales[1]. In doing this work pathology laboratories consume around 3.3% of total NHS expenditure[1]. The workload continues to rise at the rate of around 2% per annum. As in all other areas of patient care, successful laboratory investigation depends on team work; nurses are important members of that team. Good communication between nursing and laboratory staff can help to ensure that resources consumed by pathology laboratories are used to best effect for the patient.

References

(1)   Audit Commission (1993) *Critical Path. An Analysis of Pathology Services.* HMSO, London.

Further reading

Kalfayan Y. & Rimmer J. (1996) GP's use of pathology services. *Audit in General Practice* **4**: 10–12.

2 Some Principles of Laboratory Testing

Laboratory investigation of patients can be divided into three distinct phases:

■ the pretesting phase, which includes collection and transport of specimens to the laboratory
■ the analytical phase within the laboratory, and finally
■ the post-testing phase which includes reporting and interpretation of results.

In this second introductory chapter some general principles relating to pretesting procedures are discussed. Then three general topics relating to the post-testing phase are considered. They are: units of measurement, the concept of normal or reference range, and critical values.

Pretesting procedures

It is difficult to overemphasise the importance of good practice during the pretesting phase of laboratory investigation. The production of high quality, accurate results which are clinically useful depends as much on practice before the sample reaches the laboratory as it does on the analytical process within the laboratory. Aspects of the pretesting phase which need to be considered are

■ the pathology request form
■ the timing of sample collection
■ sampling technique
■ collecting the right amount of sample
■ the sample containers and labelling
■ safety during collection and transport of samples.

This chapter is concerned with principles only. The detail of pretesting will be considered again under each test heading. However, it must be remembered that practice, although based on the principles in this book, does vary between laboratories. There is no real substitute for consultation with your local laboratory.

Pathology request form

Each patient sample must be accompanied by the appropriate, fully completed pathology request form, signed by the medical officer making the request or in some instances, where that responsibility has been delegated, by the specialist nurse practitioner. Poor documentation can result at the very least in delay of pathology reports and may result in reports never being filed in patient records. Attention to detail is particularly vital for blood transfusion requests. Most cases of incompatible blood transfusion are the result of documentation errors. All pathology request forms should include the following information set:

- patient details, including full name, date of birth and hospital number
- hospital ward/clinic or GP's surgery
- nature of specimen (e.g. venous blood, urine, biopsy, etc.)
- date and time of sample collection
- name of test requested (e.g. blood glucose, full blood count, etc.)
- clinical details (these should very briefly explain why the test is being requested and may include a suspected or provisional diagnosis or symptoms)
- details of any drug therapy which might affect test or interpretation
- an indication, where relevant, of the urgency of the request
- some health authorities request details about budget cost centres.

Timing of sample collection

Wherever possible, samples should be taken to coincide with routine transport to the laboratory so that they can be processed by the laboratory without undue delay. It is not good practice to leave samples for more than a few hours or overnight before sending them to the laboratory; in many cases the samples will be unsuitable for analysis. For a few biochemical tests, e.g. blood hormone levels, it is vital that blood be sampled at a particular time of the day. For others (e.g. blood glucose) it is simply important to know what time the sample is collected. Some tests (e.g. blood gases) require that samples be processed immediately they are taken. These must be timed by prior agreement with the laboratory. Samples for microbiological investigation are best taken before antibiotic therapy is started, since antibiotics will inhibit the growth of bacteria in culture.

Sample collection technique

Venous blood collection

Most blood tests are performed on venous blood collected by a technique known as venepuncture, using either a needle and syringe or, more commonly these days, an evacuated tube system (Fig. 2.1).

- Patients may be anxious at the prospect of a venepuncture. A calm confident manner is important. Explain in simple terms what is involved and that mild discomfort or pain is usually felt as the needle is inserted.
- If there is a history of fainting during blood collection, take the sample with the patient lying down.
- When performing venepuncture on a patient receiving IV fluids, do not take blood from the arm used for IV administration. This avoids the risk of IV fluid contamination of the sample.
- Haemolysis, the rupture of red cells during blood collection, may render the sample unsuitable for analysis. This may occur if blood is forced at speed through narrow-gauge needles or if the sample is shaken vigorously. When using syringe and needle technique, remove needle before expelling blood into sample container.
- Prolonged use of a tourniquet can affect laboratory results. Avoid the use of a tourniquet if possible and do not collect blood if tourniquet has been in place for more than one minute. Release and try the opposite arm.
- Although the cephalic or basilic vein are the preferred site, the back of the hand or the foot are alternative sites for those with 'difficult' veins.

Capillary blood collection

Capillary blood flows through the fine capillaries just under the skin and can be recovered by a simple puncture with a lancet, usually on the fingertip or, in the case of neonates, the heel of the foot. It is useful if only very small sample volumes are required. The technique can be performed by patients themselves and is routinely used, after training, by diabetics to obtain samples for monitoring their blood glucose concentration.

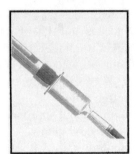

Vacutainer System comprises:
- Sterile, double ended needle
- Needle holder
- Blood collection tube containing a pre-set vacuum

Additional equipment required:
- disposable gloves
- tourniquet
- sterile alcohol-soaked swab
- cotton wool

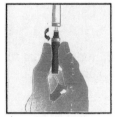

- Hold the coloured section of the needle and break the white paper seal
- Remove and discard the white plastic needle shield. DO NOT USE if paper seal already broken

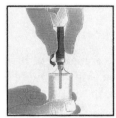

- Screw needle into needle holder and leave coloured shield on needle

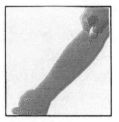

- Apply tourniquet about 10cm above elbow to make veins visible and locate a suitable site for venepuncture.
- Clean site with alcohol soaked swab. Allow to dry.

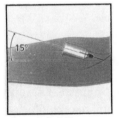

- Remove needle shield
- Ensure patients arm is supported and straight at the elbow.
- Insert needle bevelled side uppermost into the vein

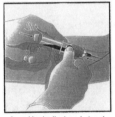

- Insert blood collection tube into the needle-holder
- Ensuring needle does not move within the vein, push tube to the end of needle holder, gently but firmly
- Release tourniquet as blood flows into tube to fill vacuum.

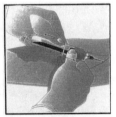

- Withdraw blood collection tube when blood flow ceases
- Continue to hold needle and needle holder in position (For further samples, insert next blood collection tube as before)

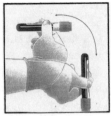

- Withdraw tube from holder
- Invert tube 8–10 times to ensure mixing of blood with any additives in tube

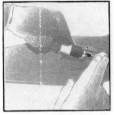

- Withdraw needle holder with needle attached.
- Cover injection site with cotton wool and apply gentle pressure for a minute or two.

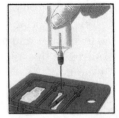

- Dispose of needle and needleholder (if disposable) in accordance with manufacturers instruction local safety policy.
- Label all tubes fully in accordance with local laboratory policy.

Fig. 2.1 Collection of venous blood with Vacutainer® system.

- The fingertip, or heel in the case of babies, is wiped with alcohol. A sterile lancet is used to puncture the cleansed skin on the side of the fingertip or heel. Puncturing the ball of the fingertip is more painful.
- Undue pressure to squeeze blood out can cause inaccurate results; blood must flow freely. Warming of the fingertip or heel before puncturing the skin will encourage free flow.
- Blood should be collected immediately into an appropriate container designated for capillary samples, and mixed gently.
- Pressure must be applied to the puncture site with a sterile gauze until blood flow ceases.

Arterial blood collection

The only test that requires sampling of blood from arteries is that for blood gases. The technique, which is more hazardous and painful than venepuncture, is described in Chapter 6.

Urine collection

Four sorts of urine collection are commonly made,

- a midstream urine (MSU)
- a catheter specimen urine (CSU)
- an early morning urine (EMU) and
- a 24-hour urine, i.e. all the urine passed during a 24-hour period.

The test requested determines which of these is appropriate. For most non-quantitative purposes, such as dipstick testing and microbiological testing, an MSU is necessary. This is a small 10–15 ml sample of urine collected part way through micturition, which can be collected at any time of the day. A CSU is the urine sample collected from a patient who has an indwelling urinary catheter. The detail of collecting an MSU or CSU for microbiological examination is given in Chapter 20.

The first urine passed in the day, the so-called EMU, is the most concentrated and an EMU provides the best method of detecting substances in the urine which are present only in low concentration. An example of its use is pregnancy testing. The urine pregnancy test is based on detection of a hormone, human chorionic gonadotrophin (HCG), which is not normally present in urine but is excreted in increasing concentration during the first few months of pregnancy. Early in pregnancy the concentration is so low that unless a concentrated urine (i.e. an EMU) is used, the result may be falsely negative.

Sometimes it is useful to know on a daily basis exactly how much of a particular substance (e.g. sodium, potassium) is being lost from the body in urine. Quantitation of this urinary loss can only be made by collecting all the urine passed during a 24-hour period. The detail of collecting a 24-hour urine is provided in Chapter 5.

Sputum, swab collection

All these specimens are destined for microbiological examination and the object is to sample only from infected sites whilst avoiding bacterial contamination from other sites on the body or from the environment. For example, a sputum specimen is intended to reflect the environment of the respiratory tract, not the mouth. Saliva is not sputum. Sputum is best collected first thing in the morning and must be coughed up from deep in the lungs. Washing out the mouth before sampling reduces the risk of salivary contamination.

When collecting throat swabs it is important to ensure that the swab does not come into contact with the tongue or sides of the mouth. This can be avoided by use of a tongue depressor. The swab should be gently rubbed only over the area at the back of the mouth (pharynx) and tonsils, especially inflamed areas.

Wound swabs are obtained by sampling the affected site only, avoiding contact with surrounding normal skin or tissue. When collecting any microbiological specimen it is important to minimise environmental contamination by using aseptic technique and replacing swabs back in sterile containers or transport medium immediately.

Tissue (biopsy) collection

A very brief reference to tissue sampling techniques, necessary for histopathological examination, has already been made (Chapter 1). Such sampling is always the responsibility of doctors and is beyond the scope of this book. Nurses are, however, involved in sampling of cervical cells for the cervical smear test (Chapter 22).

Collecting the right amount of sample

The amount of blood required for laboratory testing is governed largely by local laboratory equipment and is therefore a matter for local laboratory policy. In general, continuing technological advances serve to significantly reduce the amount of blood required for many tests. The comment, 'Insufficient sample – please repeat', recorded on laboratory reports, is now less common than it once was. All laboratories supply a list of tests with the minimum blood volume requirements. Anyone responsible for blood collection must become familiar with this local list. Some blood specimen bottles contain pre-weighed amounts of chemical preservatives and/or anticoagulants which determine the optimum volume of blood which the bottle should contain. This volume is stated on the side of the bottle. Erroneous results may occur if these blood volume instructions are not observed. Whilst the volume of urine collected for MSU and CSU is not critical, it is vital, when collecting 24-hour urines, that all the urine passed in the collection period is collected even if a second collection bottle is required.

In general, the size or amount of sample is important for successful isolation of bacteria. For example, it is more likely that bacteria will be isolated from a large specimen of sputum than from a small specimen. Aspiration of pus with a needle and syringe is more likely to result in isolation of the causative organism than a swab of the pus. Falsely negative blood culture results can occur if insufficient blood is added to culture bottles.

Sample containers

Pathology laboratories supply a bewildering array of sample bottles and containers. Each container has specific uses; it is vital for accurate results that the correct container be used for the test requested. Some blood containers contain chemicals (Table 2.1) either in liquid or powder form.

These chemicals serve two purposes: they prevent the blood from clotting and preserve either blood cell structure or the concentration of some blood constituent. It is important that these chemicals are mixed with the blood sample.

A preservative may be necessary to preserve urine during collection of 24-hour urine. The need for a preservative is determined by the substance in urine to be measured.

All sample containers for microbiological examination, e.g. urine, swabs, blood culture bottles, etc. are sterile and should not be used if seals are broken. Some bacteria will only survive outside the body if preserved in special transport media.

The structure of tissue samples needs to be preserved by 'fixing' the tissue in formalin. Biopsy sample containers contain this preservative.

All sample containers must be fully labelled including patient's full name, date of birth and location of patient (ward, clinic or GP). Laboratories receive many hundreds of specimens every day, which may include specimens from two or more patients with the same name. If results are to find their way back to the correct patient's records, it is vital that specimen labels accurately and fully identify the patient.

Table 2.1 Some common additives present in blood collection tubes.

Ethylene diamine tetraacetate (EDTA)	An anticoagulant which prevents blood from clotting by binding to and effectively removing the calcium present in blood plasma (calcium is required for clotting to occur). EDTA also preserves the structure of blood cells. Present in bottles (usually purple/lavender tops) for full blood count and some other haematology tests
Heparin (present as either the sodium or potassium salt of this acid, i.e. sodium or potassium heparin)	An anticoagulant which prevents blood from clotting by inhibiting the formation of thrombin from prothrombin. Present in bottles (usually dark green or orange tops) for chemistry tests that require blood plasma. The anticoagulant properties of heparin are used therapeutically (p. 245)
Citrate (present as the sodium salt of this acid, i.e. sodium citrate)	An anticoagulant, which prevents blood from clotting by precipitating calcium (similar in action to EDTA). Present in bottles (usually light blue top) reserved for coagulation studies
Oxalate (present as either the sodium or ammonium salt of this acid, i.e. sodium or ammonium oxalate)	An anticoagulant which prevents blood from clotting by precipitating calcium (similar in action to EDTA). Used with sodium fluoride (see below) in bottles specifically for blood glucose estimation (usually yellow or grey tops)
Sodium fluoride	This is an enzyme poison and prevents the continued metabolism of glucose in blood after collection, i.e. it preserves blood glucose concentration. Use with oxalate in bottles specifically for blood glucose (usually yellow or grey tops)

Inadequately labelled specimens may be rejected by the laboratory, resulting in the need for the patient to be retested: an entirely avoidable waste of time and resources to both patient and staff.

Safety during sample collection and transport

All laboratories have a locally written safety policy relating to the safe collection and transport of patient specimens, based on the premise that all patient specimens are potentially hazardous. Anyone involved in sample collection should be familiar with this policy. Among the many hazards which may be present in pathological specimens are the viruses which cause AIDS and hepatitis, both of which can be transmitted by contact with infected blood. Tuberculosis can be transmitted by contact with infected sputum, and gastrointestinal infections by contact with infected faeces. Good practice can have a major impact in reducing the risk to all staff and patients. The detail of good practice should be included in local safety policy. Some general points are included here.

- Disposable surgical gloves should be used during sample collection to reduce the risk of infection spread. Open sores offer an entry for viral and bacterial pathogens.
- Safe disposal of syringe and needles is vital. Needle-stick injuries provide an excellent way of inoculating yourself with patient's blood which may contain an infective virus.
- Leaking specimens present a major and surprisingly frequent potential hazard. This can be prevented by the simple expedient of ensuring sample bottles are not overfilled and tops are well secured. Most laboratories have a policy of discarding leaking specimens.
- Specimens should be transported in specially designed plastic bags which include a separate compartment for the accompanying pathology request form.
- Specimen spillages should be dealt with in accordance with local policy.
- The use of additional protection (eye goggles, disposable gown) should be considered when collecting samples from patients known to be infected with the AIDS virus, HIV, or a virus which causes hepatitis. Specimens from such patients should be clearly identified in some way, according to locally agreed policy.

Topics relating to interpretation of laboratory results

The diversity of techniques used to examine patient samples results in many types of laboratory report. Anyone who has filed pathology reports in patient case notes will have noticed that test results may be expressed *quantitatively*, *semiquantitatively* or *qualitatively*. All reports from the histopathological laboratory, for example, are qualitative; they take the form of highly technical written text describing the appearance of tissue samples when viewed microscopically. The text will include a summary of the clinical significance of any deviations in appearance from that of normal tissue. Microbiological reports tend to be either qualitative or semiquantitative. Text describes which pathogenic microorganisms have been detected, but the sensitivity of these microorganisms to antibiotics tested are reported semiquantitatively. In contrast most reports from clinical chemistry and haematology laboratories are quantitative: they take the form of numerical results. As with any other numerical measurement (e.g. body weight, temperature, pulse), all quantitative results reported by clinical laboratories are defined by the unit of measurement.

Units of measurement used in clinical laboratories

Système Internationale d'Unites (SI units)

Since the 1970s all units of scientific and clinical measurement in the UK have been based, wherever possible, on the SI system devised in 1960. In the United States non-SI units continue to be used in the reporting of clinical laboratory results, so that extreme care must be taken when interpreting laboratory results reported in US medical and nursing journals. Of the seven basic SI units (Table 2.2) only three are relevant to clinical laboratories. They are:

- the metre (m)
- the kilogram (kg)
- the mole (mol)

Although everyone is familiar with the metre as a unit of length and the kilogram as a unit of mass or weight, the mole may require some explanation.

Table 2.2   Basic SI units of measurement

Basic SI unit	Measure of	Abbreviation or symbol
metre	length	m
kilogram	mass (weight)*	kg
second	time	s
ampere	electric current	A
kelvin	temperature	K
mole	amount of a substance	mol
candela	luminous intensity	cd

*For the purposes of this text, mass and weight are regarded as equivalent.

What is the mole (mol)?

The mole is defined as the quantity of a substance whose mass in grams is equal to its particle (i.e. molecular or atomic) weight. This is a useful measure because 1 mole of any substance contains the same number of particles, i.e. 6.023×10^{23}. This is known as Avogadro's number.

Examples

What is 1 mole of sodium (Na)?
Sodium is an element (single atom) whose atomic weight is 23
Therefore 1 mole of sodium is 23 g of sodium.

What is 1 mole of water (H_2O)?
Water is a molecule composed of 2 atoms of hydrogen and 1 atom of oxygen.
The atomic weight of hydrogen is 1
The atomic weight of oxygen is 16
Therefore the molecular weight of water is $(2 \times 1) + 16 = 18$
Therefore 1 mole of water is 18 g of water.

What is 1 mole of glucose?
A molecule of glucose is composed of 6 carbon atoms, 12 hydrogen atoms and 6 oxygen atoms.
The molecular formula of glucose is written $C_6H_{12}O_6$
The atomic weight of carbon is 12
The atomic weight of hydrogen is 1
The atomic weight of oxygen is 16
Therefore the molecular weight of glucose is

$$
\begin{array}{rl}
6 \times 12 = & 72 \text{ plus} \\
12 \times 1 = & 12 \text{ plus} \\
6 \times 16 = & \underline{96} \\
& 180
\end{array}
$$

Therefore 1 mole of glucose is 180 g glucose.

Thus 23 g of sodium, 18 g of water and 180 g of glucose all contain 6.023×10^{23} particles, either atoms in the case of sodium or molecules in the case of water and glucose. Knowing the molecular formula of any substance allows the use of the mole as a unit of amount. For some molecular complex chemicals present in blood, e.g. proteins, the precise molecular weight cannot be defined. The unit of amount (mole) cannot be used when measuring such substances.

Multiples and fractions of basic SI units

When the basic SI unit (metre, kilogram or mole) is too large or too small for the measurement being made, it is convenient to use secondary units which are multiples or fractions of the basic unit. The SI system is decimal so that SI secondary units are expressed as powers of ten of the basic unit. Table 2.3 describes the most commonly used secondary SI units of length, mass(weight) and amount used in clinical and laboratory medicine.

Units for measuring volume

Strictly speaking the SI unit of volume should be based on the metre, i.e. cubic metre (m^3), cubic centimetre (cm^3), cubic millimetre (mm^3), etc.

However, when the SI system was devised it was decided to retain the litre as a measure of fluid volume because it was already in use and is almost exactly the same as $1000\,cm^3$. In fact 1 litre = $1000.028\,cm^3$.

The litre (L or l), then is the basic 'SI' unit of volume. From this are derived the following secondary units of volume used in clinical and laboratory medicine:

decilitre (dL or dl) is 1/10 (one-tenth or 10^{-1}) of a litre
centilitre (cL or cl) is 1/100 (one-hundredth or 10^{-2}) of a litre
millilitre (mL or ml) is 1/1000 (one-thousandth or 10^{-3}) of a litre
microlitre (μL or μl) is 1/1 000 000) (one-millionth or 10^{-6}) of a litre
Note: $1\,ml = 1.028\,cm^3$.

Units of concentration

Nearly all quantitative analysis of patient specimens involves determination of the concentration of a substance in blood or urine. Concentration may be defined as the amount or mass (weight) of a substance that is contained in a specified volume of fluid. Units of concentration then comprise two elements: the unit of amount or mass (weight) and the unit of volume. For example, if we weigh out 20 g (mass) of salt and dissolve it in 1 litre (volume) of water, we have a solution of salt whose concentration is 20 g per litre. In this case the unit of mass (weight) is the gram, the unit of volume is the litre and the SI unit of concentration is gram per litre or g/l. Where the molecular weight of the substance being measured is precisely defined, as it is for many of the blood-borne chemicals measured in clinical laboratories, the mole (unit of amount) is used.

Table 2.3 Secondary SI units of length, mass(weight) and amount used in laboratory medicine

---

Basic unit of length: metre (m)

Secondary unit

centimetre (cm) is 1/100 (one hundredth, i.e. 10^{-2}) of a metre
100 cm = 1 m

millimetre (mm) is 1/1000 (one thousandth, i.e. 10^{-3}) of a metre
1000 mm = 1 m   10 mm = 1 cm

micrometre (mm) is 1/1 000 000 (one millionth, i.e. 10^{-6}) of a metre
1 000 000 μm = 1 m   10 000 μm = 1 cm   1000 μm = 1 mm

nanometre (nm) is 1/1 000 000 000 (one thousand millionth) of a metre
1 000 000 000 nm = 1 m   10 000 000 nm = 1 cm   1 000 000 nm = 1 mm   1000 nm = 1 μm

Basic unit of mass (weight): kilogram (kg)

Secondary units

gram (g) is 1/1000 (one thousandth, i.e. 10^{-3}) of a kilogram
1000 g = 1 kg

milligram (mg) is 1/1000 (one thousandth, i.e. 10^{-3}) of a gram
1000 mg = 1 g   1 000 000 mg = 1 kg

microgram (μg) is 1/1000 (one thousandth, i.e. 10^{-3}) of a milligram
1000 μg = 1 mg   1 000 000 μg = 1 g   1 000 000 000 μg = 1 kg

nanogram (ng) is 1/1000 (one thousandth, i.e. 10^{-3}) of a microgram
1000 ng = 1 μg   1 000 000 ng = mg   1 000 000 000 ng = 1 g   1 000 000 000 000 ng = 1 kg

picogram (pg) is 1/1000 (one thousandth, i.e. 10^{-3}) of a nanogram
1000 pg = 1 ng   1 000 000 pg = 1 μg   1 000 000 000 pg = 1 mg   1 000 000 000 000 pg = 1 g

Basic unit of amount mole (mol)

Secondary units

millimole (mmol) is 1/1000 (one thousandth, i.e. 10^{-3}) of a mole
1000 mmol = 1 mol

micromole (μmol) is 1/1000 (one thousandth, i.e. 10^{-3}) of a millimole
1000 μmol = 1 mmol   1 000 000 μmol = 1 mol

nanomole (nmol) is 1/1000 (one thousandth, i.e. 10^{-3}) of a micromole
1000 nmol = 1 μmol   1 000 000 nmol = 1 mmol   1 000 000 000 nmol = 1 mol

picomole (pmol) is 1/1000 (one thousandth, i.e. 10^{-3}) of a nanomole
1000 pmol = 1 nmol   1 000 000 pmol = 1 μmol   1 000 000 000 pmol = 1 mmol

---

The following 'real' examples demonstrate some of the variety of units used in the chemical analysis of blood.

What does the result 'plasma sodium 144 mmol/l' mean?

Every litre of blood plasma contains 144 mmol of sodium.

What does the result 'plasma albumin 23 g/l' mean?

There are 23 g of albumin in every litre of blood plasma.

What does the result 'plasma iron – 9 μmol/l' mean?

Every litre of blood plasma contains 9 micromoles of iron.

What does the result 'plasma B_{12} – 300 ng/l' mean?

There are 300 nanograms of vitamin B_{12} in every litre of blood plasma.

Units of cell count

Much haematology testing involves counting the concentration of cells in blood. Here the unit of amount is the number of cells and the unit of volume is again the litre. Normally healthy individuals have between 4 500 000 000 000 (that is 4.5 million million) and 6 500 000 000 000 (that is 6.5 million million) red cells in every litre of blood. The unit of red cell count is the number of million million cells there are in 1 litre of blood, expressed in short notation as 10^{12} per litre or 10^{12}/l. This allows the use of manageable numbers so that in normal practice we might say a patient has a red cell count of 5.3. This does not of course mean the patient has only 5.3 red cells; rather, in every litre of blood, the patient has 5.3 million million red cells. There are far fewer white cells than red cells in blood and this is reflected in the unit of the white cell count, which is 10^9/l or the number of thousand million cells in every litre of blood.

The reference (normal) range

When making any clinical measurement, for example weighing a patient or measuring pulse rate, results are interpreted by reference to what is normal. The same is true of tests performed on patient samples. All quantitative tests have a reference range recorded alongside patient test results to aid interpretation. Biological variation determines that just as there is no clear-cut demarcation between normal and abnormal height and weight, there is no clear-cut demarcation between normal and abnormal concentration of any constituent of blood and urine. The use of the term 'reference range' in preference to normal range is a recognition of this limitation. Reference ranges are constructed by measuring the substance in question in a large population of apparently healthy 'normal' individuals.

The graph in Fig. 2.2 describes the results of measuring the concentration of hypothetical substance x in the blood of a large population of apparently healthy individuals (the reference population), and those with a hypothetical disease y.

Since the blood concentration of substance x is usually raised in those

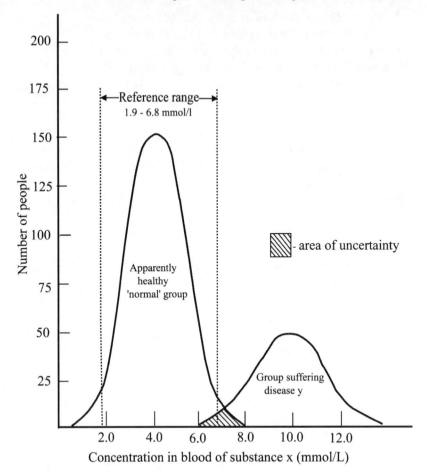

Fig. 2.2 Demonstrating reference (normal) range for theoretical substance x and the overlap in values between healthy individuals and those suffering theoretical disease y (see text for explanation).

suffering disease y, it is used as a blood test to confirm the diagnosis among those with symptoms of y. From the graph it can be seen that the concentration of x among apparently healthy individuals ranges from 1.0 to 8.0 mmol/l. The chance that a particular result is normal diminishes the further away the result is from the average or mean result of the reference population. The extreme ends of the range *may* represent abnormality. To take account of this, all reference ranges are conventionally constructed by excluding the results of 2.5% of the reference population whose results lie at either end of this range. By definition, then, a reference range is the range in concentration of 95% of the reference (healthy) population. In this case, then, the reference range is 1.9–6.8 mmol/l. Using this reference range we can identify those who are suffering disease y. Clearly there is a high degree of certainty that a patient with a blood x concentration of more than 8.0 mmol/l is suffering disease y, and that one with a concentration of less than 6 mmol/l, is not. However, there is a grey area of uncertainty for those whose blood levels lie between 6.0 and 8.0 mmol/l. The poor discriminating power near the limits of a reference range is very typical of quantitative laboratory tests and should always be taken into account when interpreting laboratory test results. For example, supposing the local reference range for serum sodium is 135–145 mmol/l, there is no doubt that a sodium concentration of 125 mmol/l is abnormal and may require treatment. By contrast an isolated sodium concentration of 134 mmol/l, although clearly outside the reference range, has no particular significance. Remember by defi-nition 5% (i.e. 1 in 20) of the healthy population have a result outside the limits of a reference range.

Factors which affect the reference range

Various quite normal physiological factors may need to be taken into account when interpreting laboratory test results. Test results may be affected by

- age of the patient
- sex of the patient
- pregnancy
- time of the day the sample was collected.

For example blood urea concentration rises with age, and blood hor-mone levels are different among adult males compared with adult females. Pregnancy can affect the results of laboratory tests of thyroid function. Blood glucose levels fluctuate throughout the day. Many drugs and alcohol can affect blood test results in a variety of ways. The precise nature and extent of these physiological and drug effects will be con-sidered in more detail as each test is discussed. Finally a reference range is dependent on the analytical techniques used by laboratories. When interpreting any individual patient results, it is important to use only the reference ranges constructed by the laboratory that produced the test result. Throughout this book the reference ranges quoted are a guide only but will approximate to the reference values for all laboratories unless otherwise stated.

Critical values

When a patient test result lies outside the reference range, it is useful for nursing staff to know if the result warrants immediate clinical intervention. Should the medical officer be informed urgently of this test result? The concept of critical values (inappropriately sometimes called 'panic' values) is intended to help with this area of decision making. A critical value is defined as a pathophysiological state at such variance with normal as to be life-threatening, unless something is done promptly and for which some corrective action could be taken.[1] Not all tests warrant critical values, but where appropriate throughout this book suggested critical values for each test will be recorded alongside reference range values. As with reference ranges, critical values are determined by local laboratories. Just as it is important to use locally constructed reference ranges in the interpretation of actual patient test results, so too nurses should follow existing local protocol relating to critical values.

Difference between serum and plasma

Throughout this book reference will be made to blood serum (or simply serum) and blood plasma (or simply plasma). Before leaving this introductory chapter it is important to clarify what these terms mean. Blood is composed of cells (red cells, white cells and platelets) suspended in a liquid, which is essentially an aqueous (water) solution of many different inorganic and organic chemicals. It is this liquid which is analysed in most chemistry and some haematological blood tests. The first step for all these tests is to separate and remove the liquid part from the cells. In physiology texts the liquid is called plasma. An alternative name is serum. The essential difference between serum and plasma is the sample tube into which blood is collected. If blood is collected into a plain tube containing no additives, the blood clots and the liquid recovered is serum. By contrast, if blood is collected into a tube containing an anticoagulant, the blood remains fluid (does not clot). The fluid that remains when cells have been removed from this sample is called plasma. With some important exceptions, most notably tests of blood coagulation, the results from testing either plasma or serum are virtually the same; in these circumstances it is a matter of local laboratory preference as to which is used.

Case history 1

On the second day following elective surgery, Alan Howard, a 46-year-old man, was feeling unwell. Blood was taken for a range of chemical tests and a full blood count (FBC). Among the results phoned back to the ward were the following:

		Reference range
Plasma sodium	135 mmol/l	(135–145)
Plasma potassium	8.0 mmol/l	(3.5–5.2)
Plasma bicarbonate	28 mmol/l	(25–35)
Plasma urea	5.5 mmol/l	(2.5–6.6)
Plasma calcium	1.1 mmol/l	(2.35–2.75)

The FBC results were normal. Realising that the potassium and calcium results were grossly abnormal, the patient's named nurse immediately informed the house officer, who took a second sample. Twenty minutes later the laboratory telephoned back with an entirely normal set of results. It transpired that the person who had taken the blood had overfilled the full blood count bottle and tipped blood into the bottle for chemistry tests to bring the level in the full blood count bottle down to the right mark on the label. How did this cause the abnormal potassium and calcium results?

Discussion of case history

Blood for a full blood count must be prevented from clotting. This is achieved by the presence in the bottle of a chemical anticoagulant, namely the potassium (K^+) salt of ethylene diamine tetraacetate (or, more manageably, K^+-EDTA. This is an anticoagulant which works by chelating (effectively removing) calcium from blood. (Calcium is essential for the normal clotting process.) The addition of K^+-EDTA, whilst preventing blood from clotting, has two incidental effects: it raises the potassium concentration and reduces calcium concentration. The small volume of blood which was tipped into the bottle for U&E contained sufficient K^+-EDTA to markedly reduce calcium concentration and increase potassium concentration. This case history demonstrates that a K^+-EDTA sample of blood is unsuitable for potassium and calcium estimation, and provides a graphic illustration of one of many ways in which poor sampling technique can adversely affect laboratory results. In this case the abnormal results were actually incompatible with life and therefore easily identified. Less dramatic changes, which may remain undetected and are therefore potentially more dangerous, can be caused by poor practice at the time of sample collection and transport.

Reference

(1)   Emancipator K. (1997) Critical values – ASCP Practice Parameter. *Am. J. Clin. Pathol.* **108**: 247–53.

Further reading

Campbell J. (1995) Making sense of the technique of venepuncture. *Nursing Times* **91**(31): 29–31.

Ravel R. (1995) Various factors affecting laboratory test interpretation. In *Clinical Laboratory Medicine*, 6th edn, pp. 1–8. Mosby, Missouri.

Ruth E., McCall K. & Tankersley C.M. (1998) *Phlebotomy Essentials*, 2nd edn Lippincott, Philadelphia.

3 Blood Glucose

The most significant reason for measurement of the concentration of glucose in blood is to aid diagnosis and monitoring of diabetes mellitus, a common chronic metabolic disease which affects more than 1 million people in the UK and 100 million world-wide. The incidence of diabetes is increasing both in the UK and around the world.[1,2] There is currently no cure, and to remain well many diabetic patients must monitor their blood glucose on a daily basis. As we shall see, abnormality in blood glucose concentration is not confined to those suffering diabetes.

Normal physiology

The carbohydrate present in the food we eat accounts for around 60% of our energy requirement. In the alimentary tract, complex dietary carbohydrates, starches, are broken down (digested) by enzymes to simple molecules for absorption into the bloodstream. These simple molecules are the monosaccharides, glucose, fructose and galactose. Of these, glucose is by far the most abundant, representing on average around 80% of absorbed monosaccharides. Once inside the body most of the fructose and galactose is converted to glucose. Thus, nearly all of our dietary carbohydrate is converted to glucose. Most cells in the body also have mechanisms for converting non-carbohydrates (fats and proteins) to glucose when demand for glucose is high and supply is low (starvation).

Why is glucose important?

Glucose can only function within cells, where it is the major source of energy. In every cell of the body this energy is realised by the metabolic oxidation of glucose to carbon dioxide and water. In the process the energy contained within glucose is used to form the energy-rich compound adenosine triphosphate (ATP) from adenosine diphosphate (ADP). The energy contained within ATP is in turn used to drive many chemical reactions within the cell (Fig. 3.1).

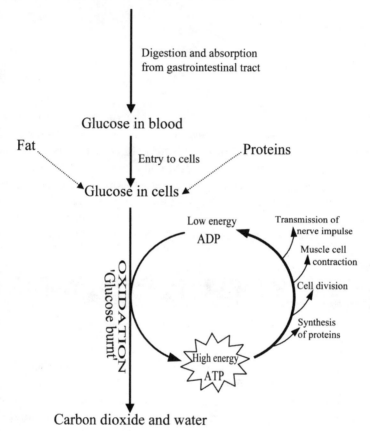

Fig. 3.1   Glucose has a central metabolic role within cells providing energy for many chemical reactions required for cell function.

The oxidation of glucose with the resulting generation of energy-rich ATP occurs in two major cellular metabolic pathways (Fig. 3.2). They are the Embden–Meyerhof pathway (often called the glycolytic pathway or simply glycolysis) and the Krebs cycle (sometimes referred to as the tricarboxylic acid cycle). The process begins with the Embden–Meyerhof pathway in which glucose is converted (oxidised) via 13 separate enzymic reactions to the tricarboxylic acid, pyruvate. The fate of

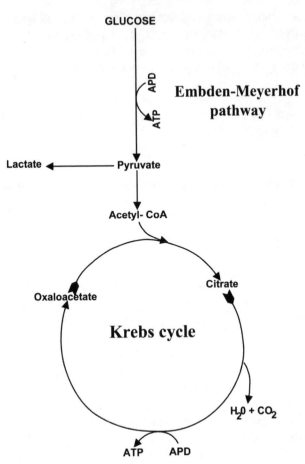

Fig. 3.2 Simplified account of the cellular oxidation of glucose.

pyruvate depends on the relative amount of tissue oxygen. In normally oxygenated tissue, pyruvate is converted to a substance called acetyl CoA which enters the Krebs cycle and joins (condenses) with another tricarboxylic acid, oxaloacetic acid, to form citric acid. In a further nine enzymic reactions, citric acid is converted back to oxaloacetic acid for condensation with more acetyl CoA generated by glycolysis.

Oxidation of one molecule of glucose in the glycolytic pathway yields two molecules of pyruvate and eight molecules of ATP. Further oxidation of the two molecules of pyruvate generated by the glycolytic pathway in the Krebs cycle yields a further 30 molecules of ATP. So, in total, oxidation of one molecule of glucose to CO_2 and H_2O yields 38 molecules of energy-rich ATP.

In the absence of sufficient oxygen, glucose can still be converted to pyruvate by the glycolytic pathway, but pyruvate cannot enter the Krebs cycle. It is converted to lactate (lactic acid). Accumulation of lactic acid in the blood (lactic acidosis) is the cause of metabolic acidosis (Chapter 6) which occurs in any pathological condition associated with poor tissue perfusion and therefore relative tissue hypoxia, and is a direct result of anaerobic glycolysis (i.e. glycolysis in tissues with relative oxygen deficiency).

Importance of maintaining normal blood glucose concentration

Unlike all other tissues the brain is unable to manufacture or store glucose and is entirely dependent on a ready supply of glucose in blood for its energy requirements. The maintenance of a minimum amount of glucose in blood is essential for normal brain function. A blood glucose concentration above around 3.0 mmol/l ensures this function. It is equally important, however, to ensure that blood glucose concentration does not rise too high. Glucose is an osmotically active substance. This means that, as the concentration of glucose in blood rises, its osmotic effect tends to draw water out of surrounding cells leaving them relatively dehydrated. In order to combat this potentially devastating effect on cells, the kidneys compensate by excreting glucose in urine when blood levels rise above a certain concentration called the renal threshold (usually around 10.0–11.0 mmol/l). However, in doing this the valuable energy resource which glucose represents is lost from the body. For good health, then, the glucose concentration of blood must not rise above a maximum level or the body's most important energy resource will be lost in urine, but it must not fall too low either or brain function will be threatened.

Glucose can be stored

Although all cells require glucose for energy, the demand may vary between cells and will vary at different times of the day. For example, muscle cell demand will be highest during exercise and lowest during sleep. Cellular demand for glucose does not always coincide with meals when glucose is available, and there is therefore a need to store dietary glucose until it is required. Most cells in the body can store limited amounts of glucose but three sorts of tissue mainly serve this function:

- liver cells
- muscle cells
- fat cells (adipose tissue).

These cells are able to remove glucose from blood when demand is low or supply is high (after meals) and release it back into blood when demand is high or supply is low (between meals).

Liver and muscle cells store glucose as the polymer molecule glycogen, which is effectively many glucose molecules joined together. The enzymic process by which glycogen is formed from glucose in these cells is called glycogenesis. The reverse process called glycogenolysis allows glucose to be recovered from this store and occurs in response to a falling blood glucose concentration. Glucose can be taken up by fat cells and converted by a process called lipogenesis to triglyceride, a fat, and stored in this form. Triglyceride can be mobilised from fat stores to provide energy by a process known as lipolysis, but this will only occur after glycogen stores are depleted. In this way glycogen provides short-term storage of glucose and fat provides long-term storage of glucose.

How is blood glucose concentration maintained within the normal range?

Despite the considerable variation in glucose intake and utilisation throughout the day, blood glucose concentration never usually rises above around 8.0 mmol/l or falls below around 3.5 mmol/l. Figure 3.3 describes the typical normal daily fluctuation.

Immediately after a meal the glucose level in blood rises as glucose present in food is absorbed from the gut. The glucose is taken up by the cells of the body until the immediate energy requirement is met. Liver and muscle cells store excess glucose as glycogen. Between meals blood glucose levels fall and glucose is mobilised from liver and muscle glycogen stores to maintain a minimum blood glucose concentration. If necessary, glucose may also be manufactured within cells from non-carbohydrate sources such as protein, by a process called gluconeogenesis. Both the uptake of glucose from blood by cells and all the metabolic pathways involved in blood glucose regulation (glycogenesis, glycogenolysis, etc.) are under the overall control of hormones, the secretion of which are governed in turn by blood glucose levels.

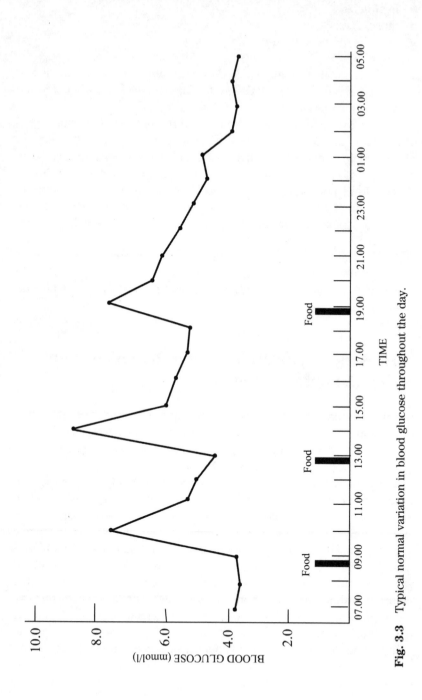

Fig. 3.3   Typical normal variation in blood glucose throughout the day.

Hormonal control of blood glucose concentration

The pancreatic hormones insulin and glucagon are the most important for regulating blood glucose levels. Insulin has the effect of reducing blood glucose levels by:

- promoting uptake of glucose by cells from blood (the uptake of glucose by cells of the liver and central nervous system is independent of insulin)
- promoting the cellular metabolism (oxidation) of glucose to pyruvate (glycolysis)
- increasing formation of glycogen from glucose in liver and muscle (glycogenesis)
- increasing formation of triglyceride from glucose in adipose cells (lipogenesis)
- inhibiting production of glucose from non-carbohydrate sources (gluconeogenesis).

Insulin is secreted by the so-called beta (β) cells of the pancreas in response to a rising blood glucose concentration and operates by binding to insulin receptors present on the surface of insulin-sensitive cells. The normal hormonal response to a rising blood glucose depends, then, on:

- adequate amounts of insulin and therefore normally functioning pancreatic β cells, and
- adequate and functioning insulin receptors on the surface of insulin-sensitive cells.

Without either of these, blood glucose concentration continues to rise.

Glucagon is an insulin antagonist secreted by the alpha (α) cells of the pancreas in response to falling blood glucose. In direct contrast to the action of insulin, glucagon has the effect of raising blood glucose levels by:

- increasing the breakdown of glycogen in the liver (glycogenolysis)
- increasing the intracellular production of glucose from non-carbohydrate sources (gluconeogenesis).

Examination of Fig. 3.3 reveals that blood glucose rises after a meal due to absorption of dietary carbohydrate. A rising blood glucose stimulates the pancreas to secrete insulin. By its various effects, insulin reduces blood glucose. Falling blood glucose levels then induce glucagon production which prevents further blood glucose reduction. By the continuous synergy of these two opposing hormonal effects, blood glucose levels are maintained within normal limits.

Three further hormones are secreted in response to a low blood glucose or stress. They are: cortisol – synthesised by the adrenal cortex; adrenalin (epinephrine) – synthesised by the adrenal medulla; and growth hormone – secreted by the anterior pituitary. These all have the effect of increasing blood glucose levels. There are, then, four hormones, glucagon, cortisol, adrenalin and growth hormone, that serve to prevent blood glucose dropping too low, but only insulin prevents blood glucose concentration from rising too high. This reflects the prime importance of maintaining an adequate minimal level of glucose in blood for normal brain function. Table 3.1 provides a summary of the hormones involved in blood glucose regulation.

LABORATORY MEASUREMENT OF BLOOD OR PLASMA GLUCOSE

PATIENT PREPARATION

If the test is to determine fasting blood glucose, no food should be taken for at least twelve hours prior to blood sampling; otherwise no particular patient preparation is necessary.

TIMING OF SAMPLE

Blood glucose concentration varies throughout the day, highest at around 1 hour after the main meal of the day and lowest first thing in the morning before food; correct interpretation demands that the time be recorded on the specimen. Samples may be random (without reference to time of food), fasting (sample taken after an overnight fast) or 2 hours post-prandial (sample taken 2 hours after a meal).

SAMPLE REQUIREMENT

Around 2 ml venous blood is collected into a special tube (most often grey or yellow top), containing the glucose preservative, sodium fluoride, and an anticoagulant, potassium oxalate. Fluoride is an enzyme poison which effectively prevents continued red cell glycolysis and therefore preserves glucose concentration. Anticoagulant prevents the sample from clotting. The blood should be mixed with these chemicals by gentle inversion. Glucose may be measured directly on the whole blood sample or on plasma, the fluid that remains when blood cells have been removed.

'cont.'

'continued'

REFERENCE RANGE

    Fasting blood glucose   3.5–5.0 mmol/l
    Random blood glucose 3.5–8.0 mmol/l
    2 hours post-prandial glucose At 2 hours after food, glucose levels should be falling towards normal fasting levels

(*Note:* Plasma glucose results are between 10–15% higher than those derived from whole blood.)

CRITICAL VALUES

Blood glucose < 2.2 mmol/l or > 25.0 mmol/l. Severe hypoglycaemia, particularly among neonates, is associated with the risk of permanent brain damage. Severe hyperglycaemia may result in the immediate life-threatening complications of diabetes mellitus, diabetic ketoacidosis or hyperosmolal (non-ketotic) coma.

TERMS USED IN INTERPRETATION OF RESULTS

- Normoglycaemia – normal blood or plasma glucose
- Hyperglycaemia – raised blood or plasma glucose
- Hypoglycaemia – low blood or plasma glucose

Table 3.1 Hormones involved in regulation of blood glucose concentration

Hormone	Site of production and release	Released in response to:	Overall effect on blood glucose concentration
Insulin	Pancreas (beta cells)	Raised blood glucose	Reduces blood glucose
Glucagon	Pancreas (alpha cells)	Reduced blood glucose	Increases blood glucose
Adrenalin (epinephrine)	Adrenal gland (medulla)	Stress	Increases blood glucose
Cortisol	Adrenal gland (cortex)	Reduced blood glucose and/or stress	Increases blood glucose
Growth hormone	Anterior pituitary gland	Reduced blood glucose and/or stress	Increases blood glucose

Causes of abnormal blood glucose

Abnormalities of blood glucose (hyper- or hypoglycaemia) are almost always the result of too little or too much of one of the hormones required for normal regulation of blood glucose. By far the most important cause of hyperglycaemia is diabetes mellitus.

Diabetes mellitus

Diabetes mellitus is characterised by hyperglycaemia due to an absolute or relative deficiency of insulin. Glucose accumulates in blood as it cannot enter cells (except those of the liver and brain) in the absence of an effective insulin response. Cells become relatively starved of glucose. There are two main types. Between 10 and 15% of diabetic patients have Type 1 (or insulin-dependent) diabetes in which hyperglycaemia is the result of insulin deficiency due to autoimmune destruction of the insulin-producing beta (β) cells of the pancreas. Nearly all of the remainder have Type 2 (or non-insulin-dependent) diabetes, in which the primary problem is not inadequate production of insulin – indeed many patients have raised blood insulin concentration – but lack of insulin effect. This is termed insulin resistance. Some of the differences between Type 1 and Type 2 diabetes are highlighted in Table 3.2.

Pregnancy is associated with many quite normal hormonal changes which predispose to hyperglycaemia and therefore diabetes. Depending on the population studied, as well as the criteria adopted for diagnosis, between 1 and 14% of women become temporarily diabetic during their pregnancy.[3] When diabetes is diagnosed during pregnancy, it is called gestational diabetes. The diagnosis does not apply to those women with Type 1 or Type 2 diabetes who subsequently become pregnant. In most cases of gestational diabetes, the abnormality disappears at the end of the pregnancy as hormonal changes induced by pregnancy revert to non-pregnant values. However, between 30 and 50% of women with a history of gestational diabetes eventually develop Type 2 diabetes.[3]

In addition to Type 1, Type 2 and gestational diabetes, there is a fourth group of diabetic patients whose diabetes is caused by some underlying, quite separate disease. This very small subset of the total diabetic population are said to be suffering secondary diabetes. Successful treatment of the underlying disease cures the diabetes in such cases. Causes of secondary diabetes mellitus are listed in Table 3.3.

Table 3.2 Major distinguishing features of Type 1 and Type 2 diabetes

Type 1 Diabetes (insulin-dependent diabetes mellitus, IDDM)	Type 2 Diabetes (non-insulin-dependent diabetes mellitus, NIDDM)
Usually diagnosed in childhood	Usually diagnosed in adulthood
Little or no insulin reserves	Insulin production normal or may be raised
Less common (10–15% of total diabetic population)	More common (around 85–90% of total diabetic population)
Genetic factors less important as a cause	Genetic factors important – very often a family history
Patients typically not obese; may be thin	Obesity common
Ketoacidosis may be presenting feature; may also arise after diagnosis.	Ketoacidosis extremely rare
Absolute need for insulin	No absolute requirement for insulin. Treatment normally dietary manipulation and blood glucose lowering tablets

Table 3.3 Most common causes of secondary diabetes

	Underlying pathology	Hormone affected	Effect on blood glucose
Acromegaly (gigantism)	Tumour of the pituitary gland	Increased growth hormone production	Increased blood glucose
Phaeochromocytoma	Usually tumour of the adrenal medulla	Increased adrenalin production	Increased blood glucose
Cushing's syndrome	Overactivity of adrenal cortex	Increased cortisol production	Increased blood glucose
Haemochromatosis	Iron accumulation in pancreas – pancreatic damage	Decreased insulin production	Increased blood glucose
Chronic pancreatitis	Inflammation of pancreas – pancreatic damage	Decreased insulin production	Increased blood glucose

Whether the disease be primary diabetes (i.e. Type 1 or Type 2), gestational diabetes or, much more rarely, secondary diabetes, all untreated diabetic patients have a raised blood glucose. A consistently normal blood glucose excludes the diagnosis.

Signs and symptoms of diabetes

At normal blood glucose levels, urine contains no glucose. When blood glucose level rises above the renal threshold, which for most people (i.e. diabetics and non-diabetics) is between 10 and 12 mmol/l, glucose begins to be lost in urine. By its strong osmotic effect glucose draws water with it, causing polyuria (increased urine volume) and potential dehydration, which stimulates thirst centres in the brain to increase fluid intake. By these mechanisms severe hyperglycaemia causes five classical symptoms of untreated diabetes:

- glucose excreted in urine (glycosuria)
- increased urination, often at night (polyuria, nocturia)
- thirst
- increased fluid intake (polydipsia)
- dehydration (only if compensatory increased fluid intake is not sufficient to replace fluid lost in urine).

Type 2 diabetes has a long subclinical period during which there are no symptoms, and the condition is often diagnosed when a raised blood glucose or glycosuria is found incidentally during a general health screen. Diabetes is associated with increased risk of certain bacterial and fungal infections, e.g. boils, urinary tract infection, and candida infection of the penis (balanitis) and female genital tract (vaginitis). Such infections may be the first sign of Type 2 diabetes.

The damage to the pancreas which causes Type 1 diabetes begins in the very early years. As the damage accumulates over several years, the insulin deficiency eventually becomes sufficient to cause clinical signs, usually in childhood or early adolescence. The first evidence of diabetes among this group may be diabetic ketoacidosis, an acute and life-threatening complication of very severe insulin deficiency triggered by infection or some other intercurrent illness.

Diabetic ketoacidosis

In the absence of insulin, glucose cannot enter cells and an alternative energy source is required if cells are to survive. Fat (triglyceride) present in adipocytes – the cells in which body fat is stored – provides such an alternative. Many of the symptoms of diabetic ketoacidosis are the result of mobilisation of fat to provide energy in the absence of intracellular glucose. The first step in realising the potential energy in fat is splitting of triglyceride (lipolysis) to release its constituent fatty acids. Fatty acids are transported from adipocytes via blood to all the cells of the body, where they are utilised as an energy source. In the liver, fatty acids are oxidised. The product of this oxidation is acetoacetate which is further metabolised to 3-hydroxybutyrate and acetone. Acetoacetate, 3-hydroxybutyrate and acetone are collectively known as ketone bodies. They are quite normal products of fat metabolism, which would normally be metabolised further. In diabetic ketoacidosis, however, the rate of production outstrips the rate of metabolism and they accumulate in blood and are excreted in urine. Some of the excess acetone is excreted by the lungs and can be smelt on the breath of a patient in ketoacidosis. The other two ketone bodies are acids (keto-acids), and their abnormal accumulation in the blood overwhelms the normal homeostatic mechanisms which maintain normal blood pH, with development of metabolic acidosis (see Chapter 6).

Increased respiration (hyperventilation) to promote removal of carbon dioxide from the blood, thereby restoring normal blood pH, is a normal compensatory mechanism in metabolic acidosis. This is seen as a deep sighing respiration (Kussmaul's breathing) in patients with ketoacidosis. To summarise, then, in addition to the symptoms already mentioned due to hyperglycaemia – glycosuria, polyuria, thirst, polydipsia and dehydration – patients in diabetic ketoacidosis also

- have ketones in blood and urine (ketonaemia, ketouria)
- have the smell of acetone on their breath
- have a metabolic acidosis (low blood pH)
- hyperventilate (exhibit Kussmaul's breathing)
- are usually hypotensive due to severe fluid and electrolyte loss in urine and vomit (vomiting is common in diabetic ketoacidosis).

Without treatment, patients become increasingly drowsy and eventually lapse into coma. Low blood volume consequent on fluid loss threatens normal perfusion of the kidney, so that acute renal failure may occur if blood volume is not restored immediately.

LABORATORY DIAGNOSIS OF DIABETES

Criteria for laboratory diagnosis of diabetes are based on World Health Organization (WHO) recommendations formulated in 1985[4], and revised in 1998 following recommendations by the American Diabetes Association[5]. The revised WHO criteria were adopted in the UK in June 2000. Diabetes is confirmed if a single fasting blood glucose is equal to or greater than 6.1 mmol/l (plasma glucose 7.0 mmol/l) or a random blood glucose is greater than 10.0 mmol/l (plasma glucose 11.1 mmol/l) on at least two occasions. For a minority of patients with symptoms suggestive of diabetes, fasting and random glucose levels are above the normal range but not sufficiently high to make the diagnosis. The glucose tolerance test (GTT) is indicated for these patients.

GLUCOSE TOLERANCE TEST

PRINCIPLE

The GTT involves measuring blood glucose before and after ingestion of a standard (75 g) glucose dose, on a fasted patient.

PATIENT PREPARATION

For at least three days prior to the test, patients must be on a normal carbohydrate diet (i.e. > 150 g/day). The test is conducted in the morning following an overnight fast of at least 12 hours. The patient may have free access to water. Smoking on the morning of the test should be prohibited.

TEST PROTOCOL

Blood is sampled for fasting glucose estimation and 75 g of glucose dissolved in 300 ml water administered by mouth (a more palatable alternative is 353 ml Lucozade). Two hours later, a second blood sample is taken for glucose estimation.

INTERPRETATION

The normal response to a glucose load is an initial increase in blood glucose, which stimulates insulin secretion. This in turn reduces blood glucose so that at 2 hours, glucose concentration has returned to near fasting levels. In both Type 1 and Type 2 diabetes, blood glucose remains high. Table 3.4 describes how the results of a GTT are used to make a diagnosis of diabetes.

   The terms impaired glucose tolerance and impaired fasting glycaemia are reserved for those patients whose results do not indicate diabetes but which are nevertheless abnormal. Such patients are at increased risk of diabetes and should be retested annually.

Table 3.4   Interpretation of glucose tolerance test results

	Fasting plasma glucose (mmol/l)	Plasma glucose at 2 hours after 75 g glucose
Diabetes mellitus unlikely	Less than 5.5 (4.9)	Less than 7.8 (6.7)
Impaired glucose tolerance	Less than 7.0 (< 6.1)	7.8–11.1 (6.7–10.0)
Impaired fasting glycaemia	6.1–7.0 (5.3–6.1)	
Diabetes mellitus	**Equal to or greater than 7.0 (6.1)**	**Equal to or greater than 11.1 (10.0)**

Note: Figures in parentheses should be used for interpretation if blood glucose rather than plasma glucose is measured.

Monitoring diabetes

Whilst treatment of the underlying disease can effect a cure of diabetes for that very tiny subset suffering secondary diabetes, there is no cure for primary diabetes. Patients with Type 1 diabetes have a lifelong need for daily insulin injections supplemented by dietary manipulation. For those with Type 2 disease, a combination of dietary manipulation and oral hypoglycaemic tablets is usually sufficient, though some may require insulin injection eventually. Whatever the treatment, one of the principal objectives is to maintain blood glucose levels as near to normal as possible. Striving to maintain reduced blood glucose concentrations of course carries with it an increased risk of hypoglycaemia, a complication of insulin therapy. The near normal goal of ideal diabetic control has been defined as a plasma glucose which never falls below 4.4 mmol/l or rises above 10.0 mmol/l.[6] Normalisation of blood glucose concentration not only removes the acute symptoms and complications of diabetes such as dehydration, polyuria, thirst, ketoacidosis and hypoglycaemia, but significantly reduces the risk of the long-term progressive complications of diabetes which include kidney disease (diabetic nephropathy), loss of vision (diabetic retinopathy) and nerve damage (diabetic neuropathy). For these reasons diabetic patients, particularly those requiring insulin therapy, are encouraged to monitor their blood glucose concentration regularly. Measurement of blood glucose outside the laboratory was first made possible by the development of glucose reagent strips and then by the development of hand-held blood glucose monitors.

Patient self-monitoring of blood glucose

There are several test strips (e.g. the BM® test) available on prescription to diabetic patients which allow blood glucose concentration to be measured on a single drop of capillary blood within a minute or two. All the systems are in principle the same. A drop of blood is placed on the reagent strip which contains the colour-sensitive reagents. A change in colour results from the reaction between the glucose in blood and reagents on the test strip. The degree of colour change is determined by blood glucose concentration. By comparing the final colour of the reagent strip with a colour chart supplied, the approximate blood glucose may be determined. Alternatively the test strip may be placed in a glucose meter (e.g. Reflolux S®), which measures the intensity of the colour change and provides a digital readout of the glucose concentration. The use of a meter provides more precise and reproducible results than visual reading of the strip. If used strictly according to the manufacturer's instructions, these systems provide results of sufficient accuracy and precision. However, poor technique can easily cause entirely erroneous results. An adequate training and a continuing quality control programme are essential for results of optimum accuracy and precision. This requires co-operation between patients, diabetic nurse specialists and laboratory staff. The manufacturers of blood glucose monitors continue to refine their products, making them increasingly user friendly, but the following points still need to be borne in mind:

- Blood must be sampled from a clean, dry finger or ear lobe.
- Whatever the sampling device used for pricking the finger, it must result in free blood flow and not be dependent on squeezing the finger unduly, which can cause falsely low results. Warming the finger can increase blood flow.
- Blood must be dropped on (not smeared or spread) and must cover the entire reagent pad. False low results can occur if only part of the reagent pad is covered.
- The timing of the reaction, which begins as soon as the drop of blood makes contact with the reagent pad, is absolutely crucial. Falsely high results will occur if the prescribed time is exceeded, and falsely low results if insufficient time is allowed.
- The reagent contained in strips can deteriorate so strips must be stored in accordance with the manufacturer's instructions. They must not be used once the printed expiry date has passed.
- Quality control is essential. Depending on the instrument, this may include calibration of the instrument using a glucose solution of known concentration. Some systems are internally calibrated. All

systems must be tested at regular intervals using an external quality control solution which tests both the machine and the continuing expertise of the patient to produce reliable results.

Urine glucose monitoring

Before methods for the estimation of blood glucose concentration outside the laboratory were available, diabetic patients monitored blood glucose by testing urine for the presence of glucose. This remains a less satisfactory alternative for those patients who are unwilling or unable to measure blood glucose. The test is performed using one of several commercially available urine glucose strips which are in principle similar to those used for measuring blood glucose. A colour change on dipping the strip in urine indicates the presence of glucose. The test is semi-quantitative, so that increasing intensity of the colour change reflects increasing concentration of glucose in urine. A positive result merely indicates that, at some time since the bladder was last emptied, blood glucose rose above the renal threshold. Since the renal threshold varies between people from as low as 6.0 mmol/l to as great as 15.0 mmol/l, the presence of glucose in urine is a poor indicator of blood glucose. The renal threshold should be determined for every diabetic who uses urine testing to monitor blood glucose levels. The test is unable to distinguish hypoglycaemia from normoglycaemia; the test is negative in both instances.

Recent developments in blood glucose monitoring

However sophisticated and 'user friendly', a blood sample is required for all currently available glucose monitors. Many patients are discouraged from regular blood glucose monitoring because of the pain and inconvenience associated with obtaining a blood sample, and researchers have long been investigating ways of monitoring blood glucose less invasively. One promising line of research is transdermal extraction of glucose.

It is possible to extract glucose across the skin by application of a small, quite painless, electrical potential to the skin surface. The amount of glucose extracted across the skin by this technique (known as reverse iontophoresis) accurately reflects blood glucose concentration.[7] Now a prototype glucose measuring 'watch' has been developed based on reverse iontophoresis. The prototype instrument is designed to be worn on the arm, allowing automatic digital readout of blood glucose concentration every 20 minutes without the need for blood sampling. Although still in development, the success of clinical trials[8] of this prototype instrument suggest that the 'bloodless' blood glucose will soon be a reality.

Glycated haemoglobin

This is a laboratory-based test of long-term blood glucose control. Around 5–8% of the haemoglobin which circulates in the red cells of blood has a glucose molecule attached and is said to be glycated. The degree of haemoglobin glycation is dependent on the concentration of glucose that red cells are exposed to during their 120-day life. At any one moment the percentage of haemoglobin which is glycated is dependent on the mean or average blood glucose during the preceding month or two, and provides an excellent overview of blood glucose control between clinic visits. The higher the glycated haemoglobin, the poorer the control.

A 2.5 ml sample of venous blood collected into a bottle containing the anticoagulant EDTA (usually purple top) is required. No particular patient preparation is necessary and the sample can be taken at any time of day. Glycated haemoglobin, HbA1, is composed of three fractions: HbA1a, HbA1b and HbA1c. In some laboratories all three fractions are measured and results expressed as HbA1, whilst in others the principal fraction of HbA1, i.e. HbA1c, is measured.

Interpretation: Approximate reference ranges

- HbA1 = 5.0–9.0% (varies according to methodology)
- HbA1c = 4.7–6.1%

Good diabetic control has been defined as an HbA1c of less than 6.5%. Results lying between 6.5 and 7.5% are borderline and all results > 7.5% represent poor glucose control.[6]

Hyperglycaemia in non-diabetics

A raised blood glucose does not necessarily indicate diabetes. A transient increase in blood glucose often accompanies severe stress because adrenalin, a hormone produced in response to stress, is one of those which tends to increase blood glucose. An example of this mechanism is the transient hyperglycaemia which often accompanies the cardiogenic shock associated with myocardial infarction (heart attack). What distinguishes these stress-related causes of hyperglycaemia from diabetes is their transitory nature. As stress resolves, blood glucose quickly returns to normal concentration.

A raised blood glucose can be treatment related. For example, administration of intravenous glucose-containing fluids and certain drugs (corticosteroids, phenytoin and some diuretics) are often associated with an increase in blood glucose concentration.

Hypoglycaemia

Hypoglycaemia is defined as a blood glucose of less than 2.2 mmol/l although symptoms may occur above this concentration. Since the brain is dependent on an adequate supply of glucose in blood, low levels cause neuroglycopaenia, that is reduced glucose within the brain and throughout the central nervous system. Hypoglycaemia also stimulates synthesis and release of the adrenal medulla hormone adrenalin to increase blood glucose. It is a combination of neuroglycopaenia and increased adrenalin secretion which causes the symptoms of hypoglycaemia.

Symptoms of hypoglycaemia

Those due to raised levels of circulating adrenalin may include

- feeling of hunger
- palpitations
- sweating
- fainting
- tremor
- feeling of anxiety.

Those due to reduced glucose in cells of the brain (neuroglycopaenia) may include

- lethargy
- headache
- confusion
- Apparent drunkenness (unsteady gait, slurred speech)
- convulsions

Untreated severe hypoglycaemia results in coma and (rarely) permanent brain damage. The condition is potentially fatal.

Causes of hypoglycaemia

An inappropriately high level of insulin is usually the cause. Accidental overdose of insulin among diabetic patient accounts for most cases of hypoglycaemia; for example, failing to eat after an insulin injection may precipitate hypoglycaemia. Exercise tends to reduce blood glucose; so less insulin is required. Excessive exercise without insulin dose reduction may precipitate a hypoglycaemia attack in the diabetic patient.

Hypoglycaemia among non-diabetics may be due to insulinoma (a tumour of the β cells of the pancreas) in which the normal control of insulin production is lost. The cells of the tumour secrete insulin despite a falling blood glucose.

A deficiency of any of the three hormones which tend to raise blood glucose and oppose the action of insulin may precipitate hypoglycaemia. For example, in Addison's disease the cells of the adrenal gland that normally produce cortisol are destroyed. The resulting cortisol deficiency is often associated with hypoglycaemia. The liver plays a central role in regulating blood glucose levels; this function remains intact during mild to moderate liver disease but hypoglycaemia may be a feature of severe liver disease. Alcohol is metabolised in the liver and inhibits the process of liver gluconeogenesis, which provides glucose during starvation. Alcoholics who are not eating adequately are particularly at risk of hypoglycaemia for this reason. Hypoglycaemia may be a feature of the neonatal period, particularly among premature babies and very early infancy. There is often no identifiable cause. However, babies born to diabetic mothers are at increased risk during the hours following birth, and a small minority of babies with hypoglycaemia on further investigation turn out to have inherited a genetic deficiency of one of the many enzymes involved in carbohydrate metabolism.

Case history 2

Mrs Bishop is a slightly anxious 25-year-old housewife whose older brother has recently been diagnosed as suffering Type 2 diabetes. Mrs Bishop has read that diabetes runs in families and decides to test her urine for the presence of glucose, using her brother's urine test strips. A positive result convinces her that, although she is well, she has diabetes. She goes to see her GP, who takes blood for glucose estimation. The random blood glucose result is well within the reference range at 6.2 mmol/l but, despite attempts at reassurance, Mrs Bishop remains convinced she has diabetes. Her concern is fuelled by two subsequent urine tests which are also positive for glucose. Her GP suggests a glucose tolerance test. The results are: fasting plasma glucose 4.8 mmol/l and 2-hour post-glucose load, plasma glucose 7.5 mmol/l.

(1) Is Mrs Bishop right to be concerned?
(2) Does she have diabetes?
(3) What is the significance of the positive urine test for glucose?

Discussion of case history

(1) Mrs Bishop is justified in her concern. It is possible to inherit a predisposition to diabetes; in around a third of Type 2 diabetes cases there is a family history of the condition. Furthermore the presence of glucose in urine is a presenting feature of diabetes. The lack of symptoms is not an argument against the diagnosis. Many cases are discovered before symptoms develop, when blood or urine is tested for occupational or insurance health examinations.
(2) The results of Mrs Bishop's glucose tolerance test are entirely normal (see Table 3.4) and the diagnosis can be excluded on the basis of these results.
(3) Glycosuria, the presence of glucose in urine, usually only occurs when blood glucose concentration is high and is therefore suggestive of diabetes. The renal threshold is the blood glucose concentration above which glucose is detectable in urine. Normally this is around 10–12 mmol/l. For some people, however, the renal threshold is significantly lower and glucose may appear in urine at normal blood glucose concentration. Mrs Bishop is among this group. The term 'renal glycosuria' is used to describe this entirely benign defect of kidney function. Although the finding of glucose in urine should never be ignored, it does not necessarily indicate diabetes.

References
(1) King H., Aubert R.E. & Hermann W.H. (1998) Global burden of diabetes 1995–2025. Prevalence, numerical estimates and projections. *Diabetes Care* **21**(9): 1414–31.
(2) Gardiner S., Bingley B., Sawtell P. *et al.* (1997) Rising incidence of IDDM in children aged 5 years in Oxford region: time trend analysis. *BMJ* **315:** 713–17.
(3) Fischer U., Spinas G., Huch A. & Lehmann R. (1999) Using fasting glucose concentrations to screen for gestational diabetes mellitus: prospective population based study. *BMJ* **319**: 812–15.
(4) World Health Organization (1985) Study Group: Diabetes Mellitus. *WHO Tech. Rep. Ser.* **721**: 1–104.
(5) Expert Committee on Diagnosis and Classification of Diabetes Mellitus (1997) Report of the Expert Committee on Diagnosis and Classification of Diabetes Mellitus. *Diabetes Care* **20**: 1057–58.

(6)   British Diabetic Association (1997) *Recommendations for the Management of Diabetes in Primary Care*, 2nd edn. British Diabetic Association, London.

(7)   Tamada J., Bohannon N. & Potts R. (1995) Measurement of glucose in diabetic subjects using non invasive transdermal extraction. *Nature Med.* **11**: 1198–1201.

(8)   Garg S., Potts R., Ackerman N. *et al.* (1999) Correlation of fingerstick blood glucose measurements with GlucoWatch Biographer Glucose results in young subjects with Type 1 diabetes. *Diabetes Care* **22**: 1708–14.

Further reading

Coates V. (1994) Monitoring diabetic control. *J. Clin. Nursing* **3**: 263–9.

Diabetes Control and Complications Trial Research Group (DCCT) (1993) The effect of intensive treatment of diabetes on the development and progression of long-term complications of diabetes. *New Engl. J. Med.* **329**: 977–86.

Gallichan M. (1997) Self monitoring of glucose by people with diabetes. *BMJ* **314**: 964–8.

Hart S.P. & Frier B. (1998) Causes, management and morbidity of acute hypoglycaemia in adults requiring hospital admission. *Q.J. Med.* **91**: 505–10.

Mandrup–Poulsen T. (1998) Diabetes. *BMJ* **316**: 1221–25.

Weiner K. (1992) The diagnosis of diabetes mellitus including gestational diabetes. *Ann. Clin. Biochem.* **29**: 481–93.

Serum Sodium and Potassium

The most frequently requested test of blood chemistry is urea and electrolytes (U&E). This is not one but five tests performed simulta- neously on the serum or plasma recovered from one sample of blood. They are: serum or plasma concentration of sodium, potassium, bicar- bonate, urea and creatinine. The first three are electrolytes, that is, positively or negatively charged ions in solution. This chapter con- cerns the positively charged ions (cations), sodium (Na^+) and potas- sium (K^+). Bicarbonate, a negatively charged ion (anion), is considered in Chapter 6. Urea and creatinine are considered in Chapter 5.

Normal physiology – sodium

Sodium is required for nerve cell conduction and bone formation but its principal function is maintenance of extracellular fluid volume. This function reflects the fact that sodium and water metabolism are inex- tricably linked. As will become clear, careful monitoring of water intake and output (fluid balance) is as important as measuring sodium concentration in elucidating the cause and monitoring treatment of electrolyte disturbances.

Distribution of body water

Around 60% of body weight is water; for an average adult weighing 70 kg this represents around 40 litres of water. Approximately 25 litres are contained within the cells of the body (the intracellular fluid, ICF), and 14 litres outside cells (the extracellular fluid, ECF). The ECF comprises approximately 3.5 litres of plasma, the fluid part of the blood contained

within the vascular system and 10.5 litres of interstitial fluid which fills
the microscopic space between tissue cells (Fig. 4.1)

It is vital for health that both the total amount of water in the body and
its distribution between these compartments is constant. The passage of
water across cell membranes, that is, between the ECF and ICF, is

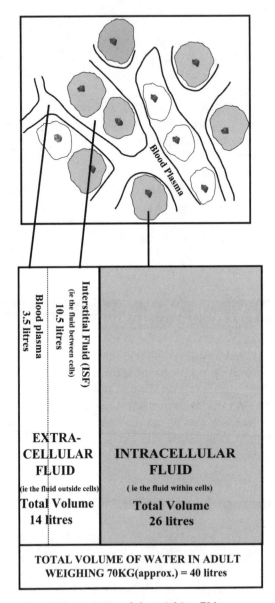

Fig. 4.1 Distribution of water in an adult weighing 70 kg.

largely dependent on the osmolarity on either side of the membrane; so long as this is equal, water will not pass and the volumes of each compartment are maintained.

How does sodium determine ECF volume?

The osmolarity of any solution is determined by the total concentration of dissolved solutes. Because they are present in relatively high concentrations in body fluids (i.e. ECF and ICF) compared with other solutes, electrolytes are the major determinants of osmolarity. Figure 4.2 describes the distribution of electrolytes between the ECF and ICF.

Within cells, the predominant cation is potassium; there is very little sodium within cells. By contrast the ECF has a high concentration of sodium and very little potassium; these different electrolyte concentrations on either side of the cell membrane must be maintained by active transport. This active transport is achieved by the so-called sodium–potassium pump (Fig. 4.3), an energy-requiring system present in the membrane of all cells; sodium is pumped out of cells in exchange for potassium.

Without such active transport, sodium and potassium would diffuse passively across cell membranes until concentrations of ECF and ICF were equal. The active transport of sodium out of cells ensures its high concentration in the ECF and therefore its predominant effect on overall osmolarity of the ECF. Since osmolarity determines the distribution of water between the ICF and ECF, sodium concentration determines ECF volume.

Control of water balance

To avoid dehydration or overhydration, water intake and output must be the same. A minimum urine volume (i.e. water loss) of 500 ml per day is required for excretion of the waste products of metabolism by the kidneys. To this must be added the water lost via the lungs in respired air (400 ml), via the skin in sweat (500 ml), and in faeces (100 ml). Thus a minimum of 1500 ml of water is lost from the body each day. Around 400 ml of water is produced by the body each day, a by-product of cellular metabolism. To maintain normal balance, then, a minimum intake of around 1100 ml is required. In practice fluid intake is greater than this minimum, but the kidneys are easily able to excrete an increased volume of water to balance intake. In fact on average most people excrete between 1200 and 1500 ml of urine every day, and the kidneys have the capacity to produce a urine volume far in excess of this if required.

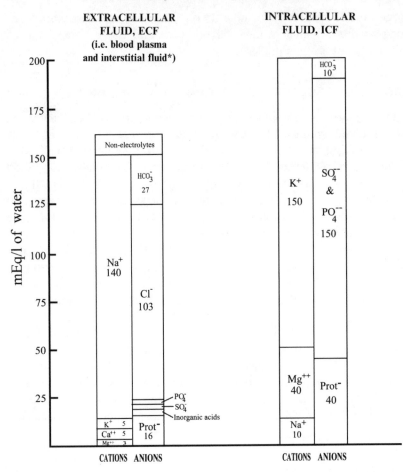

Fig. 4.2 Comparison of the solute concentration in ECF and ICF.

Note: mEq/l = mmol/l for monovalent ions (e.g. sodium, Na, and potassium, K, but mEq/l must be divided by 2 to convert to mmol/l for divalent ions (e.g. calcium, Ca, and magnesium, Mg).

*Figures for ECF refer specifically to blood plasma; interstitial fluid very similar except it has a lower protein and higher chloride concentration.

Water intake and urine loss are controlled by plasma osmolarity. If, for example, water is being lost from the body without adequate replacement, the ECF volume decreases and osmolarity rises. This causes water to pass from cells into the ECF, restoring ECF volume and osmolarity to some extent. This internal movement of water can, however, be only a

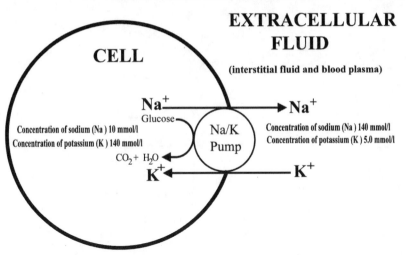

Fig. 4.3 Maintenance of sodium and potassium concentration in cells and surrounding fluid.

short-term corrective. As cells become relatively dehydrated, more water is required.

The normal response to this water deficit is described in Fig. 4.4. As blood with plasma of high osmolarity passes through the hypothalamus in the brain, special cells (osmoreceptors) respond to low osmolarity, with two simultaneous outcomes: the thirst response is invoked and the pituitary gland secretes antidiuretic hormone (ADH). Thirst of course induces increased water intake. ADH conserves body water by its action on the kidney. ADH increases water reabsorption from the distal tubules and collecting ducts of the kidney. A concentrated urine of relatively low volume is excreted.

If too much water is ingested, ECF osmolarity falls. Osmoreceptors are not stimulated and the thirst stimulus and ADH secretion cease. A dilute urine of relatively high volume is excreted, correcting the effective water overload. It must be remembered that around 8000 ml of water are secreted into the gastrointestinal tract each day as saliva, gastric juice, bile, and pancreatic and intestinal juice. In health 99% of this water is reabsorbed and just 100 ml is lost in faeces. However, failure to conserve the water contained in these secretions can result in severe water imbalance. Maintenance of normal water balance is dependent, then, on:

- an intact thirst response, which requires consciousness
- a normally functioning hypothalamus and pituitary gland

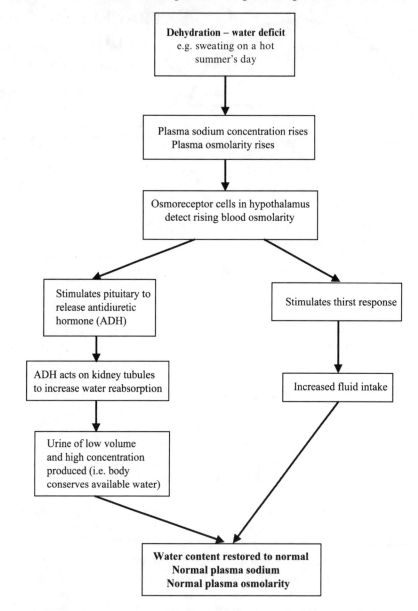

Fig. 4.4   Normal water balance is dependent on intact hypothalamic–pituitary axis; adequate ADH, thirst response and normal renal function.

■ normal kidney function
■ a normally functioning gastrointestinal tract.

Control of sodium balance

Just as health demands a balance between water intake and loss, the same is true of sodium. An adult normally contains around 3000 mmol of sodium, most of which, as we have seen, is present in the ECF (i.e. blood plasma and interstitial fluid) at a concentration of around 140 mmol/l. A minimum of 10 mmol/day is lost in urine, sweat and faeces and this must be replaced to remain in balance. In fact, we ingest far more than this minimum; the average diet contains on average between 100 and 200 mmol per day, mostly as salt flavouring. Excess sodium is excreted by the kidneys in urine. It is kidney regulation of sodium excretion which ensures normal sodium balance, despite wide variation in intake. Sodium excretion by the kidneys is dependent first on the glomerular filtration rate (GFR) (see Chapter 5). A relatively high GFR increases sodium excretion, and a low GFR increases sodium retention. Most (95–99%) of the sodium filtered at the glomerulus is actively reabsorbed during passage through the proximal convoluted tubule. By the time the ultrafiltrate arrives in the distal convoluted tubule just 1–5% of sodium filtered at the glomerulus remains. The fate of this sodium, that is whether it is to be excreted in urine or reabsorbed into the bloodstream, is largely dependent on the blood concentration of the adrenal hormone, aldosterone. This hormone acts on the cells of the distal tubule to enhance sodium reabsorption in exchange for potassium or hydrogen ions. Thus in the presence of high levels of aldosterone most of the remaining sodium in the distal tubule is reabsorbed; in its absence no more is reabsorbed and a urine of relatively high sodium concentration is excreted.

Aldosterone secretion by the adrenal cortex is controlled by the renin–angiotensin system (Fig. 4.5). Renin is an enzyme produced by and secreted from the cells of the juxtaglomerulus of the kidney when blood flow through the glomerulus falls. Since the rate of blood flow through the kidneys (indeed any organ) is dependent on blood volume and therefore sodium concentration, it follows that renin is secreted from the kidneys when plasma sodium is relatively low.

Renin enzymically splits a protein known as renin substrate which circulates in the blood; one of the products of this enzymic action is a small peptide of ten amino acids called angiotensin I. A second enzyme, called angiotensin converting enzyme (ACE), produced predominantly

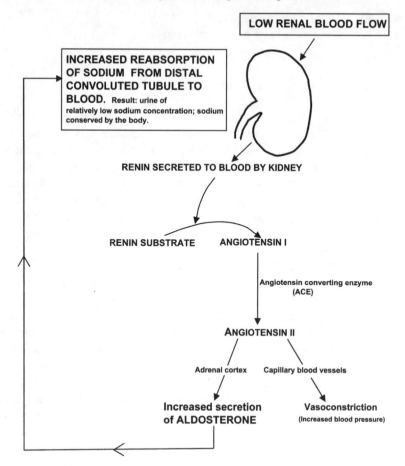

LOW RENAL BLOOD FLOW

INCREASED REABSORPTION OF SODIUM FROM DISTAL CONVOLUTED TUBULE TO BLOOD. Result: urine of relatively low sodium concentration; sodium conserved by the body.

RENIN SECRETED TO BLOOD BY KIDNEY

RENIN SUBSTRATE   **ANGIOTENSIN I**

Angiotensin converting enzyme (ACE)

ANGIOTENSIN II

Adrenal cortex   Capillary blood vessels

Increased secretion of ALDOSTERONE   **Vasoconstriction** (Increased blood pressure)

Fig. 4.5   Renin–angiotensin system.

in the lung, then splits two amino acids from angiotensin I. The remaining eight amino acid peptide is the hormone angiotensin II. This hormone has two important effects:

- It causes capillary blood vessels to narrow (a process called vaso-constriction), increasing blood pressure and thereby helping to restore normal renal blood flow.
- It also stimulates the cells of the adrenal cortex to synthesise and secrete aldosterone, the effect of which, as described above, is reabsorption of sodium and thereby restoration of normal blood volume and renal blood flow.

An additional hormone, atrial natriuretic peptide (ANP), released by the atrial cells of the heart in response to rising blood pressure and volume, has an antagonistic effect to that of aldosterone. The effect of rising blood levels of ANP is reduced sodium reabsorption from the distal tubule and excretion of a urine of relatively high sodium concentration.

Around 1500 mmol of sodium is excreted into the gastrointestinal tract along with water every day (see above). Normally, all save around 10 mmol which is excreted in faeces is reabsorbed. Failure of gastrointestinal sodium reabsorption inevitably leads to potential sodium deficit which becomes real if renal compensation is incomplete. Sodium balance is chiefly dependent on

- normal kidney function
- appropriate secretion of aldosterone by the adrenal cortex gland
- normal gastrointestinal function.

Normal physiology – potassium

Potassium is required for the action of many metabolic enzymes, for electrical transmission of nerve impulses and for muscle contraction. Virtually all the body's 3000 mmol of potassium is within cells. Just 0.4% is in plasma where it can be measured, so that plasma potassium is a poor indicator of total body potassium. The maintenance of a normal plasma potassium level is, however, essential for health and this is dependent on maintaining overall potassium balance.

Normal control of potassium balance

A minimum of around 40 mmol of potassium is lost from the body every day in urine, faeces and sweat. This must be replaced in order to maintain balance. Normal dietary intake is of the order of 100 mmol/day, obtained from citrus fruits, leafy vegetables, potatoes and bread. The kidneys ensure that sufficient potassium is excreted in urine to match that ingested. As with sodium, most of the potassium filtered at the glomerulus of the kidney is reabsorbed in the first (proximal) part of the kidney tubule. Fine regulation occurs in the distal part of the tubule and collecting ducts. Potassium can be either secreted into the tubule in exchange for sodium ions, or reabsorbed at this point. Sodium–potassium exchange is enhanced by the renin–angiotensin–aldosterone system so that under the influence of aldosterone, as sodium is reabsorbed, potassium is lost in urine. The amount of potassium lost in urine is also affected by the kidney's role in maintaining the pH of blood within normal limits. Under circumstances of acidity, for example, excess hydrogen ions must be secreted in urine. This is achieved by exchange with sodium ions so that less sodium is available for potassium exchange. Overall this means that in acidosis less potassium is lost in urine; the reverse is the case in alkalosis. As we shall see, there are other ways in which potassium and acid–base balance affect each other. Around 60 mmol of potassium is normally secreted into the gastro-intestinal tract every day, but less than 10 mmol is lost in faeces: the remainder is normally reabsorbed. Potassium deficit can occur if this reabsorption is defective.

Movement of potassium across cell membranes

The high concentration of ICF potassium and the low concentration of ECF (plasma) potassium are maintained by the sodium–potassium pump. Increased and decreased activity of this pump can have a profound effect on the plasma potassium level as potassium shifts between the ECF and ICF. In addition since hydrogen ions compete with potassium for exchange across the cell membranes, disturbances of acid–base balance may affect the plasma potassium concentration. An abnormal increase or decrease in plasma potassium concentration does not necessarily mean an overall body deficit or excess: it may simply reflect a shift of potassium into or out of cells. Maintenance of a normal plasma potassium level is dependent then on

- adequate dietary intake of potassium
- normal renal function
- normal gastrointestinal tract function
- normal production of aldosterone by adrenal glands
- maintenance of normal acid–base balance
- normal action of the sodium–potassium pump.

LABORATORY MEASUREMENT OF SODIUM AND POTASSIUM

PATIENT PREPARATION

No particular patient preparation is necessary. Sodium and potassium measurements are frequently requested on patients receiving fluids intravenously. Sampling blood from an arm into which iv fluid is being administered may cause errors and should be avoided.

TIMING OF SAMPLE

Blood may be sampled at any time for sodium and potassium, but as these estimations may be made more than once a day on the same patient it is important to record the time the sample was collected.

SAMPLE REQUIREMENTS

Around 5 ml of venous blood is required. Measurement may be made on the serum or plasma recovered from a blood sample. If local policy is to use serum, then blood must be collected into a collection tube without anticoagulant. Plasma estimation requires collection into a tube containing the anticoagulant lithium heparin. No other anticoagulant is suitable for sodium and potassium estimation.

Poor technique during blood collection may cause damage to the membrane of blood cells (haemolysis), resulting in erroneously high potassium levels. This is because potassium is present in such high concentration within cells compared with plasma (Fig. 4.2); damage to (red and white) cells results in a massive influx of potassium (and other cell contents) from cells into plasma. Haemolysis has relatively little effect on serum/plasma sodium concentration because its concentration in cells is low compared with that of plasma. Haemoglobin released from haemolysed red cells changes the colour of serum/plasma from straw coloured to red, providing laboratory staff with a means of identifying haemolysed samples. Haemolysis may occur if blood is forced at pressure through syringe needles, or if blood is shaken violently or frozen. It is a frequent occurrence if there has been any difficulty in collecting blood. Haemolysed samples are unsuitable for potassium analysis.

Some sodium and potassium analysers including those sited in intensive care units or recovery rooms allow immediate analysis of whole blood without the need to separate serum or plasma. Blood must be collected into a syringe or bottle containing the anticoagulant lithium heparin. There is no way of knowing if such samples are haemolysed.

'cont.'

'continued'

EFFECTS OF STORAGE

When blood is removed from the body, the available energy source, glucose, for normal maintenance of the sodium pump, is soon used up and the sodium–potassium pump begins to fail. At this point potassium begins to leak from cells into plasma, and sodium passes from plasma into cells. As with haemolysis, the effects are greater for potassium, and erroneously high serum/plasma potassium levels are seen in samples left for more than a few hours. Blood for potassium estimation must be transported to the laboratory within an hour or so. Samples are best left at room temperature during any delay in transport. Blood left for more than three hours before transport to the laboratory is unsuitable for potassium analysis.

INTERPRETATION OF RESULTS

REFERENCE RANGE:

Serum/plasma sodium   135–145 mmol/l
Serum potassium   3.5–5.2 mmol/l

(Plasma potassium is slightly lower than serum potassium.)

CRITICAL VALUES:

Serum/plasma sodium   < 120 mmol/l or > 160 mmol/l
Serum/plasma potassium < 2.5 mmol/l or > 6.0 mmol/l

TERMS USED IN INTERPRETATION:

Hyponatraemia – reduced plasma/serum sodium concentration, i.e. sodium < 135 mmol/l

Hypernatraemia – raised plasma/serum sodium concentration, i.e. sodium > 145 mmol/l

Hypokalaemia – reduced plasma/serum potassium concentration, i.e. potassium < 3.5 mmol/l

Hyperkalaemia – raised plasma/serum potassium concentration, i.e. potassium > 5.2 mmol/l

Causes of hyponatraemia

As we have seen, sodium and water metabolism are inextricably linked. Sodium concentration is dependent on two variables: the amount of sodium in the ECF and the ECF volume, that is, the amount of water in the ECF. Hyponatraemia, a frequent finding in many common illnesses, may develop if sodium is lost from the body (sodium depletion) in excess of water or if there is an abnormal excess of ECF water relative to sodium (sodium dilution). It is important to remember that serum sodium concentration is a poor indicator of total body sodium; hyponatraemia can be present even if total body sodium is normal, raised or decreased.

Sodium depletion

Abnormal losses of both sodium and water via the gastrointestinal tract occur during protracted vomiting and diarrhoea and from the skin during profuse sweating or as a result of burns. Haemorrhage also represents a loss of both sodium and water. The effect that these losses have on serum sodium concentration depends on the concentration of the fluid lost compared with that of plasma. Excessive vomiting, diarrhoea or sweating result in predominant water deficiency and therefore a tendency for serum sodium to rise. However, if these conditions are treated with fluid relatively deficient of sodium (i.e. hypotonic solutions), hyponatraemia will develop. This is a common cause of hyponatraemia.

Fluid lost during extensive burns and during haemorrhage has the same concentration as that of serum and in these cases, despite being sodium depleted, patients have a near normal sodium concentration. However, hyponatraemia will again develop if the fluid used to replace losses is relatively deficient of sodium.

Excessive losses of sodium in urine are the cause of the hyponatraemia which often accompanies diuretic therapy and may contribute to the hyponatraemia seen in renal failure. The hormone aldosterone regulates sodium loss in urine. A deficiency of the hormone results in increased inappropriate losses of sodium in urine. Addison's disease is characterised by destruction of the adrenal gland; the resulting deficiency of aldosterone causes hyponatraemia.

Excess ECF water

Mild hyponatraemia is a frequent finding among any population suffering disease (the mean sodium concentration of hospital in-patients is 3–5 mmol lower than that of a control population in good health). The sick cell syndrome is thought to be the cause of this non-specific mild hyponatraemia frequently seen in generalised illness. The sick cell is one in which reduced cellular energy causes an abnormal increase in cell membrane permeability. This allows a slight abnormal shift of water from the ICF to the ECF, effectively diluting plasma sodium. This transient slight fall in serum sodium concentration requires no treatment and resolves as the underlying illness is treated.

Untreated diabetes mellitus is often associated with hyponatraemia. Glucose is an osmotically active substance. If its concentration in blood rises, as in diabetes, water flows from cells into the ECF to correct the rising ECF osmolality. The increased ECF volume which results from this shift of water effectively dilutes sodium. This tendency to hypona-traemia in diabetes is compounded by the sodium loss in urine which accompanies the osmotic diuresis as excess glucose is excreted in urine.

As we have seen, hormones are involved in the renal regulation of sodium and water loss. The syndrome of inappropriate antidiuretic hormone (SIADH) results in abnormal retention of water, with dilution of sodium and therefore hyponatraemia. SIADH may complicate the course of many serious pathologies including some lung cancers, infectious disease of the lungs, head injury, brain tumours and Guillain Barré syndrome. Some drugs can also precipitate SIADH.

Water and sodium excess is a feature of oedema, i.e. accumulation of fluid in the interstitial space. Such fluid accumulation occurs in liver disease (cirrhosis), cardiac failure and renal failure. Despite increased total body sodium, water excess usually predominates in oedema, causing hyponatraemia. Sodium replacement therapy is of course not indicated in this subset of hyponatraemic patients who have sufficent sodium but are retaining abnormal amounts of water. The causes of hyponatraemia are summarised in Table 4.1.

Causes of hypernatraemia

Hypernatraemia is much less common than hyponatraemia. Although excess sodium can cause hypernatraemia, relative water depletion is more often the cause.

Excess sodium

Hypernatraemia may occur during over-vigorous sodium replacement therapy among patients with sodium depletion.

Uncontrolled secretion of aldosterone by a tumour of the adrenal gland is the cause of sodium retention of Conn's syndrome (primary hyperaldosteronism). The kidneys respond to high plasma sodium by excreting less water; this tends to restore plasma sodium concentration towards normal but is usually insufficient, and slight hypernatraemia is a common finding in Conn's syndrome. Excess cortisol (another hormone which affects renal loss of sodium) is a feature of Cushing's syndrome and has a similar effect.

Water deficit

Despite maintenance of normal amounts of sodium, hypernatraemia will develop if water output in urine, sweat, faeces and expired air exceeds water intake. Inability of the kidneys to retain water may cause hypernatraemia in chronic renal failure. Abnormal loss of fluid of relatively low sodium concentration is a feature of protracted vomiting, diarrhoea and sweating. All result in hypernatraemia if fluid intake is not increased to replace losses.

The thirst response is essential for adequate intake. A minimum loss of water from the body each day is inevitable. Under normal circumstances the thirst response ensures that we take sufficient water to replace these losses. Unconscious patients and those who have sustained head injury involving damage to hypothalamic thirst centres within the brain are at increased risk of water depletion and therefore hypernatraemia because they are unable to experience thirst.

The ability of the kidneys to conserve water when necessary, by excreting urine of low volume and high concentration, is dependent on adequate amounts of ADH (see Fig. 4.4). A deficiency of ADH, or in some cases lack of ADH effect on the kidney tubules, is the cause of diabetes insipidus. This syndrome results in water depletion as urine of inappropriately high volume and low concentration is excreted. Failure of the pituitary to secrete ADH can be due to damage to the hypothalamus or the pituitary (e.g. head injury, neurosurgery). Some rather rare invasive tumours of the hypothalamus and pituitary can cause diabetes insipidus. Infections of the central nervous system (meningitis and encephalitis) sometimes precipitate diabetes insipidus. In some cases of diabetes insipidus, ADH production and secretion are normal, but the kidney tubules are unable to respond normally. This so-called nephrogenic diabetes insipidus can be inherited, or precipitated by the action of some drugs (lithium, used in the treatment of manic depressive disorders, is the most widely documented). The causes of hypernatraemia are summarised in Table 4.1.

Causes of hypokalaemia

Inadequate intake rarely causes hypokalaemia but may be a feature of chronic starvation, for example in anorexia nervosa. Most cases are the result of increased losses from the body. Increased loss of potassium in urine is an unwanted side effect of some diuretic drugs (e.g. frusemide, Lasix). Diuretic therapy is probably the most common cause of hypokalaemia. Potassium supplements may need to be prescribed for patients receiving diuretic therapy.

The adrenal cortex hormone aldosterone regulates potassium excretion in urine. Excess of this hormone causes abnormally high urinary losses of potassium with resulting hypokalaemia and is a feature of Conn's syndrome, in which there is excessive aldosterone secretion by an adrenal tumour. Raised levels of aldosterone in part account for the severe hypokalaemia which occurs in the very rare Bartter's syndrome and in a similar condition precipitated by liquorice abuse!

Like sodium, potassium can be lost in abnormally high amounts from the gastrointestinal tract; for example, severe acute diarrhoea and the chronic diarrhoea associated with purgative abuse can result in sufficient potassium being lost from the body to cause hypokalaemia. Vomiting is not usually associated with significant potassium depletion except in the case of pyloric stenosis in which the projectile vomiting of acid contents of the stomach causes alkalosis.

Hypokalaemia may be caused not by loss of potassium from the body but by a shift of potassium from the ECF into cells. Such an abnormal shift occurs for one of two reasons: increased activity of the sodium–potassium pump or if there is a hydrogen ion deficit, i.e. raised blood pH (alkalosis). In the first case potassium passes into cells in exchange for sodium; in the second potassium passes into cells in exchange for hydrogen ions (to correct ECF pH). The pancreatic hormone insulin increases the activity of the sodium–potassium pump, so that a shift of potassium from ECF to cells occurs during insulin therapy for diabetic ketoacidosis. This contributes to the hypokalaemia that often occurs as diabetic ketoacidosis is treated. Incidentally this action of insulin is used therapeutically to reduce plasma potassium in those with severe hyperkalaemia, whatever the cause.

The passage of potassium from ECF to cells in exchange for hydrogen ions is a feature of alkalosis and is the reason for the hypokalaemia of pyloric stenosis. This tendency to hypokalaemia during alkalosis is potentiated by increased renal excretion of potassium as hydrogen ions are conserved in an attempt to raise blood pH. Other causes of alkalosis which may be associated with hypokalaemia are considered in Chapter 6. The causes of hypokalaemia are summarised in Table 4.1.

Causes of hyperkalaemia

Excessive intake of potassium during treatment with potassium supplements to correct potassium depletion may cause hyperkalaemia but most cases of hyperkalaemia are the result of reduced potassium excretion by the kidneys. As kidneys fail they lose the ability to excrete potassium in urine; acute renal failure is probably the most common cause of hyperkalaemia.

Autoimmune destruction of the adrenal glands, i.e. Addison's disease, results in a deficiency of aldosterone, the hormone which regulates renal excretion of potassium. The hormone deficiency results in reduced potassium excretion and therefore hyperkalaemia.

Most of the body's potassium is contained within cells; widespread damage to cells results in release of potassium into the ECF. For example, severe trauma may result in hyperkalaemia as may the massive cell destruction associated with cytotoxic therapy for the treatment of leukaemia. This tendency to hyperkalaemia due to tissue destruction will be potentiated by any degree of renal dysfunction.

Potassium passes from cells into the ECF in exchange for hydrogen ions if blood is abnormally acidic. For this reason acidosis is often associated with hyperkalaemia. The causes of acidosis are outlined in Chapter 6. However, special mention is made here of the acidosis associated with untreated diabetes. Untreated diabetic ketoacidosis is usually associated with hyperkalaemia although whole body potassium is depleted. Potassium depletion occurs due to increased urinary losses of potassium during the osmotic diuresis caused by urinary excretion of glucose. This potassium depletion is masked, however, by movement of potassium out of cells into the ECF due to acidosis, and by dehydration consequent on the massive amounts of water lost during the osmotic diuresis. Although severely depleted of potassium, serum levels are normal or high. The potassium depletion soon becomes apparent as the acidosis and dehydration are corrected; hypokalaemia develops as potassium returns to cells and rehydration is effected.

It is as well to emphasise the possibility that a raised potassium level might be due solely or partially to poor practice during collection, storage and transport of specimens (see sample collection). This so-called 'pseudo'-hyperkalaemia is quite a common finding and must be considered as a possible cause in all cases of hyperkalaemia. The causes of hyperkalaemia are summarised in Table 4.1.

Table 4.1   Summary of some significant causes of abnormal serum sodium and potassium

Causes of low serum sodium	*Causes of raised serum sodium*
Heart failure	Protracted vomiting or diarrhoea
Cirrhosis	Chronic renal failure
Diabetic ketoacidosis	Failure of thirst response
Acute renal failure	(e.g. unconsciousness, head trauma)
SIADH	Diabetes insipidus
Addison's disease	Conn's syndrome
Diuretic therapy	Cushing's syndrome
Fluid replacement therapy for vomiting	Over-vigorous sodium replacement therapy
diarrhoea, burns, etc.	Lithium therapy

Causes of low serum potassium	*Causes of raised serum potassium*
Inadequate intake (chronic starvation)	Renal failure
Diuretic therapy	Excessive potassium administration
Severe or chronic diarrhoea or vomiting	Severe tissue damage (trauma, major
During treatment of diabetic ketoacidosis	surgery)
Pyloric stenosis	Acidosis including diabetic ketoacidosis
Alkalosis, Conn's syndrome	Addison's disease
Bartter's syndrome	Poor specimen handling (e.g. blood cells
Liquorice and purgative abuse	haemolysed, untimely transport to the
	laboratory)

Effects of abnormalities in serum/plasma sodium and potassium concentration

Signs and symptoms of hyponatraemia

The clinical effect of a low serum sodium depends on the cause, the magnitude of the abnormality, and the rapidity of onset. Mild hyponatraemia (130–135 mmol/l) is not usually associated with symptoms. However, most patients with a plasma sodium of less than 125 mmol/l will experience some symptoms; these will be more severe if the decrease is rapid. As we have seen, most cases of severe hyponatraemia are due to relative water excess. Symptoms result from over-hydration of cells; the cells of the brain are particularly sensitive to this water excess and neurologic symptoms predominate. Headache, lethargy, mental depression and confusion may develop. Severe hyponatraemia (plasma sodium < 115 mmol/l), particularly of rapid onset, is associated with convulsions and coma; if left untreated, severe hyponatraemia can be fatal. If hyponatraemia is due to both sodium and water depletion as in, say, late Addison's disease, symptoms of low ECF volume (circulatory shock) predominate; these include reduced blood pressure, tachy-cardia and dizziness. If, on the other hand, hyponatraemia is associated with sodium and water excess, symptoms associated with increased ECF volume predominate; these include weight gain, oedema, hyper-tension and breathlessness on exertion (pulmonary oedema).

Signs and symptoms of hypernatraemia

Most cases of hypernatraemia result from a water deficit of both the ECF and ICF. The rapidity of changes increases the severity of symptoms which are those associated with dehydration. These include thirst, dry mouth, difficulty in swallowing and red swollen tongue. Cerebral cell dehydration causes neurological symptoms including confusion and lethargy, increased neuromuscular activity (twitching) and eventually coma. Like hyponatraemia, severe hypernatraemia can be fatal.

Signs and symptoms of hypokalaemia

Symptoms of hypokalaemia do not usually arise until potassium con-centration falls below 3.0 mmol/l but when they do arise are related to the function of potassium in transmission of nerve impulses to muscle. Muscular weakness associated with general lethargy is the most common symptom. Constipation due to impaired muscle tone of the gastrointestinal tract may be a problem. In severe potassium depletion muscular paralysis may occur. Cardiac muscle is frequently affected resulting in cardiac arrhythmias including tachycardia and sinus bradycardia. Typical ECG changes which can be used to diagnose hypokalaemia include prolongation of the P–R interval and depression of the S–T segment. The toxic effects of digoxin therapy on cardiac muscle are potentiated by hypokalaemia. The metabolic alkalosis (Chapter 6) which often accompanies hypokalaemia may result in symptoms of tetany.

Signs and symptoms of hyperkalaemia

Hyperkalaemia may be accompanied by vague feelings of muscle weakness not as pronounced as those which are characteristic of hypokalaemia. Affected patients may be apathetic or even confused. Slurred speech is occasionally evident. The most significant effect of hyperkalaemia, however, is life-threatening changes in cardiac muscle contraction. As serum potassium rises above 7.0 mmol/l there is a real risk of cardiac arrest and sudden death. Characteristic changes in an ECG trace during severe hyperkalaemia include tall, peaked T waves, low or missing P waves and broadening of the QRS complex. Urgent potassium lowering therapy is required for patients with severe hyperkalaemia.

Case History 3

Mark Andrews is a very healthy 22-year-old athlete who represents his US college at a high level in inter-collegiate American-style football. After a particularly intense training session he reported to the team doctor complaining of muscle cramps. The doctor diagnosed dehydration and ordered IV fluid replacement therapy. Over a period of 5 hours Mark received 5 litres of hypotonic saline in 5% dextrose; a further 3 litres of fluid was taken by mouth. Within an hour or so of receiving the IV fluids, Mark appeared acutely ill and was admitted to the emergency room at his local hospital in a confused and disoriented state, unable to follow the simplest of instructions. He was having trouble breathing. Blood was taken for U&E; among the results the laboratory reported was:

Serum sodium 121 mmol/l

(1) Is the serum sodium low, normal or raised?
(2) Could the sodium result explain Mark's clinical state?
(3) Why were iv fluids administered?
(4) What would be the principle of treatment in this case?

Discussion of case history

(1) The serum sodium is significantly reduced. Mark was hyponatraemic on admission.
(2) Yes. Most cases of hyponatraemia including the one under discussion are due not to a deficit of sodium but to fluid (water) excess. Because the sodium is effectively diluted in this water excess, this form of hyponatraemia is sometimes referred to as 'dilutional hyponatraemia'. The excess water in the ECF results in a shift of water from ECF across cell membranes so that cells become relatively over-hydrated or waterlogged. The cells of the brain are particularly sensitive to this excess water; the symptoms of confusion and lack of mental agility are due to the excess water in the cells of Mark's brain. Accumulation of water in the lungs

results in pulmonary oedema, the cause of Mark's breathlessness.

(3) Hypotonic saline (i.e. a salt solution with a sodium concentration less than that of plasma) was administered to correct the fluid deficit (dehydration) which was assumed to have occurred during training. The fluid replacement was clearly over-vigorous in this case.

(4) When Mark was admitted he simply had too much water in his body. The principle of treatment is water restriction and diuretic therapy to increase the rate of water loss via the kidneys, i.e. increase urine volume.

Further reading

Inerarity S. & Stark J. (1997) *Fluids and Electrolytes*, 3rd edn. Springhouse Corporation, Springhouse, Pennsylvania.

Laureno R. & Karp B. (1997) Myelinosis after correction of hyponatraemia. *Annals Intern. Med.* **126**: 57–62.

Perez A. (1995) Hyperkalaemia. *RN* November, 33–35.

Perez A. (1995) Hypokalaemia. *RN* December, 33–35.

Marshall W. (1995) Water and sodium. In *Clinical Chemistry*, 3rd edn, pp. 10–36. Gower Medical, London.

5 Urea, Creatinine and Creatinine Clearance

Measurement of the serum or plasma concentration of urea and creatinine is included in the most commonly requested profile of blood chemistry, 'urea and electrolytes' (U&E). They are both tests of kidney function. Creatinine clearance is not included in a U&E profile, but is another test of kidney function; it involves measuring the creatinine concentration of a 24-hour urine collection as well as the concentration of creatinine in plasma.

Normal physiology

What are urea and creatinine?

Normal cellular metabolism of amino acids and proteins results in production of ammonia (NH_3). This toxic by-product of metabolism is transported in the blood to the liver where it is safely converted to urea by an enzymic process known as the urea cycle (Fig. 5.1).

Urea itself has no metabolic function; as a waste product of normal metabolism it must be eliminated from the body. Once synthesised in the liver it is transported via the blood to the kidney where it is excreted in urine.

Creatinine has a similar fate; like urea it is a waste product of metabolism, more precisely muscle metabolism; it is released into the blood from contracting muscle cells and is transported to the kidneys where it is excreted in urine along with urea. If the ability of the kidneys to excrete urea and creatinine is compromised, they accumulate in the blood; the serum concentration of both rises.

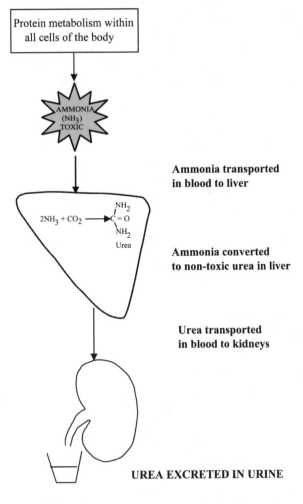

Fig. 5.1 Production and fate of urea.

Formation of urine by the kidneys: what is GFR?

The kidneys are sophisticated blood filters ridding the body of unwanted products of metabolism (including urea and creatinine) along with other substances surplus to the body's needs. Urine, the product of kidney filtration, is an aqueous solution of these unwanted chemicals. By its ability to vary both the volume and composition of urine, the kidney plays a major role in maintaining the constancy of both blood plasma and the interstitial fluid surrounding all the cells of the body. This constant internal environment is essential for normal cell function; life depends upon it.

The functional unit of the kidney is the nephron (Fig. 5.2) which consists of the glomerulus and the kidney tubule.

There are around 1 million nephrons in each kidney. Formation of urine begins at the glomeruli where blood is presented at the rate of around 1.25 litres every minute. The net filtration pressure within the capillary bed allows the passage of water and all other substances of medium and low molecular weight present in blood (including urea and creatinine) to pass from the blood into the Bowman's capsule. The so-called glomerular filtrate formed is essentially protein-free blood plasma (the protein and cells of blood are too large to pass through the filter).

The rate at which this filtrate is formed is called the glomerular filtration rate (GFR). In health the GFR is around 125 ml/minute or 180 litres per day. If there were no way of reabsorbing the product of glomerular filtration, the whole of the blood volume would be lost within a few hours! In fact the composition and volume of the glomerular filtrate is greatly modified as it passes through the tubule. Around 99% of

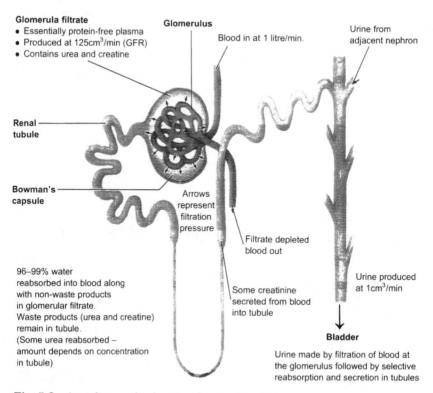

Glomerula filtrate
- Essentially protein-free plasma
- Produced at 125cm³/min (GFR)
- Contains urea and creatine

Glomerulus

Blood in at 1 litre/min.

Urine from adjacent nephron

Renal tubule

Bowman's capsule

Arrows represent filtration pressure

Filtrate depleted blood out

96–99% water reabsorbed into blood along with non-waste products in glomerular filtrate. Waste products (urea and creatine) remain in tubule. (Some urea reabsorbed – amount depends on concentration in tubule)

Some creatinine secreted from blood into tubule

Urine produced at 1cm³/min

Bladder

Urine made by filtration of blood at the glomerulus followed by selective reabsorption and secretion in tubules

Fig. 5.2 A nephron – the functional unit of the kidney.

the filtered water and essential constituents of blood, e.g. electrolytes, amino acids, glucose, etc. are reabsorbed back into the blood. There is capacity in the kidney for a few substances to be secreted from the blood into the tubule during final regulation of urine composition. The exact amount of water and nutrients reabsorbed depends upon the body's requirement at the time but urine, the final product of, first, filtration then tubular reabsorption and secretion, is produced at the rate of around 1 ml per minute, i.e. 1.5 litres a day.

Renal handling of urea and creatinine

Both urea and creatinine are filtered from blood at the glomerulus. Since both are waste products of metabolism, there is no reason for either to be reabsorbed. However, a very small proportion of filtered urea is reabsorbed and this tendency to reabsorption is greater if the urea concentration of the filtrate is particularly high. No creatinine is re-absorbed, but a small amount is normally secreted from blood into the tubule. Notwithstanding these two minimal effects, the amount of urea and creatinine excreted in urine is dependent on the glomerular filtration rate; as GFR falls, so does urea and creatinine excretion. As excretion falls, blood levels rise.

Creatinine clearance – a more sensitive measure of GFR

Although plasma concentration of urea and creatinine concentration are affected by and are a reflection of the GFR, they are not a direct measure. No increase in concentration of either occurs until around 50% of kidney function is lost so that they are poor indicators of early renal disease. Although the test has shortcomings, the creatinine clearance is the best, routinely available, direct measurement of GFR and is therefore a more sensitive and specific measure of early renal disease than either blood urea or creatinine. In essence creatinine clearance measures the volume of blood plasma which is cleared of creatinine during passage through the kidneys in one minute. The higher the clearance the more effective are the kidneys at removing creatinine from blood and excreting it in urine.

LABORATORY MEASUREMENT OF SERUM/PLASMA UREA AND CREATININE CONCENTRATION

PATIENT PREPARATION

No particular patient preparation is necessary.

TIMING OF SAMPLE

Blood may be sampled at any time of the day unless the blood is being sampled for creatinine clearance (see below).

SAMPLE REQUIREMENTS

These two tests are usually performed as part of the U&E screen. Around 5 ml of venous blood is required for U&E. Measurement may be made on either the serum or plasma recovered from a blood sample. If local policy is to use serum, then blood must be collected into a collection tube without anticoagulant. Plasma estimation requires collection into a collection tube containing the anticoagulant, lithium heparin.

EFFECTS OF STORAGE

Unlike the other parameters measured in a U&E screen, urea and creatinine concentrations remain stable when stored for up to 24 hours at room temperature.

LABORATORY MEASUREMENT OF CREATININE CLEARANCE

Creatinine clearance involves measurement of the concentration of creatinine in blood and an aliquot recovered from a well mixed 24-hour urine collection. Measurement of the total 24-hour urine volume is also required. From these measurements the clearance is calculated using the formula UV/P where U = urine creatinine concentration (mmol/l), V = urine flow (ml per minute) and P = plasma (serum) creatinine concentration (mmol). Gross inaccuracies can occur if the 24-hour urine collection is not complete.

PATIENT PREPARATION

Some laboratories recommend that patients should be on a meat-free diet to minimise dietary-related changes in serum creatinine. A correction is often made to creatinine clearance results to take account of muscle mass. If local laboratory policy is to make this correction, patient's height and weight must be recorded on the request card.

'cont.'

'continued'

SAMPLE REQUIREMENTS

- A 24-hour urine collection (Table 5.1). Some laboratories require that urine for creatinine clearance be collected into a bottle containing an acid preservative.
- A 5 ml venous blood sample for serum/plasma creatinine estimation.

TIMING OF SAMPLING

The 24-hour urine collection may be started at any time of the day but it is essential that *all* urine passed during the 24-hour period be collected. Blood must be collected at some time during that 24-hour period, preferably just before a meal.

INTERPRETATION OF RESULTS

APPROXIMATE REFERENCE RANGES

Serum/plasma urea concentration	2.5–6.5 mmol/l
Serum/plasma creatinine concentration	55–105 µmol/l
Creatinine clearance	70–130 ml/min

CRITICAL VALUES

Serum/plasma urea	> 28.0 mmol/l
Serum/plasma creatinine	> 400 µmol/l

Old age is associated with gradual deterioration in renal function, so that urea increases with increasing age. The tendency for creatinine concentration to increase due to reduced renal excretion in old age is offset by decreased production due to age-related reduction in muscle mass. Creatinine clearance gradually decreases with increasing age.

The concentration of urea in blood is a reflection of the balance between rate of liver synthesis and the rate of renal excretion. The concentration of creatinine in blood is a reflection of the balance between production by contracting muscle cells and the rate of renal excretion. If synthesis/production increases and/or excretion decreases, blood plasma concentration rises. If synthesis/production decreases and/or excretion increases, blood plasma concentration falls.

Table 5.1 Protocol for collection of 24-hour urine

Clinical diagnosis and monitoring are occasionally aided by measurement of the rate of urinary excretion of a substance normally present in urine. This requires collection of a timed (usually a 24-hour) urine sample.

The validity of the results derived from a 24-hour urine collection depends crucially on an accurately timed sample. The object is to collect *all* the urine passed during a 24-hour period.

- Obtain a 24-hour urine container for the test requested from the laboratory. Some tests require a container with an acid preservative. This may be a corrosive acid, e.g. concentrated hydrochloric acid, so care must be taken.
- Label the bottle with patient details and the date and time of the start of the urine collection.
- Explain to the patient that all the urine passed during the 24-hour collection period must be saved.
- At a convenient time (usually 9.00 AM) any urine in the bladder is voided and discarded.
- *All* the urine passed after 9.00 AM must be collected into the container.
- At 9.00 AM on the following day the bladder is again emptied. This last sample must be added to the collection. No urine passed after 9.00 AM on the second day should be included.
- The urine collection along with relevant test request form should be transported to the laboratory as soon as possible.

Notes

Sometimes the 24-hour urine volume exceeds the 2 litre capacity of the collection container. If this is the case a second urine container must be obtained to complete the collection. *All* the urine passed *must* be collected.

If the patient inadvertently discards some urine during the collection period, all the urine collected to that point must be discarded, a new bottle obtained from the laboratory and collection restarted.

The urine container should be stored in the sample fridge during the collection period.

Causes of reduced plasma/serum urea concentration

- Pregnancy is normally associated with an increased glomerular filtration rate (GFR) and therefore increased rate of urea excretion; pregnant women typically have lower urea levels than non-pregnant women.
- Low protein diet. Urea synthesis is a function of amino acid and protein metabolism which in turn is affected by dietary intake of proteins. Those on a very low protein diet synthesise less urea than those on a normal diet.
- Liver disease. Urea synthesis occurs in the liver. Although this function is not usually affected in mild to moderate liver disease, liver failure is associated with decreased urea synthesis and accumulation of toxic ammonia.

Causes of reduced plasma/serum creatinine

- Pregnancy is associated with increased excretion of creatinine.
- Creatinine is produced by contracting muscle. Any disease associated with significant decrease in muscle mass (e.g. muscular dystrophy) may result in abnormally low plasma creatinine levels.

Causes of an increased plasma/serum urea and creatinine concentration

Renal causes

Both urea and creatinine concentration of blood are raised if GFR, that is, renal function, is significantly reduced. The glomerulus is analogous to any other filtration system where the rate of filtration depends on three factors:

- the rate at which the liquid (blood in this case) to be filtered is presented to the filter
- the patency of the filter (a 'blocked' filter will result in a slower filtration rate)
- any opposing pressure on the other side of the filter, reducing filtration rate.

Extending this analogy to the many causes of renal failure allows a simplified classification of renal disease into pre-renal (reduced blood flow to kidneys), renal (damage to the filter itself) and post-renal (obstruction to urine flow) renal disease. Table 5.2 describes such an approach emphasising that a low GFR and therefore a raised concentration of urea and creatinine can be a feature of all causes of renal dysfunction. These tests provide no information about the cause of renal dysfunction. However, they are good markers of renal disease progression because, as renal function (GFR) falls, urea and creatinine concentrations rise.

It must be remembered that a normal urea and creatinine concentration does not exclude early renal disease; levels only begin to rise reliably after considerable loss of renal function. Figure 5.3 illustrates this point; plasma urea and creatinine concentrations do not rise above normal until the GFR has fallen to around 40 ml/min, less than 50% of its normal value.

Although a marked increase in urea concentration (i.e. a level greater than around 10.0 mmol/l) always indicates renal damage, a slight to moderate increase in urea (from around 6.5 to around 10.0 mmol/l) may

Table 5.2 Low GFR and therefore raised serum urea and creatinine are a feature of all causes of renal dysfunction

PRE-RENAL (RENAL) DISEASE	RENAL DISEASE	POST-RENAL RENAL DISEASE
Low GFR due to reduced blood volume being presented to the glomerulus for filtration. Kidneys structurally normal but functionally compromised	Low GFR due to damage to filter (glomerulus) i.e. 'blocked filter'. Kidney structurally abnormal and therefore functionally compromised	Low GFR due to blockage on the distal side of the glomerulus opposing filtration pressure.
Principal causes ■ Any condition which results in low blood volume (hypovolaemia), i.e. hypovolaemic shock ■ Major haemorrhage (e.g. trauma, major surgery) ■ Significant salt and water depletion (e.g. severe diarrhoea and vomiting, extensive burns) ■ Septicaemic shock (a complication of septicaemia) ■ Cardiogenic shock, i.e. reduction in cardiac output due to myocardial infarction, heart failure	**Principal causes** ■ Glomerulonephritis due to inflammation or infection ■ Diabetic nephropathy (a complication of longstanding diabetes) ■ Polycystic kidney disease ■ Gout ■ Toxic damage (drugs, heavy metals)	**Principal causes** ■ Any condition which results in urine retention: renal or ureteric stones; tumours that obstruct urine flow (e.g. carcinoma of the bladder, prostate)

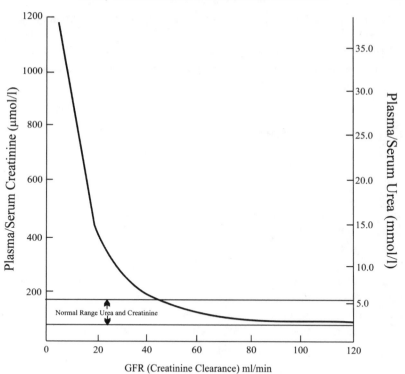

Fig. 5.3 Relationship between glomerular filtration rate (GFR) and plasma concentration of urea and creatinine. *Note:* Plasma concentration of urea and creatinine remains normal until GFR is reduced by more than 50%.

be the result of some other pathology. In these cases creatinine levels remain normal. A marginally raised urea accompanied by a normal plasma creatinine concentration result is likely to be due to non-renal causes. A marginally raised urea accompanied by an equivalent rise in creatinine indicates renal dysfunction.

Non-renal causes of raised urea

- Diet very rich in protein. Urea synthesis is increased among those on a very high protein diet.
- Chronic starvation is accompanied by increased protein catabolism as the body uses its energy reserves for survival; increased protein catabolism results in increased urea synthesis.
- Gastrointestinal bleeding from ulcers, malignancy, etc. are associated with increased protein absorption (blood within the gut is

effectively a protein-rich meal!) and therefore increased urea synthesis.

■ Dehydration: the amount of urea reabsorbed into the blood by the kidney tubules after glomerular filtration is increased in those who are dehydrated.

Causes of reduced creatinine clearance

Since creatinine clearance is a direct measure of GFR, its value decreases as GFR falls. A reduction in creatinine clearance indicates renal damage. The actual level provides an estimate of the extent of that damage, but provides no information about its cause since a reduced GFR may be a feature of all causes of renal failure. Interpretation of creatinine clearance tests is a little more difficult in the elderly because the ageing process is associated with a progressive fall in GFR; creatinine clearance may be up to 30% reduced in elderly patients without renal disease. Creatinine clearance is a more sensitive indicator of early renal disease than either plasma urea or plasma creatinine measurement. The accuracy of creatinine clearance results depends crucially on the accuracy of the 24-hour urine collection.

Effects of increased plasma urea and creatinine concentration

Although it is clear that renal failure, whatever the cause, is associated with abnormal amounts of urea and creatinine in blood and that the actual levels provide useful clinical information about severity, there is no evidence that the symptoms of renal disease are a direct result of either a raised plasma urea or creatinine concentration. However, those with a raised plasma urea and creatinine concentration may suffer any of the following major signs and symptoms of renal disease:

■ renal pain, i.e. low back pain
■ failure to maintain normal urine flow of 1000–2000 ml/day:
    anuria, no urine flow
    oliguria < 500 ml/day
    polyuria > 2000 ml/day
■ raised blood pressure
■ accumulation of fluid in tissues (oedema)
■ presence of blood and/or protein in urine (haematuria/proteinuria).

Uraemic syndrome

Uraemic syndrome is the constellation of symptoms that arise in those who have a marked reduction in GFR to below 30% (i.e. a creatinine clearance of less than around 30 ml/min). This degree of renal dysfunction is always associated with raised urea and creatinine concentration. It was once thought that the symptoms were due to a toxic effect of urea, hence the name, but it has become clear that this is not the case. Symptoms increase as urea/creatinine levels rise and creatinine clearance falls. They include:

■ progressive fatigue, impairment of thought, confusion, fits and eventually coma
■ loss of appetite, nausea, vomiting and diarrhoea
■ breathlessness
■ anaemia.

Consideration for dialysis or renal transplantation is made as urea rises above 35.0 mmol/l, creatinine levels rise above 1200 μmol/l and creatinine clearance falls to < 10 ml/min. Decline in renal function to this point may take many years for patients with chronic renal failure. By contrast, acute renal failure is associated with rapid deterioration in renal function over a period of hours or days.

Case history 4

Jane Redbridge, a 48-year-old housewife, was brought by ambulance to the local accident and emergency department, having collapsed while out shopping. She reported feeling very tired recently, and was concerned that she had been passing black stools, a sign (called melaena) that indicates the presence of blood in the gastrointestinal tract. On examination she appeared clinically anaemic and hypotensive; a provisional diagnosis of gastrointestinal bleed of unknown cause was made. Blood was sampled for full blood count (FBC) and urea and electrolytes (U&E). The following results were obtained:

Sodium	139 mmol/l
Potassium	4.1 mmol/l
Bicarbonate	24 mmol/l
Urea	9.2 mmol/l
Creatinine	78 μmol/l

(1) Are the urea and creatinine results normal?
(2) Do the urea and creatinine results indicate renal disease?
(3) Do the results support the provisional diagnosis?
(4) Are there other conditions which may be suggested by this pattern of urea and creatinine results?
(5) Would you expect Mrs Redbridge to have a normal creatinine clearance?

Discussion of case history

(1) Mrs Redbridge's plasma urea concentration is raised but her creatinine is well within the reference range.
(2) A urea concentration of 9.2 mmol/l is consistent with considerable loss of renal function. Tiredness and anaemia incidentally may also be a feature of kidney disease. However, a normal creatinine level suggests that Mrs Redbridge's kidneys are functioning normally, and therefore consideration should be given to non-renal causes of raised urea.
(3) Yes. Bleeding into the gut results in a marked increase in protein absorption as the blood is 'digested' by gut enzymes. Such a high protein intake increases urea production. If urea production exceeds urinary excretion, urea accumulates in blood. Creatinine is produced by contracting muscle cells, and blood levels are unaffected by increased protein intake. The combination of raised urea and normal creatinine supports the provisional diagnosis.
(4) Whilst a raised plasma creatinine concentration nearly always indicates renal disease, there are several non-renal causes including gastrointestinal bleeding for a marginally raised plasma urea concentration. Chronic starvation, dehydration and a very high protein diet may result in a similar pattern of urea and creatinine levels exhibited by Mrs Redbridge.
(5) If, as seems likely from laboratory results, Mrs Redbridge has normally functioning kidneys, then her creatinine clearance would be normal.

Further reading

de Wardene H.L. (1985) *The Kidney: an Outline of Normal and Abnormal Function.* Churchill Livingstone, Edinburgh.

Ravel R. (1995) Renal function tests. In: *Clinical Laboratory Medicine*, 6th edn. Mosby, Missouri.

Valtin H. (1979) Clinical assessment of renal function. In: *Renal Dysfunction: Mechanisms Involved in Fluid and Solute Imbalance.* Little, Brown & Co, Boston.

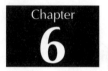

Blood Gases

The use of the term blood gases does not fully describe this test. This is because, although it includes measurement of the two physiologically important gases present in blood, oxygen (O_2) and carbon dioxide (CO_2), it also includes measurement of the pH of blood along with several other parameters of acid–base balance. The test is principally, although not exclusively, reserved for the monitoring of critically ill patients. Significant changes in the measured parameters of blood gases can occur over very short periods of time in such patients, so that, for example, intensive care patients may require blood gas measurement every few hours. For this reason blood gas analysers are often sited where critically ill patients are being cared for. In these circumstances responsibility for analysis of blood gases frequently falls upon nursing staff. It is the only blood test which requires sampling of arterial blood; all other blood tests are performed on venous blood.

Normal physiology

Normal cellular metabolism is associated with continuous production of carbon dioxide (CO_2) and hydrogen ions (H^+), as oxygen (O_2) is consumed. The rates of production and consumption vary according to the level of metabolic activity. Health demands that, despite this variation in production and consumption, the blood content of all three be maintained within narrow limits by a complex synergy of action between the lungs, kidneys and chemical buffers present in blood. The test for blood gases monitors the ability of the body to maintain these mechanisms, and an appreciation of test results depends on a basic understanding of respiratory physiology and normal acid–base balance. Although interrelated, these two topics are treated separately here for convenience only.

Respiratory physiology

The object of respiration is to supply oxygen, present in inspired air, to the tissues, and eliminate carbon dioxide, a waste product of tissue metabolism, in expired air. Venous blood returning from the tissues is low in oxygen and loaded with carbon dioxide (see Fig. 6.1). It is mixed in the right side of the heart and pumped to the lungs via the pulmonary artery. In the lungs, carbon dioxide passes from blood in exchange for oxygen. The blood, now with less carbon dioxide but loaded with oxygen, is pumped back to the heart via the pulmonary vein and out via the aorta through the arterial system for delivery of oxygen to the tissues.

Basic principles of gases in physiological systems: units of measurement and diffusion

The amount of a gas present in systems, including biological systems, is defined by the pressure it exerts, traditionally measured as the height in millimetres of a column of mercury (Hg). For example, the pressure of atmospheric air (i.e. barometric pressure) at sea level is 760 mmHg. This means that at sea level the gases contained in the air we breathe have a combined pressure sufficient to support a column of mercury 760 mm high. In a mixture of gases the total pressure is simply the sum of the partial pressures (represented by the symbol P) of each gas. So, since air is composed of 21% oxygen, 0.03% carbon dioxide and 78% nitrogen, the partial pressure of oxygen (PO_2) in inspired air at sea level is equal to 21% of total atmospheric pressure (i.e. $21/100 \times 760$) or 150 mmHg and partial pressure of carbon dioxide (PCO_2) = $0.03/100 \times 760$ or 0.2 mmHg. In clinical laboratories the Système Internationale (SI) unit of pressure, the kiloPascal (kPa) has replaced mmHg as the unit of choice when measuring partial pressures of gases. Pressure is defined as force per unit area. The SI unit of force is the Newton (N) and the SI unit of area is the square metre (m^2). Thus the derived SI unit of pressure, the Pascal (named after the 17th century physicist), is defined as 1 Newton per square metre ($1 N/m^2$). The kiloPascal (kPa) is 1000 Pascals (i.e. 1000 N/m^2). Some physiology texts continue to express the partial pressure of gases in blood in mmHg. To convert mmHg to kPa, simply multiply by 0.133. Figure 6.1 describes the PO_2 and PCO_2 of inspired air, alveolar air (the air deep within the lungs), venous blood, arterial blood and tissues.

The rate of diffusion of a gas across a physiological membrane is determined by the partial pressure of that gas on either side of the membrane. Gas diffuses from high partial pressure to low partial pressure. The greater the difference on either side of the membrane, the faster the gas diffuses. The significance of this simple principle will

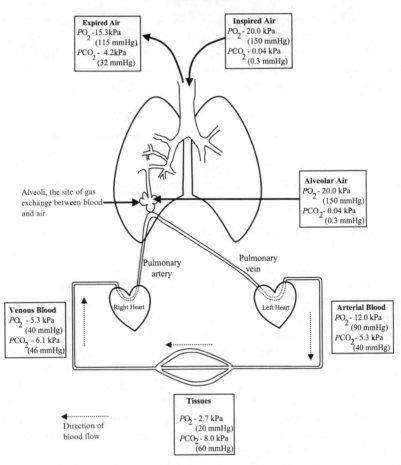

Expired Air
PO_2 -15.3kPa
(115 mmHg)
PCO_2 - 4.2kPa
(32 mmHg)

Inspired Air
PO_2 - 20.0 kPa
(150 mmHg)
PCO_2 - 0.04 kPa
(0.3 mmHg)

Alveolar Air
PO_2 - 20.0 kPa
(150 mmHg)
PCO_2- 0.04 kPa
(0.3 mmHg)

Alveoli, the site of gas exchange between blood and air

Pulmonary artery

Pulmonary vein

Right Heart

Left Heart

Venous Blood
PO_2 - 5.3 kPa
(40 mmHg)
PCO_2 - 6.1 kPa
(46 mmHg)

Arterial Blood
PO_2 - 12.0 kPa
(90 mmHg)
PCO_2 - 5.3 kPa
(40 mmHg)

Direction of blood flow

Tissues
PO_2 - 2.7 kPa
(20 mmHg)
PCO_2 - 8.0 kPa
(60 mmHg)

Fig. 6.1 Gas content within the lungs, systemic (venous and arterial) circulation and tissues.

become apparent as the exchange of gases between blood and lungs, and between blood and tissues, is examined more closely.

Gas exchange at the lungs

The site of gas exchange between blood and lungs is the alveolar membrane, the thin lining of the tiny cul de sacs of lung structure called alveoli. The millions of alveoli provide a massive alveolar membrane surface area for gas exchange: 80 square metres in the adult lung. On one side of the membrane is alveolar air. On the other are blood capillaries so small that only one blood cell can pass through. Gases diffuse across this membrane in an attempt to equalise the amount of each gas on either side of the membrane. Thus oxygen diffuses from the alveoli (PO_2 13.3 kPa) to the blood (PO_2 5.3 kPa) and carbon dioxide diffuses from the blood (PCO_2 6.1 kPa) to alveoli (PCO_2 4.8 kPa). Successful gas exchange between the lungs and blood is dependent on:

- Adequate alveolar ventilation by lungs. This is the mechanical process due to the elastic recoil of lungs which ensures movement of air in and out of alveoli.
- Normal numbers of functioning alveoli.
- Sufficient blood flow through the pulmonary capillaries.

Transport of oxygen in blood

Oxygen passes across the alveolar membrane into the blood flowing through pulmonary capillaries. In the blood a small proportion of the oxygen is dissolved in blood plasma, but most is transported bound to haemoglobin contained within red blood cells. In fact four molecules of oxygen combine with one molecule of haemoglobin to form the product oxyhaemoglobin, allowing much more oxygen to be transported in blood than could possibly be transported by simply dissolving in blood.

The extent to which oxygen combines with haemoglobin is dependent on the PO_2 (Fig. 6.2). At the high PO_2 which prevails in arterial blood, haemoglobin is almost 100% saturated with oxygen. By contrast at low PO_2 (in venous blood and tissues) haemoglobin has much less oxygen attached to it, i.e. the % haemoglobin saturation is much lower. This relationship is crucial for maximum loading of oxygen on to haemoglobin in the arterial blood leaving the lungs and unloading of oxygen from haemoglobin at the tissues. Oxygen is released from oxyhaemoglobin at the tissues because the PO_2 is so low. This tissue release of oxygen from oxyhaemoglobin is potentiated by the relatively high PCO_2 and low pH which also prevail in the tissues. For adequate oxygenation of tissues, then:

- there must be normal amounts of haemoglobin
- that haemoglobin must be 95% saturated with oxygen in arterial blood
- to achieve 95% oxygen saturation arterial blood PO_2 must be > 10 kPa (Fig 6.2).
- maintenance of arterial PO_2 above 10 KPa is dependent on the factors required for normal gas exchange between lungs and blood (see above).

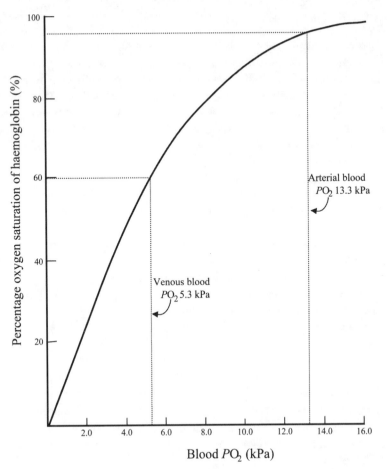

Fig. 6.2 Relationship between the amount of oxygen in blood (PO_2) and the amount of oxygen that can be carried by haemoglobin (i.e. % Hb saturation).

Acid–base balance: maintenance of normal blood pH

Normal cellular metabolism requires that blood pH be maintained within the range 7.35–7.45 despite continuous production of hydrogen ions which tend to reduce pH. Even slight excursions outside this range have deleterious effects and a pH of less than 6.8 or greater than 7.8 is considered incompatible with life. A brief review of some basic concepts are required for an understanding of acid–base balance in the body.

What is pH?

pH is a logarithmic scale (0 to 14) of acidity and alkalinity. Pure water has a pH of 7 and by convention is neutral (i.e. neither acidic nor alkaline). pH above 7 is alkaline and pH less than 7 is acidic. The term pH is an abbreviation of puissance hydrogen (*puissance* is French for power). It is thus a measure of hydrogen ion activity or concentration. pH is defined as the negative log to the base 10 (i.e. $\log_{10}$) of the hydrogen ion concentration in mol/litre or:

$$pH = -\log_{10} [H^+] \qquad\qquad\qquad \text{Eqn 1}$$

where $[H^+]$ = hydrogen ion concentration in moles per litre.

From this equation:

pH 7.4 = H^+ concentration of 40 nmol/l
pH 7.0 = H^+ concentration of 100 nmol/l
pH 6.0 = H^+ concentration of 1000 nmol/l

It is evident that:

- the two parameters change inversely; as hydrogen ion concentration increases, pH falls
- due to the logarithmic nature of the pH scale, an apparently small change in pH is in fact a large change in hydrogen ion concentration. A doubling of hydrogen ion concentration, for example, results in a fall of only 0.3 of a pH unit.

Some laboratories report hydrogen ion concentration (reported as nmol/l) in preference to pH.

What is an acid and what is a base?

An acid is a substance which dissociates in solution to *release* hydrogen ions. A base *accepts* hydrogen ions.

For example, hydrochloric acid (HCl) dissociates to hydrogen ions and chlorine ions:

$$HCl \longrightarrow H^+ + Cl^- \qquad\qquad\qquad \text{Eqn 2}$$

whereas bicarbonate (HCO_3^-), a base, accepts hydrogen ion to form carbonic acid:

$$HCO_3^- + H^+ \longrightarrow H_2CO_3 \qquad \text{Eqn 3}$$

A strong acid like hydrochloric acid dissociates easily, yielding many hydrogen ions; it therefore has a very low pH. A weak acid by contrast dissociates less easily, yielding fewer hydrogen ions and therefore a relatively higher pH than a strong acid.

What is a buffer?

Buffers are chemical compounds in solution which resist changes in pH caused by addition of an acid by 'mopping up' hydrogen ions resulting from acid dissociation. A buffer is the conjugate base of any weak acid. Because of its prime physiological importance for the maintenance of blood pH, the bicarbonate buffer system will be used as an example (there are several other buffer systems in blood). The buffer in this instance is bicarbonate, the conjugate base of the weak acid, carbonic acid. When a strong acid, e.g. hydrochloric acid, is added to a solution of sodium bicarbonate (the buffer), the hydrogen ions from the strongly dissociating hydrochloric acid are incorporated into carbonic acid, a weakly dissociating acid:

$$\underset{\substack{\text{(Hydrochloric acid)} \\ \text{a strong acid}}}{H^+ Cl^-} + \underset{\substack{\text{(Sodium bicarbonate)} \\ \text{the buffer}}}{NaHCO_3} \longrightarrow \underset{\substack{\text{(Carbonic acid)} \\ \text{a weak acid}}}{H_2CO_3} + NaCl \qquad \text{Eqn 4}$$

The important point here is that because the hydrogen ions from hydrochloric acid have been incorporated into a weak acid which does not dissociate easily, the total number of hydrogen ions in solution and therefore the pH do not change as much as would have occurred without the presence of the buffer. Although a buffer minimises changes in pH due to addition of hydrogen ions, it cannot entirely eliminate them because even weak acids dissociate to some extent. A very useful (if at first sight daunting!) equation defines the pH of all buffer systems in terms of the concentrations of their weak acid and conjugate base. This is called the Henderson–Hasselbach equation. For the bicarbonate buffer system, then, this equation is:

$$pH = 6.1 + \log\frac{[HCO_3]}{[H_2CO_3]} \qquad \text{Eqn 5}$$

where $[HCO_3]$ is the concentration of the conjugate base, bicarbonate, and $[H_2CO_3]$ is the concentration of the weak acid, carbonic acid.

The important point here is that pH is governed by the ratio of the concentration of the two parts of the buffer system. As hydrogen ions are added to bicarbonate (the buffer), the concentration of bicarbonate falls as it is converted to carbonic acid and the concentration of carbonic acid rises (Eqn 3), causing a fall in pH. However, if H_2CO_3 could be continuously removed from the system and bicarbonate continuously regenerated, the ratio and therefore the pH would remain unaltered despite continuous addition of hydrogen ions. We shall see as we apply these concepts to the physiology of acid–base balance in the body that this is exactly what happens. In broad terms the lungs ensure elimination of carbonic acid (as carbon dioxide) and the kidneys ensure continuous regeneration of bicarbonate.

Lungs and maintenance of normal blood pH

The main contribution of the lungs to the maintenance of a normal pH is control of the amount of carbon dioxide (CO_2) in blood. A normal amount of CO_2 in blood reflects a balance between that produced by cellular metabolism and that eliminated by the lungs in expired air during respiration. The sequence of events from CO_2 production in the tissues to elimination in expired air is as follows (Fig. 6.3):

- CO_2 diffuses from the tissues (high CO_2 content) to the blood.
- In the red cells of blood, CO_2 is converted to carbonic acid by the enzyme carbonic anhydrase. Carbonic acid dissociates to form bicarbonate and hydrogen ions:

$$H_2CO_3 \longleftrightarrow HCO_3^- + H^+ \qquad \text{Eqn 6}$$

- As bicarbonate concentration rises, some diffuses out of the red cells into surrounding plasma. Hydrogen ions (which if allowed to accumulate would result in a dramatic fall in pH) combine with haemoglobin which has released its oxygen to tissues. (Haemoglobin in this instance is acting as a buffer.)
- When blood reaches the lungs the reverse reaction occurs. Oxygen in inspired air diffuses across the alveoli of the lungs and combines with haemoglobin, which releases the hydrogen ion it has been buffering.
- The released hydrogen ions are buffered by bicarbonate to produce carbonic acid which is converted to CO_2 and water.

$$H^+ + HCO_3^- \longleftrightarrow H_2CO_3 \longleftrightarrow H_2O + CO_2 \qquad \text{Eqn 7}$$

- CO_2 diffuses from a high concentration in blood to a low concentration in the alveoli and is lost from the body in expired air.

From Eqn 7 it can be seen that the rate of removal of CO_2 affects the hydrogen ion concentration and therefore the pH of blood. If, for

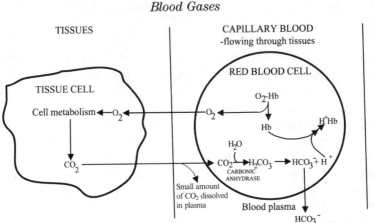

Fig. 6.3a Delivery of O_2 to tissues and first step in the elimination of CO_2.

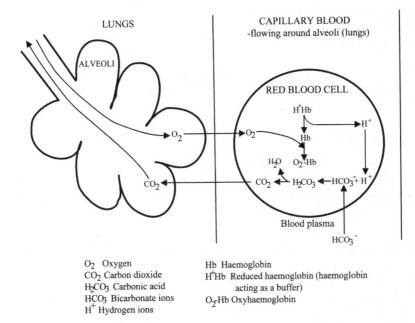

O$_2$ Oxygen	Hb Haemoglobin
CO$_2$ Carbon dioxide	H$^+$Hb Reduced haemoglobin (haemoglobin
H$_2$CO$_3$ Carbonic acid	acting as a buffer)
HCO$_3$ Bicarbonate ions	O$_2$Hb Oxyhaemoglobin
H$^+$ Hydrogen ions	

Fig. 6.3b At the lungs bicarbonate is converted back to CO_2 and eliminated by the lungs.

example, CO_2 accumulates in blood, the reaction in the lungs cannot proceed as fast and hydrogen ions accumulate, decreasing pH. Conversely, if CO_2 is eliminated at an abnormally high rate, the reaction equilibrium shifts to the right, decreasing hydrogen ion concentration (i.e. raising pH). The maintenance of normal blood pH depends, then, on normal respiration rate which in turn is dependent on a functioning respiratory centre in the brain.

The kidneys and maintenance of normal blood pH

Normal cellular metabolism results in continuous production of hydrogen ions which, without the buffering power of bicarbonate in blood, would result in a marked and dangerous decrease in the pH of blood. However, buffering does not remove hydrogen ions from the body, and maintenance of normal blood pH depends ultimately on the ability of the body to eliminate hydrogen ions. At the same time it is important to continuously replenish the bicarbonate used in buffering. These two tasks, elimination of hydrogen ions and replenishment of bicarbonate, are performed by the kidneys. Excess hydrogen ions are excreted by the kidneys, buffered by phosphate and ammonia present in the urine. The renal tubule cells of the kidneys are rich in the enzyme carbonic anhydrase which catalyses the production of carbonic acid from carbon dioxide and water. The carbonic acid dissociates into bicarbonate, which is returned to the blood, and hydrogen ions, which are excreted in urine.

In renal tubule cells, then:

$$CO_2 + H_2O \longleftrightarrow \underset{\substack{\text{Carbonic}\\\text{anhydrase}}}{H_2CO_3} \longleftrightarrow \underset{\substack{\text{Bicarbonate}\\\text{returned to blood}}}{HCO_3^-} + \underset{\substack{\text{Hydrogen ions}\\\text{excreted in urine}}}{H^+}$$

Summary

Maintenance of normal blood pH is dependent on:

- maintenance of normal CO_2 content of blood (regulated by the depth and rate of lung respiration)
- a normally functioning respiratory centre in the brain
- maintenance of a normal amount of bicarbonate in blood (regulated by the kidneys)
- the ability of the kidneys to regulate the loss of hydrogen ions.

LABORATORY MEASUREMENT OF BLOOD GASES

PATIENT PREPARATION

Changes in oxygen and mechanical ventilation therapy will affect results. It is preferable to allow the effects of these changes to stabilise for 30 minutes before sampling blood. The patient should be well rested and warned that arterial sampling may be more painful than venepuncture.

'cont.'

'continued'

TIMING OF SAMPLING

Apart from the advice provided above, the timing of sampling is not important. Some laboratories prefer to be informed by phone before sampling to ensure that analysis is performed immediately the sample arrives. Blood gases are frequently ordered more than once daily on the same patient, so it is important to record the time of blood sampling on the accompanying request card.

SAMPLE REQUIREMENTS

Around 2 ml of heparinised arterial blood is required. An arterial puncture (Table 6.1) is potentially more hazardous and usually more painful than venepuncture. Blood must be collected into a syringe which contains heparin to prevent the blood from clotting. Small clots can form, preventing analysis, if blood is not mixed adequately with the heparin. The metabolic activity of blood cells continues after blood sampling with consumption of oxygen and production of carbon dioxide. For this reason blood for blood gases should be analysed immediately after sampling. If there is to be any delay (more than 10 min), the syringe must be packed in ice to inhibit blood cell metabolism. Any air present in the syringe after blood collection will equilibrate with blood, giving falsely raised blood PO_2. It is important to expel all air from the syringe after blood collection. Arterial blood may be sampled from an indwelling arterial line. Capillary blood obtained from a finger, earlobe or heel may be used if arterial blood collection poses a problem, for example in neonates. The same principles apply: the blood sample must be heparinised, must contain no air bubbles and must be analysed without delay.

ANALYSIS

Blood is injected directly from the syringe into the blood gas analyser. Inside the analyser three separate electrodes measure pH, PCO_2 and PO_2. Using pH and PCO_2, the machine calculates several other parameters. The ones most frequently used in practice are bicarbonate and base excess. The measured and calculated parameters are printed by the machine within a minute or so after injection of the sample.

'cont.'

'continued'

INTERPRETATION OF BLOOD GAS RESULTS

REFERENCE RANGES, ADULTS

pH   7.35–7.45
(Hydrogen ion (H^+)concentration   35–45 nmol/l)
PCO_2 4.7–6.0 kPa   (or 35–45 mmHg)
PO_2 10.6–13.3 kPa   (or 80–100 mmHg)
Bicarbonate   22–28 mmol/l
Base excess/deficit − 2 to +2 mmol/l

REFERENCE RANGE, NEONATES

pH   7.30–7.40
(Hydrogen ion (H^+) concentration 40–50 nmol/l)
PCO_2 3.4–5.4   (26–40 mmHg)
$PO2$ 8.0–9.4 kPa   (60–70 mmHg)
Bicarbonate 15–25 mmol/l

CRITICAL VALUES

pH   < 7.2 or > 7.6
PCO_2 < 2.7 kPa or > 9.3 kPa
Bicarbonate < 10 mmol/l or > 40 mmol/l
PO_2 < 5.3 kPa

TERMS USED IN BLOOD GAS INTERPRETATION

■ Acidosis – low pH or raised H^+ concentration
■ Alkalosis – raised pH or low H^+ concentration
■ Hypercapnia – raised blood PCO_2
■ Hypocapnia – low blood PCO_2
■ Hypoxaemia – low Blood PO_2
■ Hypoxia – low oxygen in tissues, tissues poorly oxygenated

Table 6.1   Collection of arterial blood sample

Arterial blood is routinely sampled from the radial artery in the wrist, the femoral artery in the groin or the brachial artery in the arm.

The syringe must be loaded with the 0.5–1 ml lithium or sodium heparin solution (1000 units per ml) to prevent blood from clotting in the syringe. Pre-heparinised syringe packs specifically for arterial blood collection are usually used.

The procedure is more painful than venepuncture, and local anaesthetic is sometimes injected prior to arterial puncture.

Aseptic technique including gloved hands is required to prevent infection.

(1) Locate the injection site by feeling for pulsating artery.
(2) Prepare the site by cleaning first with alcohol and then with iodine antiseptic solution. Allow to dry.
(3) Inject local anaesthetic to the site (optional).
(4) Hold the blood gas syringe with needle attached between forefinger and thumb (like holding a dart) and with other hand relocate artery.
(5) Warn patient before inserting the needle bevel side uppermost into the skin at an angle of 45° (90° in the case of a femoral artery stab) just behind the finger locating the artery.
(6) Advance the needle in the direction of the artery.
(7) When the artery is punctured blood will automatically flow into syringe due to arterial pressure.
(8) When sufficient blood has been collected, withdraw the needle and immediately place a sterile gauze pad over the injection site. Firm finger pressure must be applied for a minimum of 5 minutes.
(9) With other hand immediately eject any air from syringe containing sample and discard needle to sharps disposable box.
(10) Cap syringe and invert it several times to ensure adequate mixing of blood with heparin solution.
(11) Immerse barrel of syringe in packed ice and arrange *immediate* transport to laboratory.

Clinical disturbances of acid–base balance

Pathologies that result in abnormal blood pH can be divided into:

- those which affect the function of the organs (lungs and kidneys) involved in the homeostatic control of blood pH, and
- those which result in an abnormal metabolic production of acids or alkalis to such a degree that normal homeostatic mechanisms are overwhelmed.

There are also therapeutic interventions which can affect acid–base balance, the most significant being mechanical ventilation and some drugs.

To understand how blood gas results can be used to identify the cause and monitor disturbances of acid–base balance we must return to the Henderson–Hasselbach equation.

$$pH = 6.1 + \log \frac{[HCO_3^-]}{[H_2CO_3]}$$
 Eqn 5

Bicarbonate (HCO_3^-) is calculated during blood gas measurement but carbonic acid (H_2CO_3) is not. However, there is a relationship between carbonic acid concentration and PCO_2, a measured parameter of blood gases, which allows restatement of the Henderson–Hasselbach equation in terms of the three most important parameters of acid–base reported following blood gas analysis, pH, PCO_2 and bicarbonate:

$$pH = 6.1 + \log \frac{[HCO_3^-]}{PCO_2 \times 0.23}$$
 Eqn 8

By removing all constants from this equation we can state that

$$pH \propto \frac{[HCO_3^-]}{PCO_2}$$
 Eqn 9

i.e. pH is proportional to the ratio of bicarbonate concentration to PCO_2. This simple relationship allows the following deductions:

- pH remains normal so long as the ratio $[HCO_3^-] : PCO_2$ remains normal.
- pH increases (alkalosis) if either bicarbonate increases or PCO_2 decreases independently.
- pH decreases (acidosis) if either bicarbonate decreases or PCO_2 increases independently.
- If both PCO_2 and bicarbonate increase by relatively the same amount, the ratio and therefore pH remain normal.
- If both PCO_2 and bicarbonate decrease by relatively the same amount, the ratio and therefore pH remain normal.

Classification of acid–base disturbances

Acid–base disturbances begin with an abnormality in either bicarbonate or PCO_2. Since PCO_2 is controlled by the lungs, a primary disturbance of PCO_2 is termed respiratory; a primary disturbance of bicarbonate is called metabolic. Using these terms all disturbances of acid–base balance can be divided into four categories:

■ If the primary disturbance is a raised PCO_2 (i.e. resulting in a low pH), the condition is called respiratory acidosis.
■ If the primary disturbance is a reduced PCO_2 (i.e. resulting in a raised pH), the condition is called respiratory alkalosis.
■ If the primary disturbance is a raised bicarbonate (i.e. resulting in a raised pH), the condition is called metabolic alkalosis.
■ If the primary disturbance is a reduced bicarbonate (i.e. resulting in a low pH), the condition is called metabolic acidosis.

Causes of the four acid–base disorders

Respiratory acidosis (primary increase in PCO_2)

Respiratory acidosis is a feature of any condition which inhibits elimination of CO_2 by the lungs. Primary disease of the lung, either acute infection (e.g. pneumonia) or severe chronic airway limitation (e.g. asthma, emphysema, chronic bronchitis), is the most common cause. Depression of the respiratory centre in the brain due to drugs (e.g. morphine, barbiturates) or trauma (head injury) may also result in reduced CO_2 elimination. Disease of or damage to chest wall muscles, for example in poliomyelitis, muscular dystrophy or severe chest injury, can compromise the mechanics of respiration sufficiently to inhibit carbon dioxide elimination. For those patients who require mechanical ventilation, respiratory acidosis may arise if ventilation is inadequate.

Respiratory alkalosis (primary decrease in blood PCO_2)

Respiratory alkalosis occurs during abnormally rapid or deep respiration (hyperventilation) causing increased elimination of CO_2. Stress-related hyperventilation, a feature of anxiety attacks and severe pain, can cause respiratory alkalosis. Hypoxia (low tissue oxygenation) and some drugs (e.g. salicylate) stimulate the respiratory centre in the brain, increasing CO_2 elimination. Excessive mechanical ventilation can cause respiratory alkalosis.

Metabolic acidosis (primary decrease in bicarbonate)

Metabolic acidosis is due to either abnormal loss of bicarbonate from the body or increased utilisation of bicarbonate in buffering abnormal amounts of acid. Bicarbonate is one of the many chemicals secreted into the lumen of the small intestine to aid digestion. Normally most of this bicarbonate is reabsorbed further down the gastrointestinal tract. If it is not reabsorbed, it is lost from the body in faeces. Any disease process which inhibits normal bicarbonate reabsorption from the intestines (e.g. severe diarrhoea) may result in losses of bicarbonate from the body sufficient to cause metabolic acidosis. Abnormal losses of bicarbonate from the body in urine, and failure of kidneys to regenerate adequate amounts of bicarbonate, both contribute to the metabolic acidosis which is a feature of renal failure.

Production of abnormally high quantities of metabolic acids – the so-called keto acids, β-hydroxybutyric acid and acetoacetic acid – is a feature of untreated or poorly controlled insulin-dependent diabetes. In this state of severe insulin deficiency called diabetic ketoacidosis (Chapter 3), the amount of bicarbonate in blood falls as it is used up in buffering these excess acids.

Cells which are severely deprived of oxygen cannot fully metabolise (oxidise) glucose; one of the metabolic consequences is production of lactic acid (see Fig. 3.2). The abnormal accumulation of lactic acid in blood accounts for the metabolic acidosis which occurs in any condition in which tissues are inadequately perfused with blood and therefore oxygen. Clinical (hypovolaemic) shock and cardiac arrest are the two most important causes of lactic acidosis; other pathologies which may be associated with lactic acidosis include renal failure, liver failure, septicaemia and leukaemia.

Metabolic alkalosis (primary increase in bicarbonate)

Metabolic alkalosis may arise during over-administration of bicarbonate. Anti-acid formulates for relief of 'acid indigestion' contain alkalis such as bicarbonate, and bicarbonate is administered iv to correct metabolic acidosis. An increase in bicarbonate occurs during potassium depletion so that metabolic alkalosis may be a feature of conditions which cause hypokalaemia (Chapter 4), most notably some diuretic drugs. Severe and prolonged vomiting of gastric juice, which is acidic, represents a loss of hydrogen ions from the body. This is the cause of metabolic alkalosis associated with pyloric stenosis, a condition (usually congenital) in which there is obstruction to passage of stomach contents into the small intestine.

Consequences of acid–base disturbances – compensation

Because of the prime importance of maintaining a normal blood pH, the body will always attempt to return an abnormal pH to normal. This process is called compensation and involves restoring the ratio of bicarbonate : PCO_2 to normal. Primary respiratory disturbances in which the PCO_2 is affected are compensated for by adjustment of the metabolic component, bicarbonate. Metabolic disturbances in which the bicarbonate is primarily affected are compensated for by adjustment of the respiratory component, PCO_2. For example, a patient with a metabolic acidosis (i.e. primary decrease in bicarbonate) will respond by increasing the rate and depth of respiration to increase CO_2 elimination and thereby reduce the amount of CO_2 in blood. The resulting reduction in PCO_2 returns the ratio of bicarbonate : PCO_2 and therefore the pH towards normal. For the patient with a primary respiratory problem (i.e. abnormal PCO_2) compensation is achieved by the kidney and erythrocyte regulation of bicarbonate concentration. If PCO_2 is high, then kidneys and erythrocyte generation of bicarbonate is increased to correct the important ratio. Conversely, if PCO_2 is low, then bicarbonate regeneration is decreased and bicarbonate level in blood falls, returning the all important ratio towards normal.

If the compensatory mechanism is sufficient to return the pH to normal, the patient is said to be fully compensated. If the compensatory mechanism is sufficient to return the pH towards normal but insufficient to actually achieve normality, the patient is said to be partially compensated. The concept of an 'acid–base balance' allows the process of compensation to be conveyed visually (Fig. 6.4).

It must be remembered that compensation, whether partial or complete, is not a state of normality; the ratio of bicarbonate : PCO_2 and therefore the pH may be normal but both bicarbonate and PCO_2 are abnormal. Only successful treatment of the primary disturbance can return PCO_2 and bicarbonate to normal. Table 6.2 describes blood gas results before, during and after compensation of acid–base disorders. Renal compensation of respiratory disorders is much slower than respiratory compensation of metabolic disorders. In the first case,

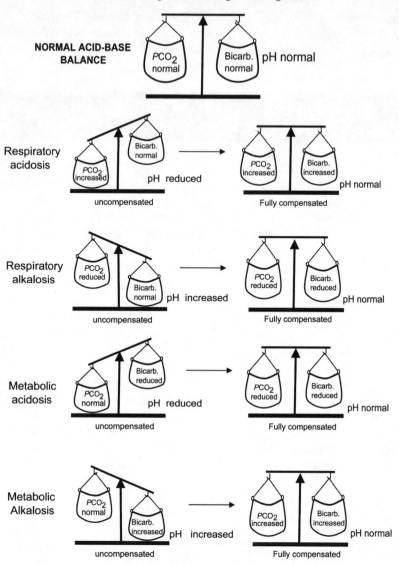

Fig. 6.4   The 'acid–base balance': compensation restores normal pH.

Table 6.2 Blood gas results in disturbances of acid–base balance

Primary disturbance	Common causes	Compensatory mechanism	Initial blood gas results (uncompensated)	Blood gas results after partial compensation	Blood gas results after full compensation
Respiratory acidosis primary increase in PCO_2	Hypoventilation Respiratory failure Lung disease Depression of brain respiratory centre	Renal and RBC: increase bicarbonate	pH decreased PCO_2 increased Bicarb. normal	pH decreased but closer to normal PCO_2 increased Bicarb. increased	pH normal PCO_2 increased Bicarb. increased
Respiratory alkalosis primary decrease in PCO_2	Hyperventilation Anxiety attacks Stimulation of brain respiratory centre	Renal and RBC: decrease bicarbonate	pH increased PCO_2 decreased Bicarb. normal	pH increased but closer to normal PCO_2 decreased Bicarb. marginally decreased	pH normal PCO_2 decreased Bicarb. decreased
Metabolic acidosis primary decrease in bicarbonate	Renal failure Diabetic ketoacidosis Circulatory failure – clinical shock	Respiratory: decrease PCO_2	pH decreased PCO_2 normal Bicarb. decreased	pH decreased but closer to normal PCO_2 marginally decreased Bicarb. decreased	pH normal PCO_2 decreased Bicarb. decreased
Metabolic alkalosis primary increase in bicarbonate	Bicarbonate administration Potassium depletion	Respiratory: but very little compensation in metabolic alkalosis	pH increased PCO_2 normal Bicarb. increased	Very little compensation in metabolic alkalosis	

compensation occurs over a period of days or weeks, but in the second, evidence of compensation is seen within hours.

Consequences of acid–base disturbances – clinical signs and symptoms

Whatever the cause, acid–base disturbances themselves result in signs and symptoms. A raised PCO_2 (hypercapnia) has non-specific effects on the central nervous system which may include confusion, headache and hand tremor. Coma may ensue if levels are particularly high. A low PCO_2 results in symptoms of light-headedness and dizziness. Acidosis can cause hyperkalaemia; patients affected may have characteristic symptoms and ECG changes (Chapter 4). Alkalosis decreases the amount of ionised (physiologically significant) calcium; this causes symptoms of tetany which include painful muscle cramps and spasm, pins and needles and paraesthesia. As we have seen, potassium depletion is an important cause of metabolic alkalosis but alkalosis can itself cause hypokalaemia so that symptoms and signs of hypokalaemia often accompany alkalosis, whatever the cause. Compensation for metabolic acidosis involves deep and rapid respiration (Kussmaul respiration) to eliminate CO_2.

Mixed acid–base disturbances

Thus far it has been assumed that any particular patient with a disturbance of acid–base balance suffers only one of the four categories of acid–base imbalance discussed. Whilst this may well be the case, patients can present with a mixture of two or even three disturbances making interpretation of results very difficult. As an example of a mixed disturbance consider a patient with a chronic respiratory disease such as emphysema who has a heart attack and suffers cardiac arrest. Before the arrest the patient has a compensated respiratory acidosis due to longstanding emphysema. The cardiac arrest causes metabolic acidosis. The results of gas analysis of blood sampled within a few hours of arrest will reflect the combined effect of both respiratory and metabolic acidosis. Having regard to the causes of single acid–base disturbances it is not difficult to imagine many other clinical situations in which a patient might be suffering more than one type of acid–base disturbance.

Causes and consequences of a low arterial blood PO_2 (hypoxaemia)

Breathing air which has relatively low PO_2 (e.g. atmospheric air at high altitude) will result in a low arterial blood PO_2 but clinically the most important causes are those in which gas exchange with blood across the alveolar membrane is compromised. Poor gas exchange is of course the cause of the raised PCO_2 which characterises respiratory acidosis so that a low PO_2 occurs in all those conditions which cause respiratory acidosis. Hypoxaemia may occur in the absence of respiratory acidosis, for example in pulmonary oedema. In the early stages of chronic lung disorders (e.g. bronchitis and emphysema) or infections (pneumonia) the so-called hypoxic drive induced by low PO_2 increases respiration (CO_2 elimination) sufficient to maintain a normal or even low PCO_2. Respiratory acidosis develops late on in the disease process when even the hypoxic drive is insufficient to prevent CO_2 retention. Finally inadvertent sampling of venous blood rather than arterial blood causes falsely low results, and this explanation should be considered if there is no clinical reason for a low PO_2.

From Fig. 6.2 it can be seen that reduction in PO_2 reduces oxygen saturation of haemoglobin and therefore oxygen delivery to the tissues. Respiratory failure (defined in adults as a PO_2 of less than 8.0 kPa) causes breathlessness, confusion, sweating, tachycardia and cyanosis. In patients with accompanying respiratory acidosis the symptoms of hypercapnia may also be present.

Case history 5

When Mr Bridges, a 70-year-old man with a ten-year history of emphysema, experienced sudden worsening of his symptoms, his wife called their GP who arranged immediate transfer to hospital. On arrival he was breathless even while lying still. He was by now drowsy and confused. Arterial blood was sampled for blood gases. The laboratory reported the following results:

pH	7.28
PCO_2	8.8 kPa
Bicarbonate	35 mmol/l
PO_2	5.4 kPa

On admission to intensive care, he was mechanically ventilated and given oxygen. After half an hour of ventilation the patient showed signs of tetany. Results of blood gases at this time were:

pH	7. 59
PCO_2	3.4 kPa
Bicarbonate	33 mmol/l
PO_2	10.9 kPa

(1) What was Mr Bridges' acid–base and oxygen status on arrival at hospital?
(2) How does emphysema result in such an acid–base disturbance?
(3) Explain the relationship between symptoms and blood gas results.
(4) What is the acid–base and oxygen status after mechanical ventilation? Explain the marked change.
(5) What are the symptoms of tetany? Why did Mr Bridges have such symptoms?

Discussion of case history

(1) On arrival at hospital Mr Bridges was acidotic (low pH). Acidosis may be respiratory (due to raised PCO_2) or metabolic (due to reduced bicarbonate). In this case the acidosis is clearly of respiratory origin. A markedly reduced PO_2, consistent with respiratory failure and the medical history, substantiates this. A raised bicarbonate indicates some degree of compensation, emphasising the longstanding nature of his condition. However, since the pH remains abnormal, compensation is incomplete. At the time of admission, then, Mr Bridges was suffering severe partially compensated respiratory acidosis and severe hypoxaemia.
(2) Emphysema is a chronic disease of the lungs in which the normal elasticity of the air sacs (alveoli) is progressively lost due to the destructive action of enzymes released from dead and dying phagocytic cells recruited to the lungs to fight infection and inflammation. In the normal lung these enzymes would be inactivated by specific blood-borne proteins, but in the emphysema patient the balance between destructive enzyme production and inactivating protein production is lost. Unopposed enzymic destruction of alveoli compromises normal transfer of oxygen and carbon dioxide between the environment and blood; blood PCO_2 level rises and blood PO_2 level falls. The rising PCO_2 in blood results in reduced blood pH (acidosis). To compensate and return pH towards

normal, the kidneys and erythrocytes regenerate more bicarbonate than usual and bicarbonate concentration increases.

(3) The cardinal symptom of emphysema is progressively worsening breathlessness due to hypoxaemia. Eventually, as in the case of Mr Bridges, the PO_2 drops so low that even at rest the patient is literally gasping for air. Marked increase in PCO_2 depresses the central nervous system and this is probably the cause of the confusion and drowsiness experienced by Mr Bridges. This state of severe hypoxaemia and hypercapnia is life threatening, and urgent mechanical ventilation to increase CO_2 elimination (i.e. decrease blood PCO_2) along with oxygen therapy to reduce the level of hypoxaemia (i.e. raise blood PO_2) is required for survival.

(4) After 30 minutes of mechanical ventilation, Mr Bridges had a raised pH (alkalosis) which may be respiratory (reduced PCO_2) or metabolic (increased bicarbonate) in origin. Since the bicarbonate level remained unchanged, it must be the marked reduction in PCO_2 brought about by mechanical ventilation which caused the alkalosis. As a result of over-enthusiastic ventilation Mr Bridges suffered respiratory alkalosis. The normal renal compensation for respiratory alkalosis is to decrease bicarbonate by renal mechanisms involving increased elimination in urine and decreased regeneration of bicarbonate. But this is a relatively slow process occurring over days rather than minutes so that in this case there was no evidence of compensation. Respiratory alkalosis due to over enthusiastic mechanical ventilation can be quickly corrected by reducing the rate of mechanical ventilation. Administration of oxygen resulted in a marked increase in PO_2, increasing the all important oxygen saturation of haemoglobin (see Fig. 6.2) and thereby improving delivery of oxygen to tissues.

(5) The symptoms of tetany, which include pins and needles, muscular spasms and rarely convulsions, are due to a reduction of ionised plasma calcium, a substance required for normal neuromuscular transmission. Calcium in blood is present in two almost equal fractions: half is bound to the protein albumin and is physiologically inactive, and the other half is free, physiologically active, ionised calcium. The proportion of total calcium which is ionised is determined in part by the pH of blood; if the pH of blood is high (i.e. alkalotic), then less calcium than normal is in the ionised physiologically active form and more is present bound to albumin and therefore physiologically inactive. As in Mr Bridges' case, tetany is a frequent finding in patients who have a raised blood pH, no matter what the cause. The symptoms of tetany disappear as the alkalosis is corrected and blood pH returns to normal.

Further reading

Courtney S., Weber K., Breakie L., Malin S. *et al.* (1990) Capillary blood gases in the neonate: a reassessment and review of the literature. *Am. J. Dis. Child.* **144**: 168–72.

Davenport H. (1974) *The ABC of Acid–Base Chemistry*, 6th edn. University of Chicago Press, Chicago.

McCall R. & Tankersley C. (1998) Arterial blood gases. In: *Phlebotomy Essentials*, 2nd edn. Lippincott, Washington.

Pilon C., Leathley M. *et al.* (1997) Practice guideline for arterial blood gas measurement in ICU decreases numbers and increases appropriateness of tests. *Crit. Care. Med.* **25**: 1308–13.

Raflin T.A. (1986) Indications for arterial blood gas analysis. *Ann. Intern. Med.* **105**: 390–98.

Venkatesh B., Clutton Brock T. & Hendry S. (1994) A multiparameter sensor for continuous intra-arterial blood gas monitoring: a prospective evaluation. *Crit. Care. Med.* **22**: 588–94.

Cholesterol and Triglycerides

The principal use of this test is to help assess an individual's risk of coronary heart disease (CHD), the leading cause of death in the western world. There is now overwhelming evidence that too much cholesterol and/or triglycerides in the blood increases the risk of CHD; the higher the level the greater is this risk. The test is also used to monitor the effectiveness of therapy (drugs and dietary manipulation) aimed at reducing the amount of cholesterol and triglyceride in blood.

Normal physiology

What are cholesterol and triglycerides?

Apart from inorganic elements such as sodium, potassium, calcium, etc., there are four broad classes of chemical present in the human body and the food we eat. They are: proteins, carbohydrates, nucleic acids and lipids (or fats). Although structurally dissimilar (Fig. 7.1), cholesterol and triglycerides are lipids. They are provided in a normal diet, both being present in meat and dairy products. Eggs are a particularly rich source of cholesterol. In addition to dietary sources, cholesterol and triglycerides are synthesised in the body, principally in the liver (both cholesterol and triglycerides) and adipose or fat tissue (triglycerides only).

Function of cholesterol and triglycerides

In common with all lipids, cholesterol and triglycerides are essential components of all cell membranes. However, their function is not confined to cell structure. In the liver, cholesterol is converted to bile acids and salts and excreted from the gall bladder into the intestinal tract in the digestive juice, bile. The presence of bile acids and salts in bile is

Cholesterol structure, like other sterols,
which include steroid hormones, Vitamin D
and bile acids, is based on the six carbon ring.

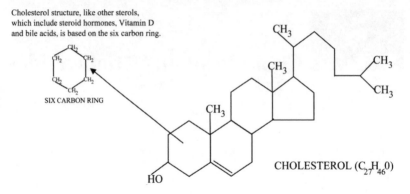

SIX CARBON RING

CHOLESTEROL ($C_{27}H_{46}O$)

Triglycerides are formed by combination of 1 molecule of glycerol and three fatty acids.

Glycerol

Fatty acid 2

Fatty acid 1

Fatty acid 3

Diagrammatic structure of a triglyceride

Glycerol

CH_2OH
$HO-CH$
CH_2OH

Fatty acids

$CH_3 - (CH_2)_n - COOH$

General formula for fatty acids
(n = number of CH_2 groups which
varies)

eg $CH_3 - (CH_2)_{14} - COOH$

Formula for palmitic acid, a fatty
acid with 14 CH_2 groups

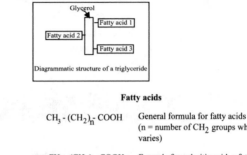

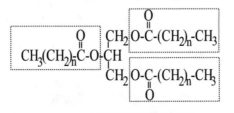

$$CH_3(CH_2)_n-\overset{O}{\overset{\|}{C}}-O-CH \quad \begin{array}{l} CH_2\text{-}O\text{-}\overset{O}{\overset{\|}{C}}\text{-}(CH_2)_n\text{-}CH_3 \\ \\ CH_2\text{-}O\text{-}\underset{O}{\underset{\|}{C}}\text{-}(CH_2)_n\text{-}CH_3 \end{array}$$

A TRIGLYCERIDE

Fig. 7.1   Structure of cholesterol and triglycerides.

essential for absorption of dietary fats. Cholesterol is the raw material
from which steroid hormones are synthesised; examples include cortisol
in the adrenal glands, progesterone in the ovaries and testosterone in the
testis. Vitamin D is synthesised in the skin from a cholesterol-derived
compound.

Triglycerides are the principal fat present in adipose (fat) tissue and as such their main function is energy storage; triglycerides provide an alternative energy source to glucose during fasting and starvation when glucose is in short supply. During these periods of relative glucose depletion, triglycerides present in adipose cells are broken down into their constituent parts by an enzyme called lipase in a process known as lipolysis. The free fatty acids which result from lipolysis are transported from adipose cells to all cells where they are oxidised (burnt), providing chemical energy. Meanwhile the other product of lipolysis, glycerol, is converted to glucose in the liver.

Blood transport of cholesterol and triglycerides

Like all lipids, cholesterol and triglycerides are insoluble in water and must be transported in blood plasma (essentially an aqueous salt solution) bound to water-soluble protein. The proteins that transport lipids are called apoproteins. The combination of lipid (including cholesterol and triglycerides) with apoprotein is called lipoprotein, which consists of a core of lipids surrounded by water-soluble apoprotein (Fig. 7.2). There are four types of lipoprotein in blood, each with differing proportions of cholesterol, triglycerides and apoproteins. They are defined by their relative density and are known as chylomicrons, very low density lipoproteins (VLDLs), low density lipoproteins (LDLs), and high density lipoproteins (HDLs). Around 70% of the cholesterol present in blood is present in LDL and most of the remainder is present in HDL. By contrast most of the triglycerides present in blood are contained within VLDL. The distinction between LDL cholesterol and HDL cholesterol is important when interpreting blood results.

LABORATORY MEASUREMENT OF CHOLESTEROL AND TRIGLYCERIDES

PATIENT PREPARATION

The concentration of cholesterol and triglycerides in blood is affected by diet, smoking, alcohol intake, intercurrent illness and even changes in posture. It is important that where possible blood is sampled under standard conditions to minimise some of these effects.

■ The patient's normal diet should be followed in the two to three weeks prior to testing

'cont.'

'continued'

- There is a transient and quantitatively unpredictable rise in blood tri- glycerides level immediately after a meal, making interpretation diffi- cult. For this reason blood for triglycerides estimation must be sampled only after an overnight fast of 12–14 hours. Fasting is not essential if blood cholesterol only is to be measured.
- The test should be deferred for three months if the patient has suffered major illness (e.g. myocardial infarction) or major surgery unless blood can be sampled within 12 hours of such an event. The test should be deferred for two to three weeks after minor illness.
- The patient should be well rested and seated for 5–10 min before blood collection.
- Use of a tourniquet for more than a minute or so before blood collection can cause erroneous results. If possible, avoid the use of a tourniquet for this test.
- It is not possible to accurately interpret results derived from samples taken while patient is receiving intravenous fluids containing lipids, e.g. 'intralipid'.

SAMPLE REQUIREMENT

Around 5 ml of venous blood is required. The test may be performed on either plasma or serum. If local policy is to use serum, then blood must be collected into a plain chemistry tube (i.e. without anticoagulant). If local policy is to use plasma, then blood must be collected into a tube containing an anticoagulant (EDTA or heparin) which prevents blood from clotting.

IN THE LABORATORY

Three measurements are made in the laboratory: concentration of total cholesterol (i.e. cholesterol contained in LDL, HDL and VLDL lipoprotein), concentration of HDL cholesterol (i.e. only the cholesterol contained in HDL lipoprotein) and concentration of triglycerides (i.e. triglycerides con- tained in VLDL, LDL and HDL). The concentration of LDL cholesterol is technically difficult to measure and in most laboratories is calculated using the results of analysis in the following equation:

LDL cholesterol = Total cholesterol $-$ (HDL cholesterol $-$ triglycerides/5)

INTERPRETATION

Reference range: Fasting triglycerides 0.45–1.80 mmol/l; Total choles- terol, HDL and LDL cholesterol

'cont.'

'continued'

Unlike most other blood tests the concept of a normal or reference range is not considered appropriate for cholesterol testing. This is because a large proportion of apparently healthy individuals from which a reference range would be constructed have blood cholesterol levels which are associated with an increased risk of coronary heart disease. In other words it is 'normal' to have an unhealthy amount of cholesterol in blood. Rather than a reference range, the concept of target values is used to interpret cholesterol results. These target values are:

serum total cholesterol < 5.2 mmol/l
serum LDL cholesterol < 3.5 mmol/l
serum HDL cholesterol > 1.1 mmol/l

TERMS USED IN INTERPRETATION

- Hyperlipidaemia: raised concentration of lipids in blood (either cholesterol > 5.2 mmol/l or triglycerides > 1.80 mmol/l
- Hypercholesterolaemia: raised concentration of total cholesterol, i.e. > 5.2 mmol/l
- Hypertriglyceridaemia: raised blood concentration of triglycerides, i.e. > 1.80 mmol/l.

Consequences of raised cholesterol or triglycerides

Coronary heart disease

Coronary heart disease (CHD), sometimes called ischaemic heart disease, is caused by atherosclerosis, the focal thickening and hardening of the normally elastic walls of the coronary arteries which supply oxygenated blood to heart muscle (myocardium). The internal diameter of the affected artery is decreased at the site of atherosclerosis, reducing normal blood flow to the myocardium. The portion of myocardium affected becomes relatively deficient of oxygen (ischaemic). The symptom of this relative oxygen deficit is angina pectoris, intermittent attacks of chest pain or discomfort precipitated by increased heart activity due to exercise or some other stress. The pain usually subsides as the increased oxygen demand is reduced by rest. However, if the artery suddenly becomes completely occluded by a thrombus (blood

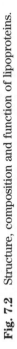

Decreasing particle size

Increasing particle density

	Chylomicrons	Very low density lipoprotein (VLDL)	Low density lipoproteins (LDL)	High density lipoproteins (HDL)
COMPOSITION	Apoprotein 2% Triglycerides 90% Cholesterol 5% Other lipids 3%	Apoprotein 10% Triglycerides 60% Cholesterol 15% Other lipids 15%	Apoprotein 25% Triglycerides 10% Cholesterol 55% Other lipids 10%	Apoprotein 50% Triglycerides 3% Cholesterol 20% Other lipids 25%
FUNCTION	Chylomicrons are synthesised in the intestine. Their function is the transport of dietary triglyceride from the intestine. The triglyceride is delivered to adipose tissue where it is stored as fat and to muscle cells where it is used as an energy source. Chylomicrons contain a small amount of dietary cholesterol which is delivered to the liver.	VLDLs are synthesised in the liver. Their function is to transport triglycerides synthesised in the liver to adipose and muscle cells. They are the precursors of LDLs.	LDLs are what remains of VLDLs when triglycerides have been delivered to adipose and muscle cells. They are the primary carriers of non-dietary cholesterol (i.e. cholesterol made in the body) to all tissues. Around 70% of cholesterol in blood is present in LDL.	HDLs are synthesised in the liver. When released to bloodstream they are composed almost entirely of apoprotein but acquire cholesterol as they circulate around the body. Principal function: transport of excess cholesterol from all non-liver cells back to the liver for excretion. Around 30% of cholesterol in blood is present in HDLs.

Protein shell (apoprotein)

Triglyceride

Cholesterol

Other lipids

Fig. 7.2   Structure, composition and function of lipoproteins.

clot) at the site of atherosclerosis, no blood can flow to the myocardium, and without an oxygen supply myocardial cells simply die. This is a myocardial infarction (MI) or heart attack. The damage to the heart may result in sudden death if it causes lethal abnormal rhythms (ventricular fibrillation). Angina, myocardial infarction and sudden death are the three most common manifestations of coronary heart disease.

Atherosclerosis is a complex and as yet not fully understood phenomenon which begins many years before symptoms of CHD develop. It is clear, however, that there are well defined risk factors (Table 7.1) which predispose people to atherosclerosis and subsequent CHD. Some, like cholesterol and triglycerides, are modifiable and some are not. All risk factors must be taken into account to make the most reliable assessment of an individual's overall risk of CHD.

Table 7.1 Major risk factors for coronary heart disease

Increasing age
Family history of CHD
Diabetes
  Diabetics have 2 to 4 times the risk of CHD compared with non-diabetics who in all other respects have a similar risk status
Cigarette smoking*
Hypertension*
Obesity*
  Defined as body mass index, BMI (i.e. weight in kg/height in metres) > 25
  Obesity associated with hypertension, raised total and LDL cholesterol and reduced HDL cholesterol
Unhealthy diet*
  High fat diet (i.e. fat more than 30% of total calorific intake) ⎫ cause increase in serum
  High intake of saturated rather than unsaturated fat   ⎬ total and LDL
  High intake of cholesterol   ⎭ cholesterol
  Diet devoid of fruit and vegetables which provide
    protective antioxidant vitamins
  High salt diet (predisposes to hypertension)
Excess alcohol*
  Although 1 or 2 drinks per day protects against heart disease, as alcohol intake rises above 21 units per week so too does risk of CHD. Excess alcohol causes hypertension
Lack of exercise*
  Exercise reduces body weight and increases serum HDL cholesterol
Abnormal concentration of blood lipids*
  Raised serum total cholesterol
  Raised serum LDL cholesterol
  Reduced serum HDL cholesterol
  High ratio serum total cholesterol : serum HDL cholesterol

---

* Modifiable risk factors

Blood lipids and coronary heart disease

To understand how the lipids in blood, particularly cholesterol, contribute to CHD it is necessary to examine in a little more detail what is known about the process of atheroma formation which leads to atherosclerosis.

Atheroma formation begins with damage to the endothelium which lines the internal surface of arteries, allowing entry of cholesterol-rich LDL particles present in blood. The damage attracts protective cells called macrophages which take up the LDL particles; LDL accumulates in these cells. At this early stage the only evidence of atheroma is a barely visible raised yellowish patch on the internal surface of the artery, known as a fatty streak. Over many years LDL cholesterol continues to accumulate within the lesion. The normal muscle cells of the artery are replaced by the fibrous protein collagen, making the vessel hard. Collagen also accumulates above the accumulating lipid, forming a hard, fibrous plaque. This is atherosclerosis. The thin and fragile endothelium covering the plaque may break, allowing blood within the plaque where a blood clot (thrombus) forms, either partially or totally occluding blood flow.

Research into the detail of this complex phenomenon continues, but some aspects are clear.

- Accumulation of cholesterol, specifically LDL cholesterol, is an important requirement for atheroma formation.
- The LDL cholesterol found in atherosclerotic plaques is derived from the blood.
- The higher the concentration of cholesterol in blood, the greater is the risk of CHD.
- It is specifically LDL cholesterol which is damaging; the higher the LDL the greater is the risk of CHD.
- By contrast HDL appears to be protective against CHD. The lower the HDL cholesterol the greater is the risk of CHD. A high level of HDL cholesterol is associated with decreased risk of CHD.
- Reducing the concentration of LDL cholesterol in a patient with raised levels is effective in reducing overall risk of CHD.
- The link between blood triglycerides and CHD is currently less clear. There is evidence that, particularly among those who have an increased LDL cholesterol or a reduced HDL cholesterol, raised blood triglycerides increases yet further the risk of CHD.
- There is little evidence, however, to suggest that reducing raised triglycerides levels decreases the risk of CHD.

It must be emphasised that blood lipid testing determines risk only; results cannot be used to diagnose or definitively predict CHD for a particular individual. Some have a raised LDL cholesterol and do not suffer CHD and there is no safe level of cholesterol or triglycerides below which one can be guaranteed not to suffer CHD. The best we can say is that the higher the level of LDL cholesterol, the greater is the risk of CHD; that risk is increased if triglycerides are also raised, and is reduced by a high HDL cholesterol level.

Other effects of raised blood lipids

There are few signs or symptoms to suggest that an individual may have an increased level of cholesterol or triglycerides and the onset of anginal pain or a heart attack is often the first indication. Lipid deposits (xanthomata) visible as nodules may form in subcutaneous tissue among those with very high levels. Lipid may also accumulate in the cornea. Severe hypertriglyceridaemia is associated with abdominal pain and acute pancreatitis.

Causes of raised cholesterol and/or triglycerides

Many genetically determined disturbances of lipid metabolism have been identified which result in either a raised cholesterol, raised triglycerides or both so that it is possible to inherit a predisposition to raised blood lipids. This in part explains why coronary heart disease runs in families. One of these inherited defects is extremely common, several are less common, and many are extremely rare. All are grouped together in the term primary hyperlipidaemias. Less commonly, a raised cholesterol or triglycerides level results not from an inherited gene defect but as a complication of another disease process; these are called secondary hyperlipidaemias. Treatment of the underlying disease often corrects secondary hyperlipidaemia.

Primary hyperlipidaemia

Most people with a raised LDL cholesterol have an inherited defect known as common 'polygenic' hypercholesterolaemia. Many genes are involved. The condition results in mild to moderate increase in LDL cholesterol, the actual level depending to a great extent on diet. Triglycerides levels are usually normal. Much higher levels of LDL cholesterol, often greater than 9.0 mmol/l, characterise a less common inherited condition known as familial hypercholesterolaemia. Affecting 1 in 500 in the UK this single gene defect is associated with high risk of myocardial infarction in middle age.

Although rare it is possible to inherit a predisposition to raised triglyceride levels. Familial hypertriglyceridaemia is the most common genetic cause of raised triglycerides. Levels are usually very high (> 10 mmol/l). Cholesterol levels are usually normal. Risk of CHD is not greatly increased for this group of patients.

Secondary hyperlipidaemia

The most common cause of secondary hyperlipidaemia is diabetes mellitus. Untreated diabetic patients tend to have a mild increase in LDL cholesterol and a moderate to severe increase in triglycerides. This is thought to be at least in part the reason why diabetic patients are at high risk of heart disease. Diabetics should have cholesterol and triglycerides levels monitored at regular intervals. Other causes of secondary hyperlipidaemia include hypothyroidism, nephrotic syndrome, cholestatic liver disease and alcohol abuse.

Case history 6

Michael Oliver, a 31-year-old accountant in good health, attended a 'well man' clinic at his GP's surgery. A family health history and lifestyle questionnaire revealed a family history of heart disease; his 61-year-old father was currently recovering from a heart attack and his grandfather had died of heart disease at the age of 71. His father's recent illness had prompted Michael to quit smoking but he took little exercise. As part of the health screen Michael was weighed, his blood pressure was taken and blood was sampled for blood glucose and lipid screen. Body weight and blood pressure were normal. Clinical examination was unremarkable.

The laboratory reported the following blood results:

Blood glucose 5.6 mmol/l
Plasma total cholesterol 5.8 mmol/l
Plasma LDL cholesterol 5.0 mmol/l
Plasma HDL cholesterol 0.98 mmol/l
Plasma triglycerides 1.0 mmol/l

Are the blood results normal? In view of his father's illness Michael was most concerned about his own risk of heart disease. Consider the advice which might be given.

Discussion of case history

Blood glucose is normal. Total and LDL cholesterol levels are slightly raised and HDL cholesterol is reduced. Triglycerides level is normal.

To advise Michael it is necessary to consider all risk factors for coronary heart disease. On the positive side Michael is young and has a normal blood pressure and body weight. However, he does have a slight increase in total cholesterol, most of which is the damaging LDL cholesterol, which increases the risk of coronary heart disease; that risk is increased yet further by a low level of the protective HDL cholesterol. Since clinical examination and blood glucose are normal, it is unlikely that the raised cholesterol is due to secondary disease, although testing for thyroid function to exclude the possibility of hypothyroidism might be indicated. In view of the family history of coronary heart disease and the slight increase in LDL cholesterol and normal triglycerides level, it seems likely that Michael has inherited common 'polygenic' hypercholesterolaemia. It would be advantageous for Michael to reduce his blood LDL cholesterol and increase his HDL cholesterol.

The options for lowering LDL cholesterol are cholesterol-lowering drugs or dietary manipulation. The increase in LDL cholesterol is only slight and it is highly unlikely that in this case drugs would be prescribed. However, a cholesterol lowering diet might well be advised. Cigarette smoking is associated with a reduction in HDL cholesterol; so long as Michael continues in his efforts to quit smoking, HDL cholesterol will probably return to normal, safer levels. Exercise also increases HDL cholesterol, so Michael should be encouraged to increase the amount of exercise he takes. Michael should be aware that he has inherited a tendency to a slight increase in LDL cholesterol. The effects of this can be minimised by attention to other risk factors and dietary manipulation. Regular (three-monthly) blood monitoring of cholesterol level might be considered necessary.

Further reading

Grundy S. (1995) Role of low density lipoproteins in atherogenesis and development of coronary heart disease. *Clinical Chemistry* **41**: 139–46.

Hu F., Stampfer M., Manson J., Rimm E. *et al.* (1997) Dietary fat intake and the risk of coronary heart disease in women. *New Engl. J. Med.* **337**: 1491–99.

Iles C. (Ed) (1999) Consensus conference on lipid lowering to prevent vascular events. *Proc. Roy. Coll. Physicians of Edinburgh.* Suppl. No. 5 **29**: 1–25.

Scandinavian Simvastatin Survival Study Group (1994) Randomised trial of cholesterol lowering in 4444 patients with coronary heart disease. *Lancet* **344**: 1383–89.

Stampfer M., Krauss R., Jing M., Blanche P. *et al.* (1996) A prospective study of triglyceride level, low density lipoprotein particle diameter, and risk of myocardial infarction. *JAMA* **276**: 882–88.

Stevens A. & Lowe J. (1995) Disease of the blood circulatory system. In *Pathology*, pp. 122–58. Mosby, Missouri.

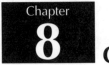

Cardiac Enzymes

This chapter is concerned with how laboratory testing contributes to the differential diagnosis of patients presenting with chest pain. A proportion of such patients will be suffering the cardiac pain associated with a heart attack or myocardial infarction (MI). Every year around 250 000 people in the UK suffer an MI[1] and around 20% die before reaching hospital. For the remaining 80%, early diagnosis and treatment can be lifesaving. Measurement of the amount of cardiac enzymes in blood plasma or serum is used to identify those patients who have suffered an MI and to exclude the diagnosis in patients whose chest pain is the result of some other pathology. The three enzymes most commonly measured in this context are creatine kinase (CK), lactate dehydrogenase (LD) and aspartate aminotransferase (AST). Two additional enzyme assays are available at some laboratories: the CK isoenzyme, CK(MB), and the LD isoenzyme hydroxybutyrate dehydrogenase, (HBD or HBDH).

Normal physiology

What are enzymes?

Enzymes are proteins which increase the rate of biological reactions without themselves being consumed; they are biocatalysts. Virtually all biologically important reactions are catalysed by enzymes. Although these reactions would theoretically occur in the absence of enzymes, the rate of reaction would be too slow to support life. Typically enzymes increase the rate of biochemical reactions by a factor of between 10^6 and 10^{12}. Enzymes are highly specific in their action, catalysing only one or a limited number of similar reactions. Cellular metabolism involves the integration of a myriad of separate reactions, each requiring its own enzyme, so that, depending on the type of tissue, between 1000 and 4000 different enzymes are present within each body cell. Although most enzymic reactions occur within tissue cells, there are exceptions; the enzymic digestion of food in the gastrointestinal tract and the blood clotting cascade provide important examples of extracellular enzyme action.

Enzyme structure

All enzymes are proteins, but they differ greatly in size and structure. The smallest are single amino acid chains (polypeptides) with a molecular weight in the range 10 000–20 000 and the largest are extremely complex particles composed of many different protein sub-units. The enzyme pyruvate dehydrogenase, for example, comprises 42 individual molecules with a total molecular weight in the order of 10×10^6. Many enzymes require co-factors, which are bound covalently to the protein. These include metals such as zinc, magnesium, iron, manganese, etc., and organic molecules, mostly derived from vitamins of the B group and pantothenic acid. For those enzymes which require a co-factor, the complete structure, enzyme plus co-factor, is called a holoenzyme; the protein without the co-factor is called an apoenzyme and has no catalytic activity.

Enzymes may be composed of one, two or more identical protein units. Within each unit are the two important functional sites of an enzyme: the binding site and the catalytic site.

Some enzymes exist in two or more structurally different forms. These are called isoenzymes. Isoenzymes are functionally identical; they combine with the same substrate and catalyse the same reaction, so the structure of the binding and catalytic site must be the same; the differences in structure of isoenzymes lie elsewhere in the enzyme.

Enzyme action

The specific substance that an enzyme reacts on is called its substrate, and the result of enzymic action is called the product. The substrate of the digestive enzyme amylase, for example, is dietary starch. Amylase catalyses the hydrolysis (splitting) of starch and the product is glucose and a mixture of dextrins. The specificity of any enzyme for its substrate is due to the particular structure of the binding site which is complementary to the structure of its particular substrate, allowing combination of enzyme only with that substrate. The binding of enzyme and substrate is analogous to the way a key fits only its complementary lock. Binding of enzyme and substrate brings the catalytic site of the enzyme in close proximity with the substrate, and a highly unstable enzyme–

product is formed which quickly dissociates, leaving the product and unchanged enzyme. The enzyme is able to react with further substrate molecules to release product many times per second. The sequence of events in the simplest of enzyme reactions is as follows:

$$\underset{\text{Binding}}{E + S \longrightarrow} \underset{\text{Catalysis}}{ES \text{ complex} \longrightarrow} \underset{\text{Dissociation}}{EP \text{ complex} \longrightarrow} E + P$$

where E = enzyme, S= substrate, and P = product.

Optimum enzyme activity is dependent on environmental factors such as pH and temperature. Normal cellular metabolism, the totality of cellular enzyme reactions, is dependent, then, on the maintenance of a constant internal environment within cells.

Enzyme nomenclature

Nearly all enzymes end in the suffix '-ase' (amyl**ase**, creatine kin**ase**, glucose-6-phosphate dehydrogen**ase** etc.). Enzyme nomenclature is based on the substrate and the type of reaction catalysed. Thus the substrate of glucose-6-phosphate dehydrogenase, a key enzyme in glucose metabolism, is glucose-6-phosphate. This enzyme specifically catalyses the dehydrogenation (i.e. removal of hydrogen) from glucose-6-phosphate, with production of gluconolactone-6-phosphate. The name of an enzyme gives important clues as to its function.

For a few enzymes which were identified long before this system of nomenclature was introduced the name adopted at the time of discovery has been retained. Many of the familiar digestive enzymes (e.g. trypsin, chymotrypsin, pepsin) fall into this group.

Clinical utility of measuring enzyme levels

General considerations

Of the more than 4000 enzymes thus far identified in the human body, probably less than 25 are routinely measured in clinical laboratories. Almost all of these are intracellular enzymes; they function only within cells. The relatively small amount normally present in blood plasma is the result of normal cell turnover; as cells die they release their contents, including intracellular enzymes, to the blood plasma. Enzymes of low molecular weight are removed from blood by kidney filtration for subsequent excretion in urine, but most are degraded by some poorly understood mechanism, probably in the reticulo-endothelial system. So long as the rate of removal from blood plasma matches the slow rate of enzyme release from tissue during normal cell turnover, the concentration of enzyme in plasma remains low and constant. However, any significant increase in cell death (necrosis) due to a disease process or injury results in increased release of intracellular enzymes to plasma, and enzyme concentration in blood plasma rises. Increased cell turnover and proliferation, as in malignant disease, will also tend to increase the plasma concentration of intracellular enzymes.

Enzymes that are routinely used as a clinical marker of cell damage are to some degree organ specific; that is, although they may be present in all or at least many tissues, they are present at highest concentration in only one or a few types of tissue. Thus raised plasma levels of a particular enzyme are indicative of damage to cells of those tissues which contain highest amounts of the enzyme.

Creatine kinase (CK)

Creatine kinase (alternative name, creatine phosphokinase, CPK) is an enzyme which catalyses the transfer of phosphate from creatine phosphate to adenosine diphosphate. The products of the reaction are creatine and the energy-rich compound adenosine triphosphate.

Creatine phosphate + adenosine diphosphate $\longrightarrow$ Creatine + adenosine triphosphate

CK is present in many types of tissue cells, but three sorts of tissue contain most of the body's CK. They are: cardiac muscle (myocardium), skeletal muscle and the brain. Creatine kinase is composed of two protein subunits, M and B, allowing three functionally identical but structurally different isoenzymes: CK(MM), CK(BB) and CK(MB). When CK is measured in plasma it is the sum of the activity of all three isoenzymes, but the individual isoenzymes can also be measured. CK isoenzymes are organ specific. Most of the CK(BB) is found in the brain. Most of the CK in skeletal muscle is present as the isoenzyme CK(MM) and cardiac muscle contains most of the body's CK(MB). In practice only CK and CK(MB) are useful for diagnosis of myocardial infarction and therefore only these are considered 'cardiac enzymes'. Since most of the body's CK(MB) is derived from cardiac muscle, it is clear that measurement of this isoenzyme is a more specific measure of cardiac muscle cell damage than CK, the sum of all isoenzymes. Some laboratories measure CK, and some measure the more specific isoenzyme, CK(MB).

Lactate dehydrogenase (LD or LDH)

This enzyme catalyses the dehydrogenation (removal of hydrogen) from lactic acid (lactate). The product of the reaction is pyruvate.

$$CH_3.\ CHOH.COOH \longleftrightarrow CH_3.CO.COOH$$
$$\text{(Lactate)} \qquad\qquad \text{(Pyruvate)}$$

This is a key reaction in anaerobic glycolysis (see Chapter 3) and may occur in any metabolically active cell, so that LD is widely distributed throughout body tissues. Highest activity is seen in skeletal muscle, liver and heart muscle, but the enzyme is also present in kidney, pancreas, erythrocytes (the red cells of blood) and lung. Like CK, lactate dehydrogenase exists in several functionally similar but structurally different forms (isoenzymes). Five isoenzymes of LD have been identified, known as LD1, LD2, etc. Also, like CK isoenzymes, these are organ specific. LD5 is the predominant form of LD to be found in liver and skeletal muscle, whilst LD1 is the predominant form of LD present in heart muscle. Unlike other LD isoenzymes, LD1 can utilise hydroxybutyrate as a substrate as well as lactate. In most laboratories total LD is measured (i.e. LD1 + LD2 + LD3, etc.) but in some the more specific isoenzyme for cardiac muscle (LD1) is measured. An alternative name for LD1, reflecting the additional substrate which it can utilise, is hydroxybutyrate dehydrogenase (HBDH).

Aspartate aminotransferase (AST)

AST catalyses the transfer of an amino group (—NH2) from the amino acid aspartic acid (aspartate) to ketoglutamic acid (ketoglutarate). The products of this reaction are the amino acid, glutamic acid (glutamate) and oxaloacetic acid (oxaloacetate)

$$
\begin{array}{ccccccc}
COOH & & COOH & & COOH & & COOH \\
| & & | & & | & & | \\
CH_2 & & CH_2 & & CH_2 & & CH_2 \\
| & & | & & | & & | \\
CH\ NH_2 & + & CH_2 & \longrightarrow & C{=}O & + & CH_2 \\
| & & | & & | & & | \\
COOH & & C{=}O & & COOH & & CH\ NH_2 \\
 & & | & & & & | \\
 & & COOH & & & & COOH \\
\end{array}
$$

Aspartate + ketoglutarate $\longrightarrow$ Oxaloacetate + glutamate

This reaction is part of amino acid metabolism and may be present in any metabolically active cell, so that AST is widely distributed throughout the tissues of the body. Heart muscle, skeletal muscle and liver tissue are particularly rich sources of AST. The enzyme is also present in the cells of the kidney and erythrocytes. A summary of enzyme function and tissue source is provided in Table 8.1.

LABORATORY MEASUREMENT OF CARDIAC ENZYMES

PATIENT PREPARATION

No particular patient preparation is necessary. Intramuscular injections can result in raised CK, complicating interpretation of results, so it is preferable to take blood either before or within an hour of such an injection.

TIMING OF BLOOD COLLECTION

It is common practice to take blood for cardiac enzymes at admission and again on the next two days, because a series of results has more diagnostic power than a single set of results. It is important to record the time of blood sampling on the accompanying request card, along with the time and date of suspected MI. Enzyme levels remain normal for 4 to 8 hours after an MI. Sampling blood too early will result in a falsely negative result.

AMOUNT AND TYPE OF SAMPLE

Around 5 ml of blood is sufficient for cardiac enzymes. The assays are performed on either plasma or serum. If local policy is to use plasma, then blood must be collected into a tube containing the anticoagulant lithium. If local policy is to use serum, then blood must be collected into a plain glass tube without any additive.

INTERPRETATION OF RESULTS

REFERENCE RANGE

The methods used to determine enzyme levels in blood vary between laboratories. This methodological variation gives rise to significant variation in reference ranges so that it would be misleading to quote even approximate reference ranges for enzyme results. It is vital in interpreting enzyme results that the reference range quoted by the laboratory performing the assay is used.

Table 8.1 Cardiac enzymes: function and tissue source

Enzyme	Function	Principal tissue source
CK	Intracellular metabolism catalyses the transfer of phosphate from creatine phosphate to ADP	Cardiac muscle (myocardium) Skeletal muscle Brain
CK(MB)	Isoenzyme of CK – same function	Cardiac muscle (myocardium) A small amount in skeletal muscle
AST	Intracellular metabolism of amino acids – catalyses the transfer of amino group from aspartate to glutamate	Cardiac muscle Liver Skeletal muscle
LDH	Intracellular metabolism catalyses the reduction of oxidation of lactic acid to pyruvic (anaerobic glycolysis)	Cardiac muscle (myocardium) Liver Skeletal muscle Pancreas Blood cells Lung Kidney
HBDH	Isoenzyme of LDH – same function. Also catalyses dehydrogenation of hydroxy-butyric acid	Cardiac muscle Blood cells

Causes of raised cardiac enzymes: myocardial infarction

Most cases of myocardial infarction are an acute manifestation of ischaemic heart disease in which a coronary artery that is already partially occluded by atherosclerosis (Chapter 7) suddenly becomes totally occluded by a thrombus (blood clot) forming at the site of atherosclerosis. Blood can no longer flow through the affected vessel, immediately depriving an area of heart muscle (myocardium) of the oxygen and nutrients that all cells require for survival. Myocardial cells die; the site and extent of this area of cell death (infarction) depends on which branch of coronary artery is occluded. As myocardial cells die, they release a myriad of biochemicals including intracellular enzymes into the bloodstream. Among these are the cardiac enzymes AST, CK, CK(MB) and LDH. Plasma concentration, measured as enzyme activity, rises.

Pattern of enzyme changes following myocardial infarction

The rise in blood plasma activity of cardiac enzymes following myocardial infarction is a transient phenomenon related to the time of the infarction. Figure 8.1 describes the typical pattern of enzyme changes in the hours and days which follow a myocardial infarction (MI).

For the first few hours no increase in any enzyme is evident. At between around 4 and 6 hours post MI, the first evidence of myocardial cell damage is seen with a rise in the amount of the isoenzyme CK(MB). This is followed by a rise in CK and AST from around 8 hours and then

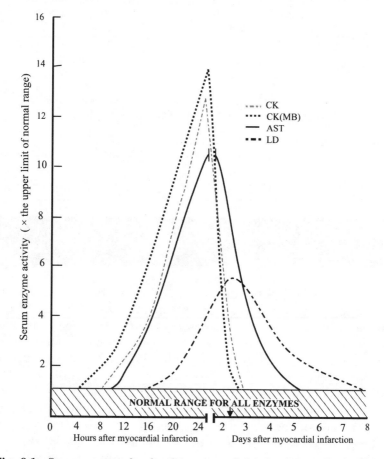

Fig. 8.1 Serum enzyme levels after myocardial infarction at time 0 hours. *Note:* Peak levels vary between patients. This variation reflects variable amount of myocardial cell damage and therefore to some extent the severity of MI.

LD along with HBDH at around 10 to 12 hours after the infarct. The most significant rise is seen in CK and CK(MB), and the least significant is LD. Although this pattern of difference between each of the peak enzyme levels is roughly the same for all patients, the actual peak levels vary greatly, reflecting to some extent the degree of myocardial cell damage. In broad terms, the more extensive the damage, the higher do all enzyme levels rise.

Levels return to normal by day 4 or 5 following the infarct. Of all the enzymes measured, LD remains abnormally high for the longest period. A secondary rise in enzyme levels after peak levels have been reached indicates that the patient has suffered a further infarct.

Role of enzyme measurement in diagnosis of myocardial infarction

In the majority of cases myocardial infarction is suggested by clinical symptoms and confirmed by characteristic electrocardiographic (ECG) changes (Table 8.2). In these circumstances cardiac enzyme measurement serves only to provide confirmatory evidence. Whilst the finding of characteristic changes to ECG, which include ST segment elevation, T wave inversion and Q wave formation, is diagnostic of a myocardial infarction, not all patients whose chest pain is the result of infarction have these diagnostic changes. In fact in around 30% of cases of myocardial infarction, ECG changes are either absent or not sufficiently typical of the condition to be diagnostic.[2] It is in the context of these difficult diagnostic cases that cardiac enzyme measurement is most useful to either confirm a diagnosis of MI, if enzyme levels rise, or to exclude the diagnosis if enzymes remain normal.

Table 8.2 Some major signs and symptoms of myocardial infarction

---

Prolonged severe chest pain which may radiate to arms, neck and jaw
Anxiety
Cold, sweaty extremities
Nausea and vomiting
Breathlessness
Changes in blood pressure
Electrocardiographic (ECG) changes which may include:
   ST segment elevation
   T wave inversion
   Q wave formation

Non-cardiac causes of raised cardiac enzymes

Although the term cardiac enzymes implies that these enzymes are derived solely from heart muscle, this is not the case. CK, AST and LD are present in other tissues, and raised levels can result from disease of these extra-cardiac tissues. This may complicate the interpretation of enzyme results when they are being used for their principal purpose, diagnosis of myocardial infarction.

Skeletal muscle is particularly rich in CK, and muscle disease (e.g. muscular dystrophy) or injury to muscle causes an increase in serum CK levels. Even an intramuscular injection or physical exertion can result in a slight increase. Significant muscle damage, such as that which may occur during surgery or accidental trauma (particularly crush injuries), commonly results in much higher levels. CK is present in brain, so that raised levels may be a feature of brain cell death associated with head injury and cerebrovascular accident. There is a small amount of CK(MB) in skeletal muscle, and levels might be raised (though not to the same extent as total CK) in very severe skeletal muscle damage or disease.

Liver cells are a particularly rich source of AST and LD, so that liver disease can result in raised levels of these two enzymes. In fact measurement of both enzymes is also used for diagnosis of liver disease (Chapter 10). Particularly high levels are seen in acute infectious hepatitis, but moderate increase of both these enzymes may be a feature of cirrhosis, obstructive liver disease and liver cancer.

Finally red blood cells (erythrocytes) contain significant amounts of LD and AST. Diseases which are characterised by an increased destruction or turnover of these cells result in raised levels particularly of LD. Such diseases include some forms of anaemia (the haemolytic anaemias), and acute leukaemia. An extremely high level of LD is a feature of megaloblastic anaemias caused by deficiency of vitamins B_{12} and folate (Chapter 17). The non-cardiac causes of raised cardiac enzymes are summarised in Table 8.3.

New blood markers of myocardial infarction

Although in 95% of cases of myocardial infarction cardiac enzymes are raised, it is evident from the above that there are many other conditions in which these enzymes may be raised. There is a need for a more specific blood test for the diagnosis of MI, that is one which is always normal in the absence of MI. Furthermore, since the introduction of thrombolytic drugs for treatment of MI, which are most effective in the first few hours following infarct, early diagnosis (within the first few hours) is crucial. With the possible exception of CK(MB), cardiac

Table 8.3 Non-cardiac causes of increased cardiac enzymes

Total creatine kinase (CK)	Creatine kinase MB isoenzyme (CKMB)
Muscle disease (e.g. muscular dystrophy) Muscle injury (trauma and surgery) Severe muscular exercise Intramuscular injections Brain injury Cerebrovascular accident (stroke)	May be slightly raised in severe muscle disease or muscle damage
Aspartate aminotransferase (AST)	**Lactate dehydrogenase (LD)**

Liver disease
  Hepatitis (very high levels)
  Cirrhosis
  Obstructive liver disease due to, for example, gallstones
  Cancer of the liver
  Infectious mononucleosis (glandular fever)
Severe haemolytic anaemia
	Disease affecting red cells (erythrocytes)
	  Haemolytic anaemias
	  Acute leukaemia
	  Lymphoma
	  Megaloblastic anaemia (particularly high levels)
	Liver disease
	  Hepatitis
	  Infectious mononucleosis
	Other
	  Pulmonary embolus
	  Malignancy of any tissue

enzymes generally do not rise until this window of therapeutic opportunity has passed.

These two factors, the need for early diagnosis and a test of greater specificity for MI, have fuelled the search for new blood markers of myocardial cell damage that are more effective than conventional cardiac enzyme measurement. Of the possible markers investigated, two proteins have shown particular promise; they are myoglobin and the troponin proteins, cardiac troponin T and cardiac troponin I.[3]

Myoglobin

Myoglobin is a protein present in all muscle cells including heart muscle cells. It has a structure similar to that of haemoglobin and like haemoglobin binds oxygen. Within two hours of myocardial infarct the concentration of myoglobin in blood plasma rises, allowing very early diagnosis. Unfortunately, since myoglobin is also present in skeletal muscle, a rise in blood levels may also be a feature of skeletal muscle damage; it is clearly not entirely specific for MI.

The troponin proteins

Troponin T, troponin I and troponin C are three sub-units of a larger troponin complex. This complex is present in all muscle tissue cells, where it functions as a regulatory protein in the interaction of myosin and actin filaments during muscular contraction. There are three isoforms of both troponin T and I. One of these is cardiac specific. Cardiac troponin T and cardiac troponin I are not normally present in blood plasma, but following myocardial cell damage they are released from myocardial cells to plasma. Blood levels begin to rise just 4 hours after a myocardial infarct. Unlike myoglobin, a rise in these proteins is highly specific for myocardial cell damage. Small dedicated analysers for the blood measurement of CK(MB), myoglobin and cardiac troponin T have now been developed. These allow fast bedside blood testing for the diagnosis of MI (results are available within 20 minutes of blood sampling).[4] Such analysers may become commonplace in the emergency room and cardiac units.

Case history 7

Henry Jarvis, a 55-year-old teacher in previously good health, suddenly felt extremely unwell whilst working in the garden. He struggled inside complaining to his wife of severe chest pain. Within an hour he arrived by ambulance at his local hospital emergency department. Clinical examination suggested a provisional diagnosis of myocardial infarction but ECG results were equivocal. At around 3 hours after admission, blood was sampled for urea and electrolytes, full blood count and cardiac enzymes. The laboratory reported the following results

    CK   80 IU/l (normal < 150)
    AST   38 IU/l (normal < 50)
    LD   155 IU/l (normal < 220)

(1) Why are AST, CK and LD usually raised following MI?
(2) As Mr Jarvis's results are all normal, can you assume that he has not suffered an MI?

Discussion of case history

(1) During an MI the cells of heart muscle (myocardium) die due to lack of oxygen. As the cells die they release their contents including

the enzymes AST, CK and LD into the bloodstream where they circulate at high levels in blood plasma.

(2)   No. These results do not exclude a diagnosis of MI, because the blood was sampled too soon after the onset of symptoms. Enzyme levels remain normal for up to 4 hours after an MI in the case of CK(MB) and even later for CK, AST and LDH (Fig. 8.1). There is little point in taking blood for these cardiac enzymes until at least 6 hours after the suspected MI. If CK(MB) is available, then blood may be taken a little earlier.

References

(1)   Melville M., Brown N., Gray D. & Young T. (1999) Outcome and use of health services four years after admission for acute myocardial infarction: case record and follow up study. *BMJ* **319**: 230–31.

(2)   Lee H., Cross S., Garthwaite P. *et al.* (1994) Comparison of the value of novel rapid measurement of myoglobin, creatine kinase and creatine kinase-MB with the electrocardiogram for the diagnosis of acute myocardial infarction. *Br. Heart J.* **71**: 311–15.

(3)   Panteghini M., Apple F.S., Christenson R.H. *et al.* (1999) Use of biochemical markers in acute coronary syndromes. IFCC Scientific Division, Committee on Standardisation of Markers of Cardiac Damage. *Clin. Chem. Lab. Med.* **37**: 687–93.

(4)   Hamm C., Goldman B. *et al.* (1997) Emergency room triage of patients with acute chest pain by means of rapid testing for cardiac troponin T or troponin I. *New Engl. J. Med.* **337**: 1648–53.

Further reading

Fox K. (1995) Cardiac enzymes. *Nursing Standard* **9**: 52–4.

Keffer J. (1997) The cardiac profile and proposed practice guideline for acute ischaemic heart disease. *Am. J. Clin. Pathol.* **107**: 398–409.

Sweeney J. & Shwartz G. (1996) Applying the results of large clinical trials in the management of acute myocardial infarction. *West. J. Med.* **164**: 238–48.

Timmis A. (1994) Will serum enzymes and other proteins find a clinical application in the early diagnosis of myocardial infarction? *Br. Heart J.* **71**: 309–10.

9   Tests of Thyroid Function

This chapter is concerned with endocrinology, that branch of medical science which is concerned with organs or parts of organs responsible for production and secretion of hormones. These hormones or 'biochemical messengers' are transported in blood to distant, target organs where they exert their various and specific effects. The thyroid gland is an endocrine organ responsible for production and secretion of thyroid hormones, thyroxine (T4) and triiodothyronine (T3). In this chapter we consider how the laboratory contributes to the diagnosis and monitoring of thyroid disorders. Thyroid function tests include the measurement of the concentration of thyroid hormones in blood. Of all endocrine disorders those involving the thyroid are the most common: disease affects around 5% of the adult population, so thyroid hormones are far and away the most frequently measured hormones in clinical laboratories.

Normal anatomy and physiology

Thyroid gland

The thyroid gland (Fig. 9.1), weighing around 20 g, is butterfly shaped and situated in the neck. The two lobes of the thyroid sit on either side of the trachea just below the larynx and are connected by a bridge of tissue, the thyroid isthmus. Thyroid enlargement (goitre), a feature of many thyroid disorders, may be visible as a swelling of the neck or at least palpable on physical examination.

The gland is composed of two types of hormone-producing cell. The bulk of the cells are so-called follicle cells which produce the two thyroid hormones, thyroxine (T4) and triiodothyronine (T3). Interspersed

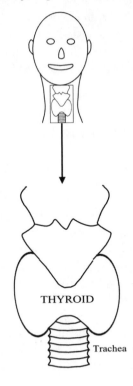

Fig. 9.1   The thyroid gland.

between these cells are the parafollicular cells or C-cells which produce the hormone calcitonin, a hormone required for normal calcium metabolism.

Function of thyroid hormones T3 and T4

Thyroid hormones are delivered via the bloodstream to every part of the body and with few exceptions have an effect on all tissues. Although T3 is the more potent of the two hormones, both increase the speed of many cellular metabolic reactions. For example, mobilisation and breakdown of body fat is increased in the presence of thyroid hormone as is the speed of many reactions involved in the metabolism of carbohydrates and proteins. This overall stimulatory effect on the body's metabolism means that thyroid hormones are essential for normal growth and development, including sexual maturation. Specific effects of thyroid hormones are evident in relation to the heart and central nervous system. Cardiac output is influenced by the concentration of thyroid hormones in blood. Mental development from birth is dependent on adequate amounts of thyroid hormone: a deficiency at this time can lead not only to impaired growth but also to severe and irreversible mental retardation.

Thyroid hormone production

Around 95% of the body's iodine is concentrated in the thyroid. This element is present in adequate amounts in a normal diet, absorbed into the blood from the small intestine and transported to the thyroid where it is required for production of the two thyroid hormones, thyroxine (T4) and triiodothyronine (T3). Hormone production, described in Fig. 9.2, begins in the thyroid follicular cells with the amino acid tyrosine.

Addition of iodine results in mono- and diiodotyrosine. Two molecules of diiodotyrosine combine to form thyroxine (T4) and one molecule of monoiodotyrosine combines with one molecule of diiodotyrosine to form triiodothyronine (T3). Both T4 and T3 are released into the blood from follicular cells, although 80% of circulating T3 is formed not in the thyroid but by enzymatic deiodination (removal of one molecule of iodine) of T4 in peripheral tissue, notably the liver and kidney. Two forms of T3 are formed in this way: physiologically active T3 and physiologically inactive reverse T3 (rT3). More than 99% of both T4 and T3 which circulates in blood is bound to specific proteins. In this protein-bound form, the hormones are inactive but serve as a reservoir or store of thyroid hormones. Just 0.05% of total T3 and T4 in blood is present in a free (i.e. unbound to protein) and therefore physiologically active form.

Control of production of thyroid hormones

It is vital for normal health that the concentration of thyroid hormone in blood is maintained within certain limits. Control of thyroid hormone production (Fig. 9.3), depends on the pituitary gland, a pea-sized organ located at the base of the brain. Among the many hormones that this tiny gland produces is thyroid stimulating hormone (TSH), which, as its name implies, stimulates secretion of thyroid hormones from the thyroid gland. The secretion of TSH is in turn controlled by thyrotrophin releasing hormone (TRH) secreted by the hypothalamus in the brain. Release of both TSH and TRH are controlled by the serum concentration of circulating thyroid hormones (T4 and T3). As thyroid hormone levels

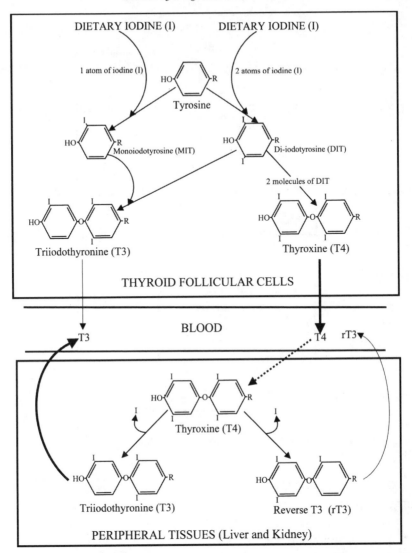

Fig. 9.2 Formation of thyroid hormones T4 and T3 and reverse T3. R = $CH_2.CHNH_2.COOH$.

fall, TRH and TSH secretion increases, stimulating the thyroid to secrete more thyroid hormone. Conversely, as thyroid hormone levels in blood rise, TRH and TSH secretion decreases and therefore thyroid hormone production decreases. By this continuing process of negative feedback, the amount of thyroid hormone in blood is maintained within normal limits.

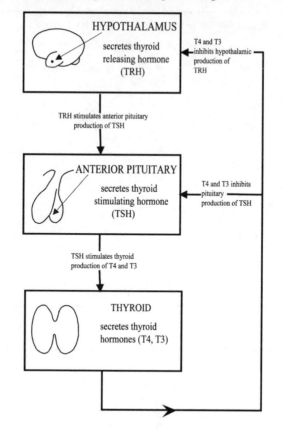

Fig. 9.3   Normal control of thyroid hormone production.

Normal concentration of thyroid hormones (T3 and T4) in blood are dependent then on:

■ a normally functioning thyroid gland
■ an adequate amount of dietary iodine for manufacture of thyroid hormones
■ adequate amounts of TSH and therefore a normally functioning pituitary gland
■ an adequate amount of TRH and therefore a normally functioning hypothalamus

LABORATORY ASSESSMENT OF THYROID FUNCTION

PATIENT PREPARATION
No particular patient preparation is necessary.

SAMPLE REQUIREMENTS
Between 5 and 10 ml of venous blood is required. The tests may be performed on blood plasma or blood serum; if local policy is to use plasma, then blood must be collected into a tube containing an anticoagulant (usually heparin) but if local policy is to use serum, blood must be collected into a plain tube (i.e. without any additive).

REQUEST CARD INFORMATION
Since drugs and pre-existing non-thyroid disease can affect interpretation, it is important to record drug and brief clinical history. In addition to its role in the diagnosis of thyroid disorders, the test may also be used to monitor the effectiveness of therapy among those already diagnosed; it is important that the reason for requesting the test and dosage of any prescribed thyroxine replacement or antithyroid drugs be recorded.

IN THE LABORATORY
The profile of tests available for first-line testing of thyroid function varies between laboratories but will usually include the following four tests.

- Total thyroxine (T4). The T4 test measures the concentration of thyroxine in blood serum. This includes both protein-bound (biologically inactive) thyroxine and free (biologically active) thyroxine.
- Free thyroxine (FT4). The FT4 test measures the concentration of free thyroxine (biologically active fraction) in blood serum.
- Total triiodothyronine (T3). The T3 test measures the concentration of total triiodothyronine in blood serum. This includes both the protein-bound (biologically inactive) fraction and the free (biologically active) fraction.
- Thyroid stimulating hormone (TSH). The TSH test measures the blood serum concentration of the pituitary hormone TSH.

Additionally some laboratories measure free T3 (FT3) and reverse T3 (rT3). These are useful in special circumstances only.

'cont.'

'continued'

INTERPRETATION OF TEST RESULTS

APPROXIMATE REFERENCE RANGES

T4   60–150 nmol/l
FT4   9–26 pmol/l
T3   1.1– 2.6 nmol/l
TSH   0.3–5.0 mIU/l

TERMS USED IN INTERPRETATION

- Euthyroid(ism) – normal thyroid activity
- Hyperthyroid(ism) – overactive thyroid gland
- Hypothyroid(ism) – underactive thyroid gland
- Goitre – enlargement of the thyroid gland. Depending on the cause, goitre may be a feature of euthyroidism, hyperthyroidism or hypothyroidism
- Thyrotoxicosis – the clinical syndrome which results from hyperthyroidism, often used as a synonym for hyperthyroidism
- Myxoedema – the clinical syndrome which results from severe hypothyroidism.

Causes of abnormal thyroid function

Overactivity of the thyroid gland is called hyperthyroidism. This may be due to disease of the thyroid gland itself, in which case the condition is known as primary hyperthyroidism or, much more rarely, arises as a result of increased secretion of TSH by the pituitary gland; this is known as secondary hyperthyroidism. Similarly, underactivity of the thyroid gland (hypothyroidism), is most commonly due to disease of the thyroid gland (primary hypothyroidism) but can result from decreased production of TSH by the pituitary gland (secondary hypothyroidism).

Primary hyperthyroidism

By far the most common cause of primary hyperthyroidism is Graves' disease, an autoimmune condition which affects around 1–2% of the adult population and is more common among women.[2] The thyroid gland of those suffering from Graves' disease is diffusely enlarged (smooth or diffuse goitre) and hyperactive, resulting in increased thyroid hormone production. The cause of this hyperactivity is an abnormal antibody produced by the immune system which acts like TSH, to stimulate the thyroid. Unlike TSH, however, the production and action of this antibody continues despite rising thyroid hormone levels.

Less common causes of primary hyperthyroidism include Plummer's disease, in which a single abnormal 'nodule' in the thyroid gland excretes increased amounts of thyroid hormone, and toxic multinodular goitre, characterised by many hypersecreting nodules. Increased secretion of thyroid hormones is also a feature of thyroiditis, a painful inflammation of the thyroid thought to be caused by viral infection. Amiodarone is an important drug-related cause of hyperthyroidism.

Whatever the cause, primary hyperthyroidism is characterised by increased thyroid hormone levels and it is this feature which accounts for the signs and symptoms (Table 9.1). Since increased thyroid hormone production suppresses pituitary secretion of TSH, a reduction in blood TSH is an important diagnostic feature of primary hyperthyroidism.

The blood results that would be expected in primary hyperthyroidism no matter what the cause are:

- serum/plasma TSH concentration always reduced (often undetectable in severe cases)
- serum/plasma T4, FT4 and T3 concentrations usually increased
- occasionally T4 and FT4 are normal and only T3 is raised (T3 thyrotoxicosis).

Table 9.1   Major signs and symptoms of primary hyperthyroidism

Thyroid hormone excess causes a general speeding of body metabolism, resulting in the following signs and symptoms:

Weight loss
Increased appetite
Intolerance of heat
Increased sweating; warm moist skin
Increased heart rate (tachycardia)
Palpitations
Diarrhoea
Nervousness
Anxiety
Inability to concentrate
Fine hand tremor
'Staring' prominent eyes (exophthalmus)
Disturbance of menstrual cycle

Secondary hyperthyroidism

Very rarely excessive thyroid hormone production is the result not of a problem within the thyroid but rather of uncontrolled secretion of TSH due to disease (overactivity) of the pituitary gland. For example, pituitary tumours secrete abnormally high amounts of TSH. In these rare cases the thyroid is responding normally to abnormal stimulation. Typical blood results in secondary hyperthyroidism are

- serum/plasma TSH concentration raised
- serum T4, FT4 and T3 concentration raised.

Primary hypothyroidism

Primary hypothyroidism affects around 2–3% of the adult population. The condition is more common among women; an estimated 1 in 10 women over the age of 45 are thought to have some degree of hypothyroidism.[3] In the UK most cases of hypothyroidism are the result of autoimmune destruction of thyroid tissue. Hashimoto's disease (sometimes called Hashimoto's thyroiditis) is the most common of these autoimmune diseases. Destruction of thyroid tissue by thyroid surgery or administration of radioactive iodine are frequently used to treat hyperthyroidism, so treatment of primary hyperthyroidism is associated with an increased risk of hypothyroidism later in life. Taken together, treatments for hyperthyroidism constitute the second most common cause of primary hypothyroidism. Some drugs, notably lithium (Chapter 13), can cause hypothyroidism.

Around 1 in 5000 babies are born with a deficiency of thyroid hormone (congenital hypothyroidism), usually due to either absence or abnormal development of the thyroid gland. If not treated with replacement hormone within the first few weeks of life, congenital hypothyroidism leads to severely impaired growth and permanent mental retardation (cretinism). All newborn babies are routinely screened for the condition soon after birth by measurement of the concentration of TSH in blood recovered from a heel prick.

Whatever the cause, primary hypothyroidism results in reduced thyroid hormone production and it is this deficiency which accounts for symptoms (Table 9.2). The normal response of the pituitary to reduced thyroid hormone production is increased production of TSH. An increased concentration of TSH in blood is the most important diagnostic feature of primary hypothyroidism. Indeed in the early stages and in mild disease this increased stimulation by the pituitary may be suffi-

Table 9.2 Major signs and symptoms of primary hypothyroidism

Deficiency of thyroid hormone causes a general slowing of body metabolism, resulting in the following signs and symptoms:

Weight gain
Puffy face, particularly below the eyes
Decreased appetite
Intolerance of cold
Dry skin, dry 'lifeless' hair
Decreased heart rate (bradycardia)
Constipation
Lethargy
Depression
Slowing of mental agility
Hoarse, 'gruff' voice

cient to maintain normal blood levels of thyroid hormones, albeit at the low end of the normal range.

The blood results that would be expected in primary hypothyroidism, whatever the cause are:

- serum/plasma TSH concentration always increased
- serum/plasma T4 concentration reduced (may be low normal in early stage of disease)
- serum/plasma FT4 concentration reduced (may be low normal in early stage of disease).

Secondary hypothyroidism

There are several very rare forms of hypothyroidism which are the result not of thyroid disease but of an inability to adequately stimulate a normal thyroid gland because of a deficiency of TSH. These are all the result of damage to or disease of the pituitary. Damage to the hypothalamus has the same effect. The blood results that would be expected in secondary hypothyroidism whatever the cause are:

- serum/plasma TSH concentration reduced
- serum/plasma T4, FT4 concentration reduced.

Non-thyroid illness

The laboratory diagnosis of hyper- and hypothyroidism is rarely a problem in otherwise well patients but interpretation of thyroid function test results is often more difficult in patients who have some pre-existing disease or who are taking certain drugs. Under these circumstances thyroid function test results may be abnormal despite normal activity of the thyroid gland (euthyroidism), providing misleading evidence of both hypo- and hyperthyroidsim. For example, a raised T4 level suggestive of hyperthyroidism is also a feature of normal pregnancy, oral contraceptive use and hepatitis, whereas a low T4, suggesting hypothyroidism, may occur in chronic liver disease (cirrhosis) and nephrotic syndrome. In these cases of non-thyroid disease, although the T4 may be abnormal, FT4 and TSH are not affected and remain normal.

Quite marked changes in thyroid function tests occur in critically ill patients no matter what the cause. The 'sick' euthyroid syndrome is used to describe these patients. Typically T4 and T3 are decreased in almost all those with 'sick' euthyroid syndrome. FT4 may remain normal but may also be low. TSH tends to be normal during critical illness but is typically transiently raised during recovery. The interpretation of thyroid function tests in the critically ill patient is difficult; results among those with 'sick' euthyroid syndrome are often suggestive of hypothyroidism. In these circumstances the reverse T3 (rT3) is useful because in hypothyroidism rT3 is abnormally low and in 'sick' euthyroid syndrome it is abnormally high.

A summary of the abnormal changes in thyroid function tests for both thyroid and non-thyroid disease is contained in Table 9.3.

Monitoring treatment of thyroid disease

The blood tests described above for the identification of patients suffering from thyroid disorders are also useful to monitor the effectiveness of therapy among those already diagnosed.

Treatment of hyperthyroidism

There are three possible treatment regimes for those with hyperthyroidism. Most patients are treated with antithyroid drugs. In the UK carbimazole, a drug which inhibits thyroid hormone production, is most often used. Typically a daily dose of carbimazole for 12 to 18 months effects a cure for around a half of patients. For those in whom drug therapy is either not indicated or unsuccessful, an alternative is radioactive iodine treatment. Like all ingested iodine, radioactive iodine is concentrated in the thyroid gland. Here the radioactivity destroys thyroid tissue. Surgical removal of thyroid tissue (partial thyroidectomy) offers a third treatment option.

Table 9.3 Summary of typical changes to thyroid function test results in thyroid and non-thyroid disease

	T4	FT4	T3	TSH
Thyroid disease				
Primary hyperthyroidism (thyrotoxicosis) Common causes: Graves' disease Rarer causes: Plummer's disease (single toxic nodule); toxic multinodular goitre; sub-acute thyroiditis	Increased (occasionally normal)	Increased (occasionally normal)	Increased	Marked decrease (may be undetectable)
Primary hypothyroidism Common causes: Hashimoto's disease; treatment of hyperthyroidism Rarer causes: congenital disease; iodine deficiency (common in some parts of the world)	Decreased (may be low end of normal range in early or mild disease)	Decreased (may be low end of normal range in early or mild disease)	Decreased (occasionally normal)	Marked increase
Non-thyroid disease				
Secondary hyperthyroidism (rare) Cause: overactivity of pituitary or hypothalamus	Increased	Increased	Increased	Increased
Secondary hypothyroidism (rare) Cause: underactivity of pituitary or hypothalamus	Decreased	Decreased	Decreased	Decreased
Euthyroid sick syndrome May be a feature of any acute, severe illness, e.g. cancer, severe liver disease, renal failure, major trauma or surgery, extensive burns, severe infection and starvation	Decreased	Normal (though may be decreased in particularly severe illness)	Decreased	Normal (may be transiently decreased during recovery)

Note 1: Normal pregnancy and hepatitis result in raised T4 suggesting hypothyroidism. However, patients are euthyroid and have normal FT4 and TSH.

Note 2: Use of many drugs affects one or more thyroid function tests. These include oral contraception, corticosteroids, propanolol, carbamazepine, phenytoin, lithium and amiodarone.

The object of therapy is to reduce thyroid hormone levels to normal (biochemical euthyroidism) and thereby remove symptoms, that is achieve a state of clinical euthyroidism. All therapies carry the risk of over-treatment, rendering patients hypothyroid, so monitoring of blood hormone levels during and after treatment is an essential part of the care of patients being treated for hyperthyroidism. The dose of antithyroid drug is adjusted in the first instance in the light of serum T4 or FT4 results; the serum TSH often remains suppressed for a month or two after treatment begins but will eventually return to normal. Since there is a long-term risk of hypothyroidism developing or recurrence of hyperthyroidism in those treated for hyperthyroidism, annual blood testing of thyroid function (T4 or FT4 and TSH) is necessary for all patients.

Treatment of primary hypothyroidism

The only treatment for primary hypothyroidism is thyroxine (T4) replacement tablets to be taken daily, usually for life. The object is to increase thyroid hormone levels (T4 and T3) to normal; this will reduce the abnormally high level of TSH secretion to normal and remove symptoms. The dosage required to achieve this state of biochemical and clinical euthyroidism varies and can only be assessed by gradually increasing dosage in the light of serum T4 or FT4 results (some authorities believe that thyroxine therapy is best monitored by measuring serum T3 levels). Too low a dose and symptoms of hypothyroidism persist; too high a dose and T4 and T3 levels rise above normal, TSH levels drop below normal and the patient develops symptoms of hyperthyroidism. Once a maintenance dose has been achieved which results in both biochemical and clinical euthyroidism, the dose usually remains the same for life and blood levels need only be checked annually.

Case history 8

Mrs Hollingsworth, a 35-year-old PE teacher, has visited her current GP only for antenatal visits during two uneventful pregnancies in her twenties and for annual 'well woman' checks over the previous five years. She now goes to see her GP because for a period of several months she has been feeling 'constantly tired and washed out' despite increasingly less activity at work and sleeping more than usual. She tells the doctor that she thinks she might be anaemic because of several 'heavy periods' over the past few months. The doctor feels that this normally lively lady appears unusually depressed. On questioning she admits feeling depressed but attributes this to tiredness and hopes that some 'iron tablets' will put things right. She also reports being frustrated at a recent increase in body weight despite eating less than normal; she feels she has lost her appetite for food. The weight gain is confirmed by comparing her current weight with measurements made at previous well woman clinics. Although there are no clinical signs of anaemia, the doctor agrees to take blood to test for anaemia but also takes a further sample for thyroid function tests.

The full blood count results are entirely normal, excluding anaemia as a cause for the tiredness.

The thyroid function test results are:

T4	55 nmol/l
FT4	8.5 pmol/l
T3	1.5 nmol/l
TSH	26 mIU/l

(1) What symptoms suggested that thyroid function tests were appropriate?
(2) Are the thyroid function results normal?
(3) What do the results suggest?

Discussion of case history

(1) As the GP suspected from clinical examination, Mrs Hollingsworth was not anaemic so there must be some other explanation for her tiredness. Tiredness, depression, excessive menstrual blood flow (menorrhagia) and weight gain without increased food intake can all result from a deficiency of thyroid hormone, i.e. hypothyroidism. The condition is particularly common in middle-aged women. The extent and severity of symptoms among patients with hypothyroidism vary greatly so that the absence of more clinical features of hypothyroidism does not exclude the diagnosis.
(2) Only T3 is within the normal range. The three remaining tests are abnormal; T4 and FT4 are both slightly low but the TSH is greatly increased.
(3) The results confirm the diagnosis of primary hypothyroidism (Table 9.3). Mrs Hollingsworth's thyroid is producing insufficient thyroid hormone despite increased secretion of TSH by the pituitary gland. In the early stages of primary hypothyroidism this pituitary stimulation of the thyroid gland is sufficient to maintain

near normal levels of thyroid hormone (T3 is actually normal in this case) but if the disease were allowed to progress without treatment (thyroid hormone replacement), more marked reduction in thyroid hormone concentration would be expected.

References

Clark J. (1993) Thyroid disease. *The Practitioner* **237**: 264–68.

Clark J. (1995) Current management of thyroid disease. *Prescriber* 5 May, 31–38.

Tunbridge W. (1977) The spectrum of thyroid disease in a community. *Clin. Endocrinology* **7**: 481–93.

Further reading

Cavalieris R. (1991) Effect of nonthyroid disease and drugs on thyroid function tests. *Med. Clin. North. Am.* **75**: 27–39.

Surks M., Chopra I., Mariash C. *et al.* (1990) American Thyroid Association Guidelines for the Use of Laboratory Tests in Thyroid Disorders. *JAMA* **263**: 1529–32.

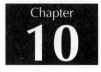

10 Liver Function Tests: Alanine transferase (ALT), gamma glutamyl transferase (GGT), alkaline phosphatase (AP), bilirubin and albumin

This chapter is concerned with the measurement of five substances present in blood plasma. Although structurally and functionally distinct they are treated together here because the blood measurement of all are used principally in identifying those patients who are suffering disease of the liver or biliary tract. The five separate tests are routinely measured together in a profile commonly known as liver function tests (LFTs). Depending on the exact nature of liver disease, one or more of these tests may be normal but it is extremely unlikely that all would be normal in any patient suffering liver or biliary tract disease. Thus, the combination of five liver function tests has more power to detect liver disease than each individual test. None of the five tests is specific for liver disease, so there are other diseases not involving the liver in which one or more of these tests might be abnormal.

Normal physiology

The liver

The liver is the largest of the body's organs weighing around 2 kg. It is located in the right upper quadrant of the abdomen, protected for the most part by the lower rib cage (Fig. 10.1). The narrower left lobe extends from the rib cage over the stomach. The liver is red–brown in colour due to its copious blood supply: the organ receives around 30% of the total cardiac output every minute from two sources, the portal vein

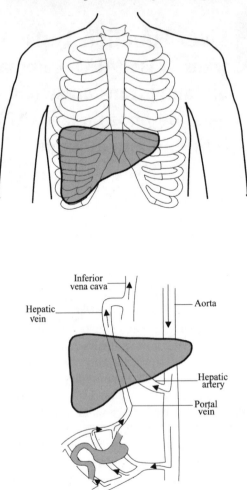

Fig. 10.1   Location of liver and hepatic circulation.

and the hepatic artery. The products of ingested food are transported to the liver directly from the gastrointestinal tract in blood via the portal vein, and oxygenated blood is supplied via the hepatic artery. Blood leaves the liver by way of the hepatic vein, draining into the inferior vena cava for return to the heart.

The cells of the liver, hepatocytes, play a central role in the metabolism of ingested carbohydrates, proteins and fats. This is why these products of digestion are transported first to the liver, via the portal vein. Large amounts of glucose derived from ingested carbohydrates are stored in hepatocytes as glycogen until required. Between meals when glucose is in short supply, these glycogen stores are mobilised. During starvation, when even glycogen stores are depleted, the liver is able to convert amino acids from ingested and body protein to glucose. By these mechanisms the liver plays an important role in regulating blood glucose concentration.

Amino acids derived from dietary proteins arrive at the liver in portal blood; some are synthesised into proteins in the liver; these include nearly all the proteins, including albumin, which are present in blood plasma. Urea, a waste product of amino acid metabolism, is synthesised in the liver before transport in blood to the kidneys where it is excreted in urine.

The liver plays a major role in the metabolism of ingested fats (lipids) by synthesising the lipoproteins necessary for transport of these fats including cholesterol and triglycerides around the body in blood.

In addition to its metabolic and synthetic functions, the liver is also responsible for production of bile, an alkaline watery yellow fluid. This fluid contains bile acids which are synthesised within the liver from cholesterol. Bile flows from the liver to the intestine via the hepatic duct, gall bladder and common bile duct. In the intestine, bile acids are required for normal digestion of dietary fats. The production of the 500 ml bile which is produced daily by the liver is not only important for digestion, but it also serves as a route for excretion of substances from the body in faeces. In this way the liver is responsible for the excretion of some drugs and waste products of metabolism which are not removed from the body by the kidneys in urine. One of these is bilirubin.

Bilirubin

Many patients suffering from liver disease have a yellow discoloration of the skin and mucous membranes, first evident in the conjunctiva of the eye. This clinical sign, known as jaundice (derived from the French word for yellow, *jaune*), which as will become clear is not confined to those suffering liver disease, is due to an abnormally high concentration in the blood of the yellow pigment bilirubin.

Bilirubin is mainly derived from haemoglobin (Fig. 10.2) the oxygen-carrying protein contained in red blood cells. At the end of their normal 120-day lifespan, red blood cells are removed from general circulation by the spleen and other parts of the reticuloendothelial (RE) system. (Incidentally, the RE system includes specialised cells in the liver called Kupffer cells which also are involved in this processing of effete red blood cells.) Within the RE system, haemoglobin released from dead red cells is split into its constituent parts, haem and globin; iron is removed from haem and recycled for production of more haemoglobin. What

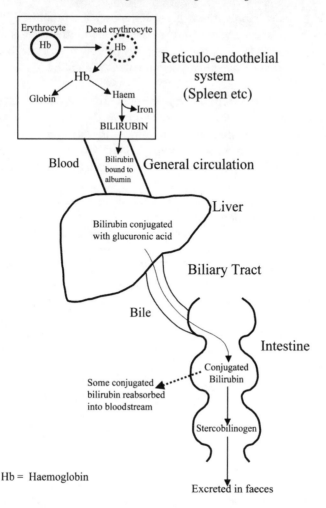

Fig. 10.2 Bilirubin production and excretion.

remains of the haem molecule is converted to bilirubin. From the reticuloendothelial system, bilirubin, now bound to albumin, is transported in the blood to the liver. On entry into hepatocytes, bilirubin is joined (conjugated) with glucuronic acid to make it water soluble for excretion in bile to the gastrointestinal tract.

Once in the gut most of the conjugated bilirubin is converted by bacteria to urobilinogen and then stercobilin, and excreted in faeces. Stercobilin is the brown pigment which contributes to the colour of faeces. Some of the urobilinogen is reabsorbed into the bloodstream and is then transported to the kidneys, where it is excreted in urine.

Albumin

Blood plasma contains a mixture of many proteins, each with its own function. These include proteins required to fight infection (immunoglobulins or antibodies), enzymes, blood clotting factors, specific transport proteins and many more. Albumin is the single most abundant protein in plasma, comprising as it does around 60% of total plasma protein; it is the most frequently measured plasma protein in clinical laboratories.

Like most other proteins present in plasma, albumin is synthesised from amino acids in the liver. It has two main functions. The first of these is as a transport protein. Many water-insoluble substances can only be transported in blood plasma when loosely bound to specific proteins. Albumin is one of these proteins and is required for transport of bilirubin and free fatty acids. Around half the calcium present in blood plasma is transported in a physiologically inactive form, bound to albumin, as are many drugs.

The other important function of albumin is maintenance of blood plasma volume. As the single most abundant protein in plasma, albumin is a major contributor to colloid osmotic pressure. This pressure opposes the tendency of fluid to escape from capillary blood vessels into the surrounding interstitial space due to blood pressure within vessels. Oedema (which may be visible as swelling) is the term used to describe an abnormal accumulation of fluid in the interstitial space, and this occurs if albumin concentration of plasma and therefore colloid osmotic pressure falls below normal.

Solution of albumin may be administered therapeutically via an intravenous line to patients who have suffered major trauma, burns or clinical shock, to restore plasma volume.

GGT, ALT and AP

GGT, ALT and AP are all enzymes (see also Chapter 8). They are present in the cells of the liver and biliary tract where they each function as catalysts of specific metabolic reactions. The liver cell death (necrosis) associated with liver disease results in increased amounts of these intracellular enzymes being released to blood plasma. The enzymes have no function in blood but the amount of enzyme in blood plasma serves as an indicator of liver cell damage, and the pattern of enzyme changes sometimes helps to elucidate the nature of the liver disease.

If the source of these enzymes was only liver tissue, then raised levels would always indicate liver cell damage. In fact, although GGT, ALT and AP are frequently referred to as 'liver enzymes', they are also present in other tissues, and damage or disease of these non-liver tissues may also be associated with a rise in serum concentration of either GGT, ALT or AP. The most significant non-liver source of GGT is the pancreas. ALT is present not only in liver but also, albeit at a far lower concentration, in kidney tissue, heart muscle (myocardium) and skeletal muscle. AP is present not only in the liver and biliary tract but also in bone, intestinal tissue and placental tissue.

LABORATORY MEASUREMENT OF LIVER FUNCTION

PATIENT PREPARATION

No particular patient preparation is necessary.

TIMING OF SAMPLE

Blood for liver function tests (LFTs) may be sampled at any time. It is, however, important that there is not undue delay (more than a few hours) in transporting specimens to the laboratory for separation of serum (or plasma) from cells.

SAMPLE REQUIREMENT

Around 5 ml of venous blood is required for LFTs. Blood should be collected into a plain tube without additives if local policy is to use serum for analysis and into a tube containing the anticoagulant lithium heparin if local policy is to use plasma. A falsely raised albumin level occurs if a tourniquet is left in position for a more than a minute or two before sampling blood. If possible the use of a tourniquet should be avoided. Bilirubin is slowly destroyed by both artificial light and sunlight, leading to falsely low results. To reduce this effect samples should be protected as far as possible from exposure to light both before and during transport to the laboratory.

NEONATAL MEASUREMENT OF BILIRUBIN ONLY

For reasons to be discussed later, newly born babies (particularly premature babies) frequently need monitoring of serum bilirubin concentration. In these cases only bilirubin need be measured, reducing the sample requirement to around 0.5 ml or less. Capillary blood obtained by a heel stab (Chapter 2) is usually used in these circumstances. Particular care is required to avoid haemolysis during blood collection, as such samples are unsuitable for bilirubin estimation. A special dark plastic container (to protect bilirubin from exposure to light) is often used for collection of blood samples for neonatal bilirubin measurement.

'cont.'

'continued'

INTERPRETATION OF RESULTS

APPROXIMATE REFERENCE RANGES

serum/plasma bilirubin $< 17\,\mu mol/l$

serum/plasma albumin $35\text{--}50\,g/l$

Serum/plasma ALT, GGT and AP. Methods used to measure enzyme levels vary between laboratories; each method has its own reference range. It would be misleading therefore to quote even approximate reference ranges for these enzyme tests. Always use local laboratory range when interpreting results. The amount of AP in serum/plasma is age dependent, being much higher in childhood and adolescence than during adulthood. Each laboratory publishes AP reference ranges for each of these age ranges. It is important that the age of the patient be taken into account when interpreting AP results. The presence of AP in placental tissue determines that AP is higher during pregnancy.

Causes of abnormal biliburin concentration

The concentration of bilirubin in serum reflects the balance between the amount produced by the normal process of red cell destruction and that removed from the blood by the liver for subsequent excretion in bile. An abnormally raised serum bilirubin occurs in three broad pathological situations. These are:

- diseases associated with increased red cell destruction and therefore increased bilirubin production (haemolytic anaemias); liver and biliary tract are normal
- diseases associated with liver cell damage and consequent inability to conjugate bilirubin before excretion in bile (liver disease)
- diseases associated with restriction of bile flow and consequent reduction in bilirubin excretion (liver or biliary tract disease)

The haemolytic anaemias are a group of conditions in which anaemia is caused by an abnormal increase in the rate of red cell destruction. The resulting increase in haemoglobin breakdown and therefore bilirubin production causes serum bilirubin concentration to rise. Generally speaking haemolytic anaemias are associated with only a slight increase in bilirubin; concentration rarely rises above $70\,\mu mol/l$. An important exception is haemolytic disease of the newborn (see later). Since the liver is functionally normal, all other LFTs are normal.

Higher serum bilirubin concentration is a feature of any disease which results in damage to liver cells and therefore reduction in the conjugation and excretion of bilirubin. For example, acute inflammation of the liver (acute hepatitis), usually the result of viral infection (Table 10.1) or alcohol abuse (alcoholic hepatitis), results in a rise in bilirubin. Peak concentrations (often greater than 300 µmol/l) are seen at around the tenth day after symptoms develop. During the 4- to 8-week recovery period, bilirubin gradually returns to a normal concentration. In some cases inflammation does not resolve and becomes chronic and progressively destructive. The term 'chronic active hepatitis' is used to describe such cases, and bilirubin, though not as high as during acute hepatitis, may remain raised. Cirrhosis, that is irreversible liver damage, most often the result of prolonged alcohol abuse or unresolved viral hepatitis (there are many rarer causes), may be associated with a near normal serum bilirubin concentration in the early stages but rises as the disease progresses over many years to liver failure. Secondary spread (metastases) of primary cancers to the liver is often associated with raised bilirubin in the later stages; jaundice is a poor prognostic sign in patients with such secondary cancer spread.

Highest serum bilirubin concentrations (up to 800 µmol/l) are seen in diseases which result in complete obstruction of bile flow (cholestasis), and therefore failure to excrete bilirubin. These are diseases not of the liver but of the biliary tract. The most common cause is gallstones that obstruct the cystic duct or common bile duct. Cancers of the common bile duct and head of the pancreas can also obstruct bile flow, causing very high serum bilirubin concentration.

A raised bilirubin during the first few weeks of life is common, particularly among premature infants whose liver and therefore ability to conjugate bilirubin are not fully mature. This is called 'physiological jaundice' because it resolves as the liver matures. The condition affects around 60% of babies to some degree during the first week or two of life. Breast feeding seems to increase the risk of physiological jaundice. Haemolytic disease of the newborn (HDN) is a quite separate and rarer cause of raised bilirubin in neonates, in which the baby's red cells are destroyed by the mother's circulating red cell antibodies (Chapter 19).

Some inherited defects of bilirubin metabolism result in raised bilirubin but all are rare except Gilbert's syndrome. This is a benign condition affecting around 5% of the population and is usually discovered quite by chance during routine blood testing. The only abnormality is a slight increase in bilirubin which rarely rises above 70 µmol/l.

Table 10.1 Viral causes of hepatitis and therefore of abnormal liver function tests

	Hepatitis A virus (HAV)	Hepatitis B virus (HBV)	Hepatitis C virus (HCV)	Hepatitis D virus (HDV)	Hepatitis E virus (HEV)	Hepatitis G virus (HGV)
Relative significance as a cause of hepatitis in the UK	Most common cause of viral hepatitis; accounts for 40% of all cases	Common cause of viral hepatitis; accounts for 35% of all cases	Less common cause of viral hepatitis; accounts for 15% of all cases	Can only occur in association with HBV infection. Never the sole cause of hepatitis	Rare. Cases are almost always the result of travel to areas where the virus is endemic, e.g. Far East, India	Newly discovered virus thought to be a rare cause of hepatitis
Mode of transmission; risk factors	Faecal–oral route; close personal contact; eating uncooked contaminated food or water	Inoculation with infected blood. Can be sexually transmitted. Those at risk include injecting drug abusers, and health care workers	As for HBV. Evidence of sexual transmission less clear cut. Blood transfusion before 1993 is a risk factor for chronic infection	As for HBV	Faecal–oral route; eating contaminated food and water in areas of the world where virus is endemic	Transmitted like HBV, HCV and HDV via infected blood. Blood transfusion an additional risk factor as blood is not tested
Symptoms of acute infection	Infection does not always result in symptoms, particularly during childhood. When they do occur, symptoms begin with a flu-like illness with fever and generalised aches and pains. This is followed a few days later by nausea, vomiting, abdominal pain and fatigue which may be extreme. For the great majority of patients symptoms gradually resolve over a period of 6–8 weeks. Rarely, acute viral hepatitis can result in liver failure				Generally speaking Hep A results in less severe symptoms.	Unclear at the present time
Long-term consequences of infection: progression to chronic liver disease (chronic active hepatitis, cirrhosis) or liver cancer	No long-term consequences	Around 5–10% of infected patients progress to chronic liver disease. Some of these subsequently develop primary liver cancer	Common. Around 70% of HCV infected patients progress to chronic liver disease, with high risk of cirrhosis and liver cancer	Risk of chronic liver disease among those infected with HBV is greater if they are also infected with HDV	No long-term consequences	Unclear at the present time

Other viral causes of hepatitis: Epstein–Barr virus, the cause of glandular fever (infectious mononucleosis); cytomegalovirus and herpes simplex virus, only in immunocompromised patients.

Causes of abnormal serum albumin concentration

Since albumin is synthesised in the liver, it might be expected that liver disease is always associated with abnormally low levels. This, however, is not the case. Albumin is reduced only in chronic liver disease (e.g. cirrhosis) and liver failure but usually remains normal if damage is acute and self-limiting (e.g. acute hepatitis). Albumin may also be reduced in conditions other than liver disease. Inadequate supply of dietary amino acids required for albumin synthesis is the cause of the low albumin associated with severe malnutrition and malabsorption. Abnormal loss of albumin from the body may also result in low levels. For example, the abnormal loss of albumin in urine accounts for the low serum albumin in diseases of the kidney (particularly marked in nephrotic syndrome). Albumin is frequently low in patients who have suffered extensive burns due to the loss of albumin through skin.

The level of hydration, although not affecting the total amount of albumin in the body, does affect the *concentration* of albumin. In dehydrated patients albumin levels (i.e. concentration) are raised and in overhydrated patients albumin levels are lower than normal.

Causes of abnormal enzyme results

Alanine transferase (ALT)

Highest ALT results (in extreme cases up to 50 or even 100 times the upper limit of normal) are seen in any disease associated with acute and massive liver cell necrosis. In acute viral hepatitis, for example, liver cell death causes ALT to rise to a peak during the first few days following development of first symptoms, usually before jaundice develops. As the disease resolves over the following 6 to 8 weeks, ALT gradually falls back to normal. A similar picture follows the liver cell death that results from acute circulatory failure (clinical shock) and that which results from ingestion of liver toxins (e.g. overdose of paracetamol in which ALT levels may be in excess of 100 times the upper limit of normal). A persistently moderately raised ALT (up to 10 times the upper limit of normal) suggests the development of chronic liver disease; chronic hepatitis, cirrhosis and primary or secondary cancer of the liver are examples of diseases usually associated with such moderate rises. ALT is usually normal or only slightly increased in diseases associated with obstruction to bile flow after it has left the liver (e.g. gallstones).

Gamma glutamyl transferase (GGT)

GGT is usually raised (up to five times the upper limit of normal) in all types of liver and biliary tract disease (acute and chronic hepatitis, cirrhosis, obstructive jaundice, etc.). The test can help to identify those with disease of the liver or biliary tract disease but is not very useful in establishing the exact nature of that disease. Measurement of GGT has however been found to be particularly useful in the management of patients who are at risk of liver disease due to alcoholism. Unlike the other two liver enzymes, GGT production is induced by alcohol, so if patients are drinking alcohol, GGT is raised even if there is no liver damage. Levels return to normal on cessation of drinking. If GGT of an alcoholic patient remains persistently high, it is likely that the patient continues to drink alcohol or that some damage to the liver has occurred (alcoholic hepatitis or cirrhosis).

GGT production is also induced by some drugs, including the anticonvulsants phenytoin, phenobarbitone, tricyclic antidepressants and paracetamol. For patients taking these and other drugs, a slight increase in GGT can be expected and does not necessarily imply any liver damage. Disease of the pancreas (e.g. acute pancreatitis) usually results in an increased GGT, and a slight increase in GGT is sometimes noted in diabetic patients.

Alkaline phosphatase (AP)

Alkaline phosphatase levels may be raised in diseases of the liver and biliary tract and in some diseases of the bone. So far as liver and biliary tract disease is concerned, highest levels are seen in diseases which obstruct the flow of bile after it has left the liver (e.g. gallstones in the common bile duct, carcinoma of the head of the pancreas). AP is also usually raised in cirrhosis and liver cancers (including liver metastases). Levels are generally only slightly raised in acute hepatitis and may be normal.

Alkaline phosphatase is present in high concentration in the osteoblastic cells of bone. The function of these cells is formation and constant remodelling of bone. Any condition associated with increased osteoblastic activity results in increased levels of alkaline phosphatase in blood. The increase in osteoblastic activity associated with growth spurts in childhood as new bone is formed accounts for the increased levels of plasma alkaline phosphatase throughout childhood. Some diseases of the bone are associated with abnormally increased osteoblastic activity. Among these are Paget's disease, a painful and bone-deforming condition usually diagnosed in middle age, and osteomalacia (called rickets in children) caused usually by vitamin D deficiency. Paget's disease is characterised by particularly high levels of plasma alkaline phosphatase. A raised AP is often seen during the healing process following bone fracture, as new bone is formed. Finally AP is raised in patients who have tumours of the bone (either primary or secondary). Primary tumours often metastasise first to the bone. An isolated raised alkaline phosphatase in a cancer patient is a poor prognostic sign as it may indicate tumour spread beyond the primary site.

Drugs and liver function tests

Liver damage can be caused by a wide spectrum of drugs, including some antibiotics (especially those used in the treatment of TB), paracetamol, aspirin, some antidepressants, cytotoxic drugs, etc. It has been estimated that 10% of cases of jaundice among hospital patients are the result of drug therapy. When trying to establish the cause of abnormally raised bilirubin, ALT, GGT or AP, a full patient drug history is important. The main causes of abnormal levels of bilirubin, albumin, ALT, GGT and AP are summarised in Tables 10.2a and 10.2b

Specific clinical effects of abnormal liver function

Bilirubin

A raised bilirubin is the cause of jaundice, although this clinical sign is not evident if the concentration is below around 50 μmol/l. At concentrations above 100 μmol/l yellow discoloration of skin and mucous membranes is evident to the untrained observer. Jaundice is very common in the neonatal period. If unconjugated bilirubin concentration rises above 300 μmol/l, as it may well do in untreated haemolytic disease of the newborn, there is an increasing risk that this lipid-soluble bilirubin is deposited in brain tissue causing a condition called kernicterus in which the deposited bilirubin damages neurones, particularly in the basal ganglia. The resulting permanent brain damage leads to spasticity and mental deficiency. Jaundiced neonates are routinely treated with UV phototherapy which destroys bilirubin in blood thus preventing kernicterus. An exchange transfusion in which blood with normal bilirubin is transfused in exchange for the affected baby's blood is sometimes indicated for those in whom the rate at which bilirubin is being formed is faster than the rate at which it can be destroyed by UV light.

Table 10.2(a)   Most common causes of abnormal bilirubin and albumin results

Increased serum/plasma bilirubin	Reduced serum/plasma albumin
Failure of liver cells to conjugate or excrete conjugated bilirubin	Failure to synthesise normal amount of albumin
■ acute/chronic hepatitis ■ cirrhosis ■ toxic liver cell damage (e.g. paracetamol overdose) ■ primary biliary cirrhosis ■ liver metastases (spread of cancer to the liver from some other primary site) ■ primary liver cancer ■ congestive cardiac failure	■ any chronic liver disease, e.g. cirrhosis, chronic hepatitis ■ malnutrition ■ diseases associated with malabsorption, e.g. Crohn's disease, coeliac disease Abnormal losses of albumin in urine: ■ nephrotic syndrome ■ chronic renal failure
Failure to excrete bilirubin due to obstruction of bile flow after it has left the liver	Movement of albumin from plasma to interstitial space (total albumin in the body remains normal)
■ gallstones obstructing the common bile duct ■ carcinoma of head of pancreas	■ any severe acute illness or tissue damage (e.g. common finding postoperatively)
Increased production of bilirubin due to abnormal rate of red cell destruction	Albumin level affected by patient's state of hydration: raised in those who are dehydrated, and reduced in those who are overhydrated
■ the haemolytic anaemias	
In neonates raised bilirubin may be due to:	
■ physiological jaundice (very common, particularly among premature babies and those being breast fed); haemolytic disease of the newborn (HDN) (less common) ■ liver disease (rare) ■ inherited metabolic defect (rare)	

Albumin

A reduced plasma albumin concentration is one of several contributory causes of oedema, the abnormal accumulation of fluid within the interstitial fluid, sometimes causing visible swelling (e.g. ankle oedema). Of particular relevance to liver disease is the abdominal swelling that complicates the course of cirrhosis in some patients. This swelling is the result of accumulation of so-called ascitic fluid in the peritoneal cavity. This form of oedema, known as ascites, is thought in part to be due to low plasma albumin concentration, a feature of cirrhosis.

Table 10.2(b) Most common cause of abnormal liver enzyme levels

Increased plasma/serum ALT	Increased serum/plasma AP	Increased serum/plasma GGT
Marked increase (up to 50 times the upper limit of normal) in all conditions associated with acute severe liver cell death ■ acute viral hepatitis, acute toxic hepatitis, e.g. paracetamol overdose ■ acute liver failure due to circulatory failure (i.e. shock) Moderate increase (up to 10 times the upper limit of normal) in other liver disease ■ cirrhosis ■ chronic hepatitis ■ primary liver cancer ■ secondary cancer spread to the liver ■ infectious mononucleosis (glandular fever) Mild increase (up to 3 times the upper limit of normal) may occur in disorders which do not affect the liver ■ severe tissue damage, e.g. major trauma or surgery ■ severe myocardial infarction ■ muscle disease	*Liver and biliary tract disease* Highest levels (up to 5 times the upper limit of normal seen in liver and biliary tract disease which obstructs the flow of bile: ■ gallstones in common bile duct ■ carcinoma of head of pancreas ■ primary biliary cirrhosis ■ primary liver cancer ■ secondary spread of cancer to the liver Moderately raised levels (up to 3 times the upper limit of normal) may be a feature of any acute or chronically active liver disease ■ acute viral hepatitis ■ acute toxic hepatitis ■ chronic active hepatitis ■ cirrhosis ■ infectious mononucleosis *Bone disease* Very high levels (may be up to 10 times the upper limit of normal) ■ Paget's disease of the bone Also raised: ■ during recovery of bone fracture ■ secondary spread of cancer to bone ■ primary bone tumour	*Liver and biliary tract disease* ■ acute hepatitis (whatever the cause) ■ infectious mononucleosis ■ gallstones ■ carcinoma of head of pancreas ■ primary liver cancer ■ secondary liver cancer *Non-liver disease* ■ pancreatitis ■ diabetes Alcohol and some drugs result in increased production of GGT ■ alcohol use ■ drugs including phenytoin and phenobarbitone

ALT, GGT and AP

There are no clinical signs or symptoms that can be directly attributable to raised liver enzymes.

Case history 9

Jamie Conrad, a 22-year-old heroin addict, attended his GP's surgery complaining of a two-day history of vomiting, abdominal pain and unusual tiredness. On questioning he revealed that he had felt unwell and feverish for a day or two a fortnight before, but those symptoms had passed. Apart from that, he judged himself to have been in good health until the current symptoms developed. The GP considered hepatitis might be the cause of his symptoms and sampled blood for LFTs. The laboratory reported the following results

Bilirubin 28 mmol/l
Albumin 42 g/l
ALT 104 U/l (laboratory normal range < 20 U/l)
AP 56 U/l (laboratory normal range < 150 U/l)
GGT 203 U/l (laboratory normal range < 50 U/l

(1) What might have persuaded the GP to investigate Jamie for possible hepatitis?
(2) What laboratory results are abnormal?
(3) Are the results consistent with a diagnosis of hepatitis?

Discussion of case history

(1) Some viruses which cause hepatitis (notably Hep B virus) can be transmitted by inoculation with infected blood. For this reason injecting drug users such as Jamie who may share syringes with those harbouring the virus are at particular risk of hepatitis. The symptoms that Jamie describes are consistent with a diagnosis of early hepatitis.
(2) The bilirubin level is raised though not sufficiently to cause visible jaundice. There is a significant increase (five times the upper limit of normal) in serum ALT. Gamma GT is also raised (four times the upper limit of normal).
(3) The results are consistent with early hepatitis. If Jamie does indeed have hepatitis then it can be expected that increases in bilirubin

and ALT particularly will become more marked over the next week to 10 days. Peak bilirubin concentration is usually sufficient to cause jaundice.

Further reading

Ravel R. (1995) Liver and biliary tract tests. In: *Clinical Laboratory Medicine*. Mosby, Missouri.

Stevens A. & Lowe J. (1995) Liver, biliary tract and pancreas. In: *Pathology*. Mosby, London.

Zilva J., Pannall P. & Mayne P. (1988) Liver disease and gallstones. In: *Clinical Chemistry in Diagnosis and Treatment*, 5th edn. Edward Arnold, London.

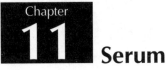

Serum Amylase

The measurement of amylase in blood serum or plasma is used almost exclusively for the differential diagnosis of acute abdominal pain, a very common symptom especially among patients admitted urgently to hospital. Acute abdominal pain is almost invariably a major presenting symptom of common surgical emergencies such as acute appendicitis, intestinal obstruction, perforated peptic ulcer and ruptured aortic aneurysm. Rapid diagnosis, sometimes with the help of blood and urine tests, is therefore important. A proportion of patients whose principal symptom is acute abdominal pain will be suffering acute pancreatitis, a potentially life-threatening inflammatory disease of the pancreas. The serum amylase test is particularly useful in identifying such patients; a marked increase in serum amylase in a patient with acute abdominal pain is strongly suggestive of acute pancreatitis.

Normal physiology

The pancreas

The pancreas is a soft, pale yellow organ around 12–15 cms in length and weighing approximately 100 g. Its shape somewhat resembles that of a tadpole, with a just recognisable 'head', 'body' and 'tail'. The organ lies transversely across the upper abdomen, with the 'head' positioned in the inner curve of the C shape formed by the first loop of the duodenum, the 'body' lying behind the stomach and the 'tail' extending from behind the stomach towards the spleen (Fig. 11.1). The micro-anatomy of the pancreas reveals two sorts of functionally distinct tissue reflecting the dual (exocrine and endocrine) role of the pancreas. Around 90% of the pancreas comprises so-called acinar (exocrine) tissue which is responsible for the production of pancreatic juice, a fluid necessary for normal

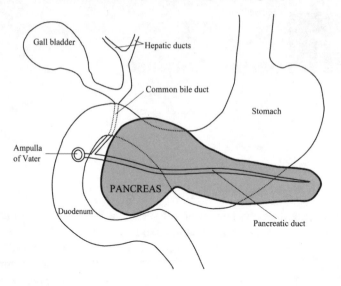

Fig. 11.1   Gross anatomy of pancreas.

intestinal digestion. Acinar cells are arranged like a bunch of grapes around a microscopical central tube or duct; acinar tissue comprises millions of these functional units. The ducts from each unit join, forming progressively larger ducts. These eventually drain all the pancreatic juice from the acinar cells into one large central duct called the duct of Wirsung running the length of the pancreas. This central duct leaves the head of the pancreas and joins with the common bile duct (carrying bile from the liver), at the ampulla of Vater in the wall of the duodenum. Here, pancreatic juice and bile drain into the duodenum through the sphincter of Oddi. Some people (around 20%) have a second pancreatic duct which drains pancreatic juice into the duodenum around 1 cm above the ampulla of Vater.

Dispersed throughout the acinar tissue of the pancreas are islands of quite distinct (endocrine) cells which have no ductal connection with the duodenum. These are the so called islets of Langerhans, which are surrounded by tiny blood capillaries and are responsible for the production of pancreatic hormones. There are at least three types of cell (alpha, beta and delta) within the islets of Langerhans, each producing a specific hormone: beta cells, by far the most numerous, produce insulin, alpha cells produce glucagon, and delta cells produce somatostatin. These pancreatic hormones are released directly into the blood flowing through the islets and have their effect on cellular metabolism throughout the body. The function of pancreatic hormones, insulin and glucagon in regulating blood glucose concentration is discussed in Chapter 3.

Pancreatic juice

The exocrine product of pancreatic acinar tissue, pancreatic juice, is a thin watery alkaline fluid (pH around 8) containing a mixture of many digestive enzymes together with electrolytes, most notably sodium, potassium, chloride and bicarbonate ions. With the exception of bicarbonate, electrolytes are present at a concentration similar to that found in blood plasma. However, bicarbonate concentration of pancreatic juice is around four times higher; this very high bicarbonate concentration accounts for the alkaline reaction of pancreatic juice. Between 1500 and 3000 ml are secreted into the duodenum every day. The function of pancreatic juice is to continue the process of enzymic digestion of food in the small intestine, already begun in the mouth, oesophagus and stomach. The many enzymes contained in pancreatic juice can be divided broadly into three groups according to the substrates in food on which they act: amylase for the digestion of carbohydrates, lipases for the digestion of fats, and proteases for the digestion of proteins. Amylase and lipases are secreted in their active form, whereas proteases (e.g. trypsin) are secreted as proenzymes (e.g. trypsinogen) capable of digesting proteins only after they have been activated within the duodenum. In health, pancreatic production and secretion of inactive proenzymes rather than their highly reactive product protects the pancreas from enzymic destruction. The alkaline pH of pancreatic juice ensures that acid chyme (partially digested food) emptying from the stomach into the duodenum is rendered sufficiently alkaline (pH 7–7.5) for optimum pancreatic enzyme activity.

The volume and content of pancreatic juice is controlled principally by hormonal pathways. Cholecystokinin–pancreozymin, a gut hormone released in response to gastric emptying of food into the duodenum, stimulates acinar cell production of digestive enzymes. Secretin, another gut hormone, promotes acinar cell production of bicarbonate. Neural pathways also affect pancreatic juice production. The vagal nerve which is stimulated by the sight, smell and thought of food as well as by the presence of food in the mouth, stimulates production of pancreatic juice. The final release of pancreatic juice into the duodenum is controlled by the sphincter of Oddi which opens when food is present in the duodenum.

By a synergy of these and other subtle hormonal and neural mechanisms, the body is able to adjust the volume, content and release of pancreatic juice to suit its digestive requirement.

Once pancreatic juice has performed its digestive function, around 99% of the water and electrolyte content of pancreatic juice is reabsorbed into the bloodstream as it passes through the large intestine.

Amylase

Amylase is just one of several digestive enzymes secreted in pancreatic juice. It is also secreted in saliva by three pairs of salivary glands in the mouth. Salivary and pancreatic amylase function only within the gastrointestinal tract, where together they are responsible for the breakdown of starch, the principal form of dietary carbohydrate. Starch is essentially many glucose molecules joined together. The product of amylase action on starch is a mixture of three sorts of molecule: the disaccharide maltose (two molecules of glucose joined together), dextrin, a short chain of around eight glucose molecules, and some single molecules of glucose. Any glucose formed by the action of amylase on starch is absorbed directly into the bloodstream by active transport across the cells of the intestinal wall, but maltose and dextrin require further enzymic degradation by the intestinal enzymes maltase and iso-maltase to single glucose molecules before absorption can occur.

Like all enzymes amylase will only work to maximum effect within a narrow pH range; for amylase the optimum pH is 7.1. Digestion of starch begins in the mouth with the action of salivary amylase during the process of chewing. As soon as food reaches the acidic medium of the stomach (pH 2–3), salivary amylase action ceases. In practice, unless food is masticated in the mouth for a prolonged period, salivary amylase contributes little to overall starch digestion and most starch is broken down in the duodenum and jejunum by pancreatic amylase.

Normally a small amount of amylase circulates in blood plasma. Most of this is of pancreatic origin; some is derived from salivary glands. Amylase has no function in blood plasma and is present there only as a result of normal pancreatic and salivary cell turnover. By comparison with most other enzymes, amylase is a small molecule. Indeed it is small enough to pass through the glomeruli of the kidneys, so that it is one of very few plasma enzymes normally found in urine.

LABORATORY MEASUREMENT OF SERUM AMYLASE

PATIENT PREPARATION
No particular patient preparation is necessary.

SAMPLE REQUIREMENTS
Between 2 and 5 ml of venous blood is required. The test is performed on either blood serum or blood plasma. If local policy is to use serum, then blood must be collected into a plain tube containing no anticoagulant. If local policy is to use plasma, then blood must be collected into a tube containing an anticoagulant (usually heparin).

TIMING OF BLOOD SAMPLING AND TRANSPORT
Blood may be collected without reference to time. In many instances the result is required urgently so must be transported to the laboratory without delay. If the request is non-urgent, the sample may be stored at room temperature before routine transport to the laboratory.

INTERPRETATION OF RESULTS

Approximate reference range: serum (plasma) amylase: 50–200 U/l
(Note: It is particularly important to use the local reference range when interpreting enzyme results.)

Terms used:
Hypoamylassaemia – serum amylase below normal
Hyperamylassaemia – serum amylase above normal

An abnormally low serum amylase is a rare finding which has little or no clinical significance. Discussion will be confined to the interpretation of a raised serum amylase.

Causes of raised serum (plasma) amylase

Acute pancreatitis

Acute pancreatitis is an acute inflammatory disease caused by premature activation of the proteolytic (protein splitting) enzymes normally produced by the pancreas in an inactive form. Activation of these enzymes within the pancreas leads to a process of 'autodigestion', in essence self-destruction of the pancreas. Temporary obstruction to the flow of pancreatic juice by gallstones transiently lodged in the ampulla of Vater is thought to be the most significant primary cause of acute pancreatitis. Alcohol abuse can also precipitate an attack. Between 80 and 90% of patients with acute pancreatitis have either gall bladder disease or a history of alcohol abuse. Other, much less common causes of acute pancreatitis include trauma to the pancreas, some drugs, over-activity of the parathyroid gland (hyperparathyroidism) and the mumps virus. Very rarely acute pancreatitis occurs as a post-operative complication following upper abdominal surgery.

The cardinal symptom of acute pancreatitis is sudden onset of severe upper abdominal pain which often radiates to the back. Vomiting and pyrexia are common. The course of acute pancreatitis is variable. Mild acute pancreatitis resolves over a few days to a week with little intervention and no long-term consequences. Severe acute pancreatitis, by contrast, is a life-threatening condition in which autodigestion of the pancreas causes widespread necrosis, inflammation and haemorrhage not only within the pancreas but also in surrounding tissues and organs. Such patients frequently present in hypovolaemic shock with severe hypotension. Complications of severe disease include cardiac failure, respiratory failure, jaundice, anaemia, hyperglycaemia and disseminated intravascular coagulation. Multiple organ failure may ensue; there is a 10% mortality associated with acute pancreatitis.

Damage to acinar cells, the central pathological feature of acute pancreatitis, results in a sudden and massive increase in release of pancreatic enzymes into the bloodstream; among these is amylase. This increase in serum amylase has no clinical consequences of itself, that is, no signs or symptoms of acute pancreatitis can be attributed to an increase in serum amylase. It does, however, provide a marker in the blood of damage to the pancreas. Serum amylase begins to rise 2 to 12 hours after the onset of symptoms and remains elevated for three to five days in most cases. An amylase level of greater then five times the upper limit of normal (i.e. > 1000 U/l) in a patient with acute abdominal pain is widely considered to be almost diagnostic of acute pancreatitis. The probability that acute pain is due to pancreatitis increases as amylase level rises above 1000 U/l. A minority of patients with acute pancreatitis do not show such a marked increase so that a serum amylase of < 1000 U/l cannot be used to exclude the diagnosis. Very rarely the serum amylase may be normal in a patient with acute pancreatitis. It might be assumed that the higher the serum amylase, the more severe the pancreatitis; this is not the case. In fact no prognostic information can be derived from measurement of serum amylase at the time of diagnosis. However, failure of amylase to return to normal following an acute attack suggests the presence of a pancreatic pseudocyst (a late complication of acute pancreatitis).

Chronic pancreatitis

Natural repair of the damage caused by the inflammation of acute pancreatitis leaves the pancreas of someone who has recovered from the disease functioning normally. By contrast, chronic pancreatitis is a chronic inflammation in which damage to the pancreas is slow but irreversibly progressive. The most common cause is long-term alcohol abuse. It may be a feature of haemochromatosis, a disease of iron overload in which excess iron is deposited in the pancreas and other organs. Continuous or at least recurrent abdominal pain is the cardinal symptom of chronic pancreatitis. Long term the condition results in malabsorption of food and consequent weight loss due to failure of pancreatic enzyme production and diabetes as a result of islet cell damage. Serum amylase may be slightly raised in the early stages but as acinar cell production of digestive enzymes (including amylase) becomes increasingly compromised, serum amylase falls to normal or even to levels below normal. Since amylase may be raised, normal or reduced, the test serves no useful purpose in the diagnosis of chronic pancreatitis.

Cancer of the pancreas

Apart from acute and chronic pancreatitis, cancer of the pancreas is the only other significant disease of the pancreas. Serum amylase is either marginally raised or normal; the test is not useful for the diagnosis of cancer of the pancreas.

Non-pancreatic disease

Serum amylase may be mildly to moderately raised (i.e. usually not greater than 1000 U/l) in some non-pancreatic disorders, e.g. perforation of peptic ulcer, intestinal obstruction, and gall bladder disease (acute cholecystitis). All these conditions are usually associated with acute abdominal pain so that a patient with a raised serum amylase in association with acute abdominal pain is not necessarily suffering acute pancreatitis. Abdominal trauma, not necessarily involving the pancreas, may result in an increased amylase; a significant minority of patients who receive abdominal surgery have a transient rise during the post-operative period.

Amylase is cleared from the blood by the kidneys. Patients in acute or chronic renal failure therefore typically have slight to moderate increases in serum amylase.

A moderate to marked increase is often a feature of diabetic ketoacidosis. Disease of or damage to the parotid glands where salivary amylase is produced may result in an increase in serum amylase. Examples include infection with the mumps virus, maxillofacial surgery, and parotid gland irradiation.

Finally, raised serum amylase is a feature of a rare and entirely benign condition called macroamylassaemia, in which amylase circulates in serum in the form of macromolecular aggregates of amylase or bound to serum proteins. Because they are so large these macromolecules cannot pass across the glomerular membrane of the kidneys and are not excreted in urine; instead they accumulate in serum.

Table 11.1 provides a summary of the principal causes of raised serum amylase.

Table 11.1   Principal causes of raised serum/plasma amylase

Acute pancreatitis
Chronic pancreatitis
Renal failure
Diabetic ketoacidosis
Intestinal obstruction
Perforated peptic ulcer
Acute cholecystitis
Abdominal trauma
Mumps
Macroamylassaemia

Case history 10

Mrs Campbell, a 40-year-old pharmacist, arrived by ambulance at the emergency department of her local hospital in considerable pain and distress, looking pale and shocked. The pain, which had only become severe 4 hours earlier, was localised in the mid-epigastric region; she described it as 'shooting through her back'. She was vomiting. Her body temperature was 100°C, her blood pressure 90/60 mmHg, and her respiratory rate 30/min. During the initial examination Mrs Campbell told the admitting doctor that she had been diagnosed as having gall-stones and was currently on a weight reduction diet in preparation for a cholecystectomy (surgical removal of gall bladder). The admitting doctor suspected Mrs Campbell might be suffering from acute pancreatitis. Blood was sampled for U&E, glucose, amylase and full blood count. The laboratory results included:

Serum amylase	1700 U/l
Blood glucose	15.6 mmol/l

(1) What suggested to the admitting doctor that Mrs Campbell might be suffering acute pancreatitis?
(2) Are the serum amylase and blood glucose normal?
(3) Do the laboratory results support the initial diagnosis?
(4) Why might a patient suffering acute pancreatitis have a raised blood glucose?

Discussion of case history

(1) The sudden onset of severe abdominal pain is the most common finding in patients with acute pancreatitis; in around a half of cases this pain is referred to the back. Vomiting is also a common symptom. Mrs Campbell was severely hypotensive, suggesting hypovolaemic shock. Loss of pancreatic secretion into the peritoneal space and haemorrhage due to vessel erosion by pancreatic enzymes can lead to hypovolaemic shock in acute pancreatitis. Finally acute pancreatitis is frequently associated with a clinical history of gall bladder disease.
(2) No. Both serum amylase and blood glucose are markedly raised; amylase is more than seven times the upper limit of normal.
(3) Yes, an increase in amylase of this degree is almost diagnostic of acute pancreatitis. Amylase may be raised in a number of non-pancreatic conditions which result in abdominal pain, but very rarely to this degree. Transient hyperglycaemia is sometimes a feature of acute pancreatitis, requiring insulin therapy and regular blood glucose monitoring.
(4) Acute pancreatitis may involve damage to the endocrine (islet) cells of the pancreas, where insulin is produced. Insulin is the principal hormone of blood glucose regulation; a deficiency of the hormone results in raised blood glucose concentration. Islet cell damage may be minimal, in which case normal insulin production and secretion continue and hyperglycaemia does not occur.

Further reading

Imrie C. (1993) Acute pancreatitis. In *Gastroenterology: Clinical Science and Practice*, Eds Bouchier L., Allan R., Hodgson H. & Keighly M. W.B. Saunders, Philadelphia.
Smith A. (1991) When the pancreas self destructs. *Amer. J. Nurs.* **91**: 38–48.

Drug Overdose: Serum salicylate and paracetamol

Clinical laboratories are often requested to analyse blood or urine samples for the presence of drugs. Such analyses are valuable in two, usually separate, clinical contexts: deliberate or accidental drug overdose and therapeutic drug monitoring. Chapter 13 is concerned principally with the latter, whilst this chapter is concerned with how laboratory measurement of serum concentration of salicylate and paracetamol contributes to the care of patients who have taken or are suspected of having taken an acute overdose of aspirin (acetylsalicylic acid) or paracetamol (acetaminophen). Presumably because of their widespread availability, aspirin and paracetamol are two of the drugs most frequently used by people intending self-harm. The incidence of paracetamol overdose has increased in recent years and now accounts for nearly half of all drug overdose cases. Every year in the UK there are around 70 000 cases of paracetamol overdose, 200 of which have a fatal outcome.[1] Overdose with aspirin is less frequent than it once was, but is still responsible for 500 hospital admissions and around 50 deaths each year.[2]

Clinical use of aspirin and paracetamol: safety of therapeutic dose

Both aspirin and paracetamol are analgesics and antipyretics, that is, they reduce pain and body temperature. They are frequently self-prescribed at doses of up to 3 g per day for the relief of temporary symptoms associated with minor viral infections (e.g. influenza, colds, etc.) and for the relief of headaches and minor muscular aches and pains. Aspirin has two further major pharmacological properties: at high dose (> 3 g/day) it has an anti-inflammatory effect and at a low dose (75–300 mg/day) an anti-thrombotic (anti-blood clotting) effect. These two properties have determined that long-term prescription of aspirin is useful in chronic inflammatory conditions such as chronic arthritis and for the prevention of myocardial infarction and strokes among high-risk patients. The use of aspirin for primary prevention of myocardial infarction and strokes is currently under investigation. There is emerging evidence that aspirin use protects against cancer of the colon.[3]

The maximum recommended dose of paracetamol for adults and children over the age of 12 is two 500 mg tablets with an interval of at least 4 hours between doses. No more than eight tablets should be taken in 24 hours (i.e. a maximum dose of 4 g/day). So long as this dose is not exceeded, paracetamol has no adverse effect and is a remarkably safe drug even if used for a prolonged period.

Long-term aspirin use, even at therapeutic dosage, is less safe. In common with other non-steroidal anti-inflammatory drugs (NSAIDs), long-term aspirin use is associated with irritation of the stomach wall lining (gastric mucosa) and the risk of gastrointestinal bleeding and stomach ulcers. Patients with a history of peptic ulcer or an increased tendency to bleed are prescribed aspirin only rarely. Some patients on long-term high-dose aspirin therapy may experience some of the symptoms of acute overdose, even if they are taking what for others is a safe therapeutic dose. There is evidence that aspirin use among children with a viral infection precipitates a serious life-threatening condition known as Reye's syndrome. For this reason aspirin is not recommended for use in children. The recommended dose for analgesic and antipyretic effect is one to two 325 mg tablets every 4 hours; no more than 12 tablets in 24 hours should be taken. For anti-inflammatory effect that dose has to be increased to around 2×500 mg tablets usually every 6 hours. Just 75–300 mg/day is sufficient for anti-thrombotic effect.

Paracetamol

Absorption, metabolism and acute toxicity

Paracetamol is quickly absorbed from the gastrointestinal tract into the blood over a period of 30 minutes to 2 hours for a therapeutic dose. A small amount (up to 5%) is eliminated unchanged in urine, but the remainder is metabolised in the liver (Fig. 12.1). Like most other drugs, paracetamol must be made more water soluble for appreciable elimination in urine. This is achieved in the liver by synthetic conjugation (joining) of paracetamol with sulphate, glucuronate, glycine and phosphate. These water-soluble conjugates of paracetamol are non-toxic. Around 90% of an ingested paracetamol dose is eliminated safely via

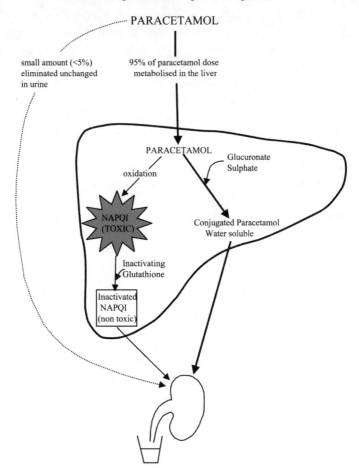

Fig. 12.1   Metabolism of paracetamol. NAPQI = N + acetyl-p-benzoquinone imine.

urine in this way. The rest of the paracetamol (between 5 and 10% of an ingested dose) is oxidised in the liver to a highly reactive and toxic free radical called N-acetyl-p-benzoquinone imine (NAPQI). It is NAPQI which is responsible for the toxic effects of paracetamol. At normal doses of paracetamol the liver is able to inactivate this potentially damaging NAPQI by reaction with a substance called glutathione, which is synthesised in the liver. The product of the reaction between NAPQI and glutathione is non-toxic and is eliminated safely in urine and bile.

If there were no limit to the rate at which the liver could synthesise glutathione, then paracetamol would not be harmful no matter how much had been taken. However, unfortunately this is not the case. If recommended dosage is exceeded, the production of NAPQI increases but the ability of the liver to synthesise the inactivating glutathione cannot keep pace and NAPQI accumulates in liver cells, disrupting cellular mechanisms and eventually causing liver cell death (necrosis). Without prompt treatment, liver cell necrosis becomes extensive, leading to liver failure. At this stage liver transplantation is the only treatment option.

A single dose of paracetamol of 150–200 mg/kg is sufficient to cause liver cell damage in adults. This means that for an adult weighing an average 70 kg, just 10 g of paracetamol (i.e. 20 tablets) may be significant. Twelve grams (24 tablets) can be fatal, and without treatment 25 g (50 tablets) is inevitably fatal. Certain drugs, notably the anticonvulsants phenytoin, carbamazepine, phenobarbitone and alcohol, result in increased production of the enzymes responsible for NAPQI production. Patients who have taken alcohol or these drugs are particularly susceptible to the toxic effects of paracetamol.

Signs and symptoms of acute overdose

The early symptoms of even potentially fatal paracetamol overdose are non-specific and unremarkable. For the first 12 hours, nausea and vomiting are the only symptoms; loss of consciousness is not an early feature. Signs and symptoms of extensive liver cell damage including jaundice, abdominal tenderness, continuing nausea and vomiting begin to develop in the 24 to 36 hours after overdose. Deterioration in liver function over the next few days leads to acute liver failure in the most severe cases. Drowsiness leading to coma is a feature at this late stage.

Principles of overdose treatment

So long as treatment is initiated early enough (i.e. within 8–10 hours), a complete recovery can be expected even after a potentially fatal dose of paracetamol. Because of the speed at which paracetamol is absorbed from the intestine, efforts aimed at reducing absorption of paracetamol, including gastric lavage and administration of charcoal, are only effective if begun within 2 hours and certainly no later than 4 hours after the overdose. The most effective treatment is early iv administration of the paracetamol antidote: N-acetylcysteine (NAC). In the body NAC is converted to glutathione, the substance required for inactivation of NAPQI, the toxic metabolite of paracetamol. NAC is successful in preventing liver damage if administered within 8–10 hours of the overdose. Although less effective after 10 hours, some benefit can be gained by administration up to 24 hours – or even 72 hours in some cases – after overdose.

Aspirin

Absorption, metabolism and acute toxicity

Absorption of aspirin from the gastrointestinal tract is dependent on the amount and formulation of the drug. Therapeutic doses of regular (non-enteric coated) aspirin are absorbed rapidly within two hours. Larger quantities (overdose) of regular aspirin, however, inhibit gastric emptying with a resulting delay of up to 6 hours in intestinal absorption. Enteric coated formulations of aspirin are designed to be impervious to the acid contact in the stomach and only begin to dissolve after arrival in the alkaline medium of the intestine; such formulations may take up to 12 hours to be completely absorbed.

After absorption, aspirin is rapidly hydrolysed to salicylic acid (salicylate). This is the substance responsible for the acute toxicity as well as many of the therapeutic effects of aspirin. Before salicylate can be eliminated in urine, it must first be conjugated with glycine to form salicyluric acid or glucuronate to form phenolic glucuronides, but the enzymes for these detoxifying reactions become rapidly saturated at even therapeutic levels. As a consequence, salicylate accumulates in tissues in a dose-dependent manner. Increased serum salicylate concentration stimulates the respiratory centre causing hyperventilation, which results in increased CO_2 elimination and respiratory alkalosis (Chapter 6). Salicylate at toxic levels has an effect on cellular metabolism which results in hyperpyrexia, sweating and abnormally high production of metabolic acids. Along with salicylate, itself an acid, these acids accumulate in blood causing a metabolic acidosis. Salicylate causes increased permeability of the vasculature in the lungs, predisposing to the development of pulmonary oedema in salicylate overdose, particularly among smokers and the elderly. Finally salicylate can adversely affect normal control of blood glucose concentration; overdose of aspirin may result in hypoglycaemia (low blood glucose) or reduced levels of glucose in the brain (neuroglycopaenia) despite normal blood glucose levels. Mild toxicity arises after a single dose of around 150 mg/kg body weight, whereas severe toxicity is associated with a single dose of greater than 500 mg/kg. For an adult of average weight (70 kg) then, just twenty 500 mg tablets or thirty 325 mg tablets are sufficient for mild toxicity.

Signs and symptoms of acute toxicity

Salicylate poisoning is much easier to recognise in the early stages than paracetamol poisoning. Mild to moderate poisoning commonly causes nausea, vomiting and tinnitus, with loss of hearing. Patients are usually hyperventilating, hyperpyrexial and sweating. Dehydration secondary to vomiting, sweating and hyperventilation is usually a feature, particularly in severe poisoning. Blood gas analysis reveals disturbance of acid–base (either respiratory alkalosis, metabolic acidosis or a combination of the two). Acidaemia (low blood pH) is a poor prognostic sign because it enhances salicylate entry into tissue cells; entry of salicylate into brain cells causes additional neurological symptoms including confusion, delirium and extreme agitation. Loss of consciousness may occur but is relatively rare.

Principles of overdose treatment

There is no antidote for the treatment of aspirin overdose as there is for paracetamol overdose. Treatment instead is based on three main objectives:

- preventing further absorption of aspirin from the gastrointestinal tract
- increasing urinary elimination of salicylate
- correction of dehydration and deranged blood chemistry (acid–base and electrolyte disturbances, and hypoglycaemia if present).

The delay in intestinal absorption of high-dose aspirin, especially enteric coated formulations, ensures that gastric lavage or repeated administration of activated charcoal are likely to be effective in reducing absorption for much longer than is the case in paracetamol overdose, although of course the sooner it is started the more effective it will be. Urinary elimination of salicylate is increased if urine is made alkaline (pH > 7.5) and urine output increased. This is achieved by administration of large volumes of sodium bicarbonate ($NaHCO_3$). Such treatment has the additional advantage of making blood more alkaline and thereby inhibiting the entry of salicylate into cells. Removal of salicylate from blood by haemodialysis or peritoneal dialysis may be considered in the most severe cases. Dextrose may be added to any iv fluid used to correct fluid and electrolyte disturbance since there is evidence that, even if blood glucose is normal, the brain is depleted of glucose in moderate to severe salicylate poisoning.

LABORATORY MEASUREMENT OF SALICYLATE AND PARACETAMOL

PATIENT PREPARATION

No particular patient preparation is necessary.

TIMING OF SAMPLE

The time of blood sampling and the time of the overdose (if known) must be recorded. Because of varying rates of paracetamol absorption, it is impossible to accurately interpret a paracetamol result of a sample taken less than 4 hours after an overdose. Blood sampling should therefore be delayed until 4 hours have elapsed since paracetamol was taken. Repeat sampling for salicylate may be required for the same reason.

SAMPLE REQUIREMENTS

Around 5 ml of venous blood is required for paracetamol and salicylate estimation. Analysis can be performed on either serum or plasma. If local policy is to use serum, blood must be collected into a plain (without additives) tube. If local policy is to use plasma, blood must be collected into a tube containing the anticoagulant lithium heparin.

TRANSPORT OF SAMPLES

The results of paracetamol and salicylate estimation are required for immediate patient management and therefore samples must be considered urgent and transported to the laboratory without delay.

INTERPRETATION OF PARACETAMOL RESULT

There seems to be no universal agreement about units of measurement for paracetamol; some laboratories report paracetamol in traditional units (mg/l or µg/ml); note that 1 mg/l = 1 µg/ml. Other laboratories use the SI unit of measurement (µmol/ml or µmol/l); note 1 µmol/ml = 1000 µmol/l. A potentially dangerous interpretation is possible if these units are confused.

Accurate interpretation of paracetamol results depends crucially on knowing the approximate time of overdose. Figure 12.2 is a widely used nomogram which allows assessment of the severity of overdose based on the paracetamol concentration in relation to the time in hours since the overdose. For example, it can be seen from the graph that a paracetamol concentration of 80 mg/l taken 4 hours after an overdose indicates that liver damage is extremely unlikely. However, the same paracetamol result in a blood sample taken 12 hours after an overdose indicates that without

'cont.'

'continued'

antidote (N-acetylcysteine) treatment, severe – even fatal – liver damage can be expected.

The graph highlights two important features of paracetamol toxicity. First, it is not possible to accurately determine the severity of a paracetamol overdose based on a serum paracetamol derived from blood sampled less than 4 hours after an overdose; a repeat sample would be advisable in these circumstances. Secondly, any measurable amounts of paracetamol in serum 24 hours or later after an overdose indicates a poor prognosis, especially as antidote treatment at this late stage is unlikely to be very effective in halting liver cell damage.

There has been a recent recommendation[4] to revise the widely used treatment nomogram depicted in Fig. 12.2. If adopted, the proposed changes would result in all patients with a serum paracetamol in excess of 150 mg/l receiving antidote treatment.

INTERPRETATION OF SALICYLATE RESULT

Again there is no consensus between laboratories about units of measurement. Most laboratories use either mg/l or mg/dl. (Note: a salicylate concentration of 10 mg/dl = 100 mg/l.)

Patients on long-term high-dose aspirin therapy for chronic inflammatory conditions such as rheumatoid arthritis typically have a serum salicylate concentration of 25–35 mg/dl (i.e. 250–350 mg/l). These levels are rarely associated with any symptoms of acute toxicity. Mild to moderate toxicity occurs with salicylate concentration in the range 40–70 mg/dl (400–700 mg/l) whilst levels greater than 70 mg/dl (700 mg/ml) are associated with severe toxicity; around 5% of patients admitted to hospital with this level of toxicity do not survive.[2] Serum salicylate levels provide an approximate and useful guide to the severity of a particular overdose but are not as reliable in this regard as serum paracetamol is in cases of paracetamol overdose. The clinical condition of the patient, along with blood gas and electrolyte results are as important as plasma salicylate results for assessment of prognosis and clinical care planning. However, some general points can be made. Nearly all patients, even those with mild toxicity, will be given gastric lavage and or activated charcoal. The likelihood that a patient will require alkalinisation of urine increases as the serum salicylate increases beyond 50 mg/dl. Finally, haemodialysis is usually reserved for those patients whose serum salicylate is well in excess of 70 mg/dl, although it may be considered the treatment of choice for all patients who have significant kidney disease.

'cont.'

'continued'

A rise in serum salicylate during treatment may indicate continuing sal-icylate absorption and/or failure to adequately increase urine elimination. A decline in serum salicylate concentration is used to confirm that treatment aimed at increased urinary elimination of salicylate has been effective. Sometimes, however, a reduction in serum concentration merely reflects haemodilution, if high volume fluids have been infused.

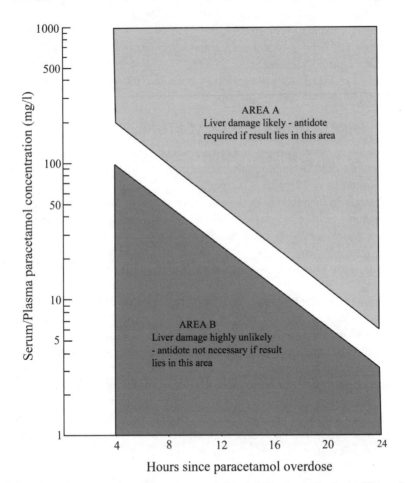

Fig. 12.2 Interpretation of paracetamol level following overdose. *Notes:* If result lies between area A and area B, antidote treatment is only necessary if patient has also taken alcohol or certain other drugs which increase the toxicity of paracetamol. It is not possible to interpret a level if blood was sampled less than 4 hours after the overdose.

Case history 11

Andrew Roberts, a 23-year-old university student, became depressed, having failed his final examinations. Following an alcoholic binge he returned to his flat, took 18 paracetamol tablets and fell asleep. On waking, early the next morning, some six hours after taking the tablets, he was feeling sick and extremely regretful about what he had done. Worried about the possible effects he rang the local hospital accident and emergency department for advice.

(1)   What would your advice be?

Discussion of case history

(1)   Andrew had taken 9 g of paracetamol, well in excess of the maximum recommended single dose which is 1 g. Assuming an average body weight of 70 kg, 9 g represents a dose of 9000/70 mg/kg (i.e. 129 mg/kg). Liver damage is unlikely if a single dose of < 150 mg/kg has been taken. However, the fact that Andrew also took alcohol must be taken into account, because alcohol increases production of the enzymes necessary for oxidation of paracetamol to the toxic metabolite NAPQI. The toxicity of paracetamol is increased if alcohol has been taken. It would be wise for Mr Roberts to attend casualty urgently so that his serum paracetamol can be checked.

Andrew took the advice given by A&E staff. Within the hour he arrived at the hospital and was seen immediately by the casualty officer who took blood for serum paracetamol estimation some 8 hours after taking the tablets. The laboratory telephoned back the result:

Serum paracetamol – 42 mg/l

(2)   Would it have been advisable for Andrew to have been given a gastric washout or charcoal on arrival?
(3)   What is the significance of the paracetamol result?

(2)   Paracetamol is absorbed from the gastrointestinal tract within a few hours of ingestion. It is highly unlikely that there would have been any paracetamol remaining in Andrew's stomach by the time he arrived in A&E. Both gastric lavage and charcoal administration would have been ineffective at this late stage.

(3) By referring to the nomogram (Fig. 12.2) it can be seen that Andrew was not at risk of liver damage and did not require antidote therapy. His physical health was considered not at risk.

References

(1) Hawton K., Ware C. & Mistry H. (1996) Paracetamol self poisoning characteristics, prevention and harm reduction. *Br. J Psychiatry* **168**: 43–48.
(2) Chapman B. & Proudfoot A. (1989) Adult salicylate poisoning: deaths and outcome in patients with high plasma salicylate concentration. *Q. J. Med* **72**: 699–707.
(3) Giovannucci E. (1999) The prevention of colorectal cancer by aspirin use. *Biomed. Pharmacother.* **53**: 303–8.
(4) Bridger S., Henderson K., Glucksman E. *et al.* (1998) Deaths from low dose paracetamol poisoning. *BMJ* **316**: 1724–25.

Further reading

Anker A. & Smilkstein M. (1994) Acetaminophen concepts and controversies. *Emer. Med. Clin. N. Amer.* **12**: 335–349.
Rumack B., Peterson, R. *et al.* (1981) Acetaminophen overdose: 662 cases with evaluation of oral acetylcysteine treatment. *Arch. Int. Med.* **141**: 380–85.
Yip L., Dart R. & Gabow P. (1994) Concepts and controversies in salicylate toxicity. *Emer. Med. Clin. N. Amer.* **12**: 351–64.

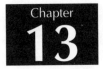

13 Therapeutic Drug Monitoring: Serum lithium, serum digoxin and serum theophylline

This chapter is concerned with how laboratory measurement of drug concentration in blood helps in determining correct drug dosage. Such an approach is either unnecessary or unsuitable for most drug therapies, but for a limited number of drugs, including lithium, digoxin and theophylline, measurement of blood serum levels is the best way of optimising dosage and preventing dangerous side effects (toxicity). Measuring blood levels also provides a means of confirming patient compliance. Other drug therapies, not discussed in this chapter, in which therapeutic drug monitoring is useful include the anticonvulsant drugs, carbamazepine, valproate and phenytoin; some drugs used to treat disturbances of cardiac rhythm (e.g. procainamide, quinidine) and a few antibiotics (e.g. gentamicin, vancomycin).

Lithium

Pharmacological action and clinical use

Although the precise mechanism of action of lithium is poorly understood, the effect of the drug is to stabilise mood; its use is confined to psychiatric patients primarily for the treatment of bipolar disorder. This common psychiatric condition, sometimes called manic depression or affective disorder, affects around 1.5–2% of the population and is characterised by cyclic episodes of depression followed by elation (mania). Normal mood is in the middle of a continuum which runs from depression at one extreme to mania at the other. Depression is associated with a lack of energy, diminished interest and ability to experience pleasure, along with feelings of despair and pessimism. During the manic phase of bipolar disease, however, symptoms are those of an abnormally expansive mood with increased mental and physical energy. Affected patients are hyperactive and have difficulty sleeping. Inflated self-esteem and false optimism are accompanied by flights of fancy and impulsive behaviour. In its most severe form, mania results in thinking that can race so fast that it becomes fragmented. Speech is fast and may be incoherent. Psychotic symptoms, including hallucinations, grandiose delusions and illusions, may be a feature of severe acute mania.

Lithium is an antimanic drug. Although used to treat acute mania and its less severe form, hypomania, among patients presenting with symptoms, the most important use of lithium is to prevent both manic and depressive episodes in patients with bipolar disorder; the result is a marked reduction in mood swings. Patients may need to take lithium for many years or even for life in order to remain well. Unfortunately, for unknown reasons, some patients with bipolar disease do not respond to lithium therapy. Lithium may also be used in conjunction with antidepressant drugs to treat severe depression which does not respond to antidepressant drugs alone.

Toxic (unwanted) side effects

All drugs have toxic, unwanted side effects and lithium is no exception. Lithium has effects in organs throughout the body. Common symptoms of toxicity include nausea, diarrhoea, vomiting, drowsiness and fine hand tremor. Lithium can affect kidney function, causing a condition known as nephrogenic diabetes insipidus which is characterised by increased urine flow (polyuria) and resulting increased thirst (polydipsia). The thyroid gland of patients on long-term lithium therapy may become underactive, with resulting symptoms of hypothyroidism (Chapter 9). This may contribute to the weight gain which is often associated with lithium use. Patients on long-term lithium therapy should have regular thyroid function tests. Special caution should be taken in prescribing lithium for pregnant women as there is an increased risk of congenital malformation of the developing foetus associated with lithium use, particularly during the first three months of pregnancy. Lithium is eliminated from the body almost entirely by the kidneys in urine. For this reason the potential for lithium toxicity is greater in older patients, whose renal function is reduced, and in patients with kidney disease. Such patients may need a lower dose of lithium than those with normally functioning kidneys if they are to avoid adverse effects.

Why and when to measure serum lithium

The lithium dose required for treatment or prevention of manic symptoms (called the therapeutic dose) is very close to that which results in toxicity. In common with all three drugs discussed in this chapter, lithium is said to have a low 'therapeutic index' or narrow 'therapeutic window'. Fortunately there is a well defined therapeutic range for serum lithium, providing a means of checking that sufficient drug is being administered for maximum therapeutic effect consistent with minimum risk of toxic side effects. Serum lithium is checked initially to determine the correct dose; if serum levels are below the therapeutic range, the dose is increased, and if higher than the therapeutic range, the dose is decreased. Once a safe and effective maintenance dose has been established, regular blood monitoring, usually once every three months or so, is usually considered sufficient. Urgent blood testing is, however, necessary if any signs or symptoms of toxicity arise and in cases of deliberate overdose (parasuicide).

Patients suffering bipolar disease may be reluctant to take their lithium regularly once initial symptoms have subsided; they may falsely believe that they do not require lithium, and stop taking tablets without consultation with their doctor. Measuring serum lithium provides a means of confirming that patients are continuing with their medication.

Digoxin

Principal pharmacological action and clinical use

Digoxin is widely used in the treatment of heart disease. It is derived from digitalis, a compound extracted from the leaves of the foxglove plant (*Digitalis lanata*). Digoxin inhibits the enzyme (ATPase) which is required for action of the sodium–potassium pump (Chapter 3) present in the membrane of all cells, which maintains the distribution of sodium and potassium between cells and surrounding extracellular fluid. The net effect of reduced sodium–potassium pump activity (and therefore digoxin administration) is an increase in sodium and calcium concentration within cells and a decrease in concentration of cellular potassium. It is the increase in calcium concentration within the muscle cells of the heart which is thought to account for the positive inotropic (increased force of muscle cell contraction) effects of digoxin. This property of digoxin is used to treat patients with chronic heart failure (CHF).

CHF is a common condition, particularly among the elderly population, in which the heart is unable to pump sufficient blood to supply the oxygen and other nutritional demands of tissues. Fatigue, lethargy and cold peripheries are the principal symptoms of this reduced blood delivery to tissues. As a result of the body's compensatory mechanisms for a failing heart, which include water and sodium retention, ankle oedema develops, causing ankle swelling. Accumulation of fluid in lungs (pulmonary oedema) contributes to the increased breathlessness, that all patients with CHF suffer, particularly on exertion and lying flat. Wheezing on inspiration may be present. More generalised oedema may develop, causing abdominal distension with associated pain and discomfort, and weight gain. CHF is currently incurable but the increased strength and vigour of heart muscle contraction which results from positive inotropic drugs such as digoxin can alleviate many of the disabling symptoms.

Apart from its positive inotropic effects, digoxin also indirectly affects the pacemaker cells of the sino-atrial (SA) and atrio-ventricular (AV) nodes in the heart which propagate electrical signals necessary for normal heart-beat rate and rhythm. For this reason digoxin is also used for the treatment of some disturbances of cardiac rhythm (known collectively as cardiac arrythmias), including probably the most common of these, atrial fibrillation.

Toxic (unwanted) side effects

Symptoms of digoxin toxicity include nausea, vomiting, diarrhoea and loss of appetite. Abnormal cardiac rhythms, which may result in either slowing of the heart rate (bradycardia) or increased heart rate (tachycardia), are common; in severe overdose, these may be life threatening. Disturbances of normal vision, including blurring of vision and loss of ability to distinguish some colour combinations, may occur. Mental effects include confusion and restlessness; rarely digoxin toxicity can precipitate acute psychoses. The primary effect of digoxin on the sodium–potassium pump determines that digoxin toxicity may be accompanied by a raised serum potassium.

Most digoxin is normally eliminated unchanged from the body by the kidneys in urine. Patients with diminished kidney function (the elderly and those with renal disease) cannot eliminate digoxin as efficiently as those with normal kidney function and are therefore at greater risk of digoxin toxicity. Abnormally low concentration of serum potassium (hypokalaemia), often the result of diuretic therapy, potentiates digoxin toxicity. A low serum magnesium and raised serum calcium have a similar effect. A few drugs, most notably the anti-arrhythmic, quinidine, increase serum digoxin concentration to toxic levels.

Why and when to measure serum digoxin

Routine monitoring of serum digoxin levels for all patients receiving digoxin is not considered necessary. However, the test is useful in certain clinical situations. Like lithium, digoxin has a low therapeutic index. The serum level required for therapeutic effect is close to that which results in toxic symptoms so that digoxin toxicity is relatively common, especially in the elderly. Unfortunately, many of the signs and symptoms of mild to moderate toxicity are non-specific and may even be due to the underlying disease which digoxin is being used to treat. The only sure way of making or excluding the diagnosis of digoxin toxicity is to measure serum digoxin concentration. A request for blood digoxin level may be made following a poor clinical response to a standard digoxin dose. If the result is below the therapeutic range, an increased dose may be safely prescribed. Finally the test can be used to assess patient compliance.

Theophylline

Principal pharmacological action and clinical use

Theophylline is a naturally occurring substance related to caffeine which is found in the leaves of the tea plant. Although the mechanism of its action is poorly understood, theophylline has three important pharmacological effects: stimulation of cardiac muscle, relaxation of smooth muscle (notably that of the lungs), and stimulation of the central nervous system. The principal clinical use of theophylline, which is derived from its effect on smooth muscle in the lung, is as a bronchodilator in the treatment of asthma.

Asthma is a common condition of the lungs, affecting up to 5% of children and 2% of adults in the UK, characterised by episodic attacks of airway constriction. Between attacks patients are usually quite well, but during attacks, which may be triggered by any number of factors including respiratory infection, environmental irritants (chemical fumes, smoke, etc.), exercise and even in some cases laughter, the bronchial airways constrict, become inflamed and produce abnormal amounts of mucus. These result in the common symptoms associated with an asthma attack: coughing, wheezing and increased breathlessness. In its most severe manifestation an asthma attack can cause respiratory failure in which normal gas exchange of oxygen and carbon dioxide is sufficiently compromised to threaten life. Although prompt hospital admission and treatment can be life-saving, around 2000 asthma patients die each year.

Theophylline is given orally as part of the ongoing drug treatment of chronic asthma to prevent attacks, and is also administered intravenously in the form of aminophylline (a salt of theophylline) for the emergency treatment of acute asthma attacks. Theophylline acts directly to relax the smooth muscles of the bronchi, effectively dilating or 'opening' the airway. The bronchodilator effect of theophylline is more pronounced if the airway is already constricted, as it is in patients with asthma.

Apart from asthma, the bronchodilating properties of theophylline are sometimes used in the treatment of chronic obstructive airways disease. A quite separate property of theophylline, the ability to stimulate the respiratory centres in the central nervous system, is thought to be the reason for its effectiveness in the treatment of apnoea of prematurity. Affected premature babies suddenly stop breathing for 20 seconds or more, threatening brain function; there is a risk of permanent brain damage. Both the frequency and duration of these so-called apnoea attacks are reduced with theophylline treatment.

Toxic (unwanted) side effects

Many patients experience minor adverse effects of theophylline therapy, and for this reason the drug is usually only prescribed for the prevention of asthma attacks after other anti-asthma drugs have failed. Nausea, vomiting and loss of appetite are the most common signs of mild toxicity. Headache, insomnia, nervousness and increased irritability reflect the effect of theophylline on the central nervous system (CNS). Whilst many patients may experience both gastrointestinal and CNS effects when they first take theophylline, a tolerance is usually acquired and symptoms disappear. Theophylline is a gastrointestinal irritant that can reactivate peptic ulcers. In addition to the gastrointestinal and CNS symptoms, marked toxicity may result in palpitations, increased pulse rate, and abnormal heart rhythms (usually sinus tachycardia). Cardiac arrest can occur in patients given a single large dose of theophylline (aminophylline) to control an acute asthma attack. Convulsions and loss of consciousness can occur during marked toxicity. Although rare, severe toxicity can be fatal.

Certain diseases (e.g. liver disease, chronic heart failure and any condition associated with persistent fever) cause a decrease in the rate that theophylline can be eliminated from the body and a consequent increase in blood theophylline to levels associated with toxic symptoms. Asthmatic patients with these additional problems require a lower dose than normal and careful monitoring if they are to avoid the effects of theophylline toxicity. Conversely, smokers eliminate theophylline more efficiently than non-smokers and so require a higher dose to achieve the same therapeutic effect. Toxicity may arise after quitting smoking if the dose is not reduced. Many drugs including alcohol and some antibiotics reduce theophylline elimination, thereby increasing toxicity at a given dosage. A full drug history must be taken into account when prescribing theophylline.

Why and when to measure serum theophylline

Theophylline has a low therapeutic index: the blood level required for therapeutic effect is close to that which results in toxic symptoms. Although the serum level for therapeutic effect has been established, the dose required to attain this therapeutic level varies so that all patients should have their serum level checked during initiation of therapy. Typically dose is increased in small increments until the blood level is within the therapeutic range. Once an effective and safe dosage regime has been established, blood levels need only be checked at 6- or 12-monthly intervals. More frequent monitoring may be considered in the following types of patient whose ability to eliminate theophylline might be diminishing. All these patient types have an increased risk of theophylline toxicity:

- the elderly
- patients with concurrent liver disease (cirrhosis, hepatitis)
- patients with concurrent congestive heart failure
- acutely ill patients (e.g. those receiving intensive care)
- those being prescribed some additional drugs.

All patients presenting with signs of toxicity should have blood level checked to decide whether a reduction in dosage or even temporary withdrawal of the drug is warranted.

Patients who seem to be failing to respond to theophylline might require a larger dose. If the blood level is below the therapeutic range, an increase in dose may be warranted.

LABORATORY MEASUREMENT OF SERUM LITHIUM, DIGOXIN AND THEOPHYLLINE

PATIENT PREPARATION

No particular patient preparation is necessary.

SAMPLE REQUIREMENTS

Around 5 ml of venous blood is required. This should be collected into a plain glass (without additives) tube.

TIMING OF SAMPLE

The concentration of any drug in blood varies in relation to the time of the last dose, so timing of sample collection is vital for accurate interpretation of routine therapeutic drug monitoring results.

- Blood for lithium should be sampled at 12 hours after the last dose.
- Blood for digoxin should be sampled at 6 hours after the last dose.
- Blood for theophylline should be sampled at 1–2 hours after the last dose.

If a patient is exhibiting signs of toxicity or a deliberate overdose is suspected, an urgent test result may be required. In these circumstances it is clearly not appropriate to wait before sampling blood, but it is important to record the time that the sample was taken and the time of the last dose or overdose, if known.

INTERPRETATION OF RESULTS

SERUM LITHIUM

Therapeutic range for those with symptoms of acute mania, 0.8–1.5 mmol/l
Therapeutic range for maintenance dose to *prevent* symptoms 0.5–0.8 mmol/l

The objective is to maintain serum levels within the therapeutic range. Patients actually suffering symptoms of acute mania can tolerate slightly higher doses of lithium than those without symptoms; hence the different therapeutic ranges. Once acute symptoms have passed and the patient has stabilised, a maintenance dose must be prescribed which results in a serum concentration within the lower therapeutic range.

'cont.'

'continued'

Symptoms of mild toxicity, diarrhoea, nausea and fine hand tremor usually arise as serum lithium rises above 1.5 mmol/l, although a minority of patients may experience lithium toxicity when their serum level is less than 1.5 mmol/l. More severe symptoms including confusion, dizziness, tinnitus, irregular heart beat and blurred vision are associated with serum levels above 2.0 mmol/l. Loss of consciousness and fatality can occur in severe overdose (serum lithium > 2.5 mmol/l) if treatment to eliminate lithium from the body is not urgently started.

SERUM DIGOXIN

Therapeutic range   1.0–2.6 nmol/l

Symptoms of toxicity are usually associated with digoxin concentration greater than 3.0 nmol/l. However, in some patients (e.g. those with hypokalaemia, hypomagnesia, hypercalcaemia and thyroid disease), there is an increased sensitivity to the effects of digoxin. For these patients, symptoms of toxicity might be present at levels lower than 3.0 nmol/l and may even occur at levels within the accepted therapeutic range. If causes of increased sensitivity can be excluded, then, for a patient whose serum digoxin level is within the therapeutic range, any symptoms suggestive of digoxin toxicity are unlikely to be due to digoxin; another cause must be sought and there is no real justification for reducing dosage. Conversely, if a patient is not responding clinically as expected to a particular dose of digoxin, a serum digoxin of less than 0.8 nmol/l (i.e. well below the lower limit of the therapeutic range) provides good objective evidence that the patient is likely to be under-digitalised and consideration can then be given to increasing the dosage.

SERUM THEOPHYLLINE

Therapeutic range for treatment of asthma   55–110 µmol/l (10–20 mg/l)
Therapeutic range for treatment of apnoea   28–44 µmol/l (8–20 mg/l)

The objective is to maintain serum level within the therapeutic range. A serum level below the therapeutic range is unlikely to be effective and one above the therapeutic range results in unwanted side effects (toxicity). Mild to moderate toxicity is associated with levels in the range 110–165 µmol/l (i.e. 20–30 mg/l). Severe toxicity with seizures and life-threatening cardiac arrhythmias do not usually occur until serum levels are in excess of 165 µmol/l (i.e. 30 mg/l).

Case history 12

Mr Anderson is 75 years old. He was first suspected of having a failing heart ten years ago when he noticed that he was becoming breathless on climbing stairs. Over the next year or two his condition gradually worsened. He became breathless when lying flat, making it difficult to sleep without additional pillows, and he developed ankle oedema. He was prescribed digoxin and oral diuretics. Although he required increasing amounts of diuretics to control oedema, his symptoms were relieved and he became much more physically active on digoxin until a month ago when his condition deteriorated. Immediately prior to hospital admission he was unable to perform any physical activity, preferring to sleep downstairs propped in a chair rather than make the effort of climbing the stairs at night. His ankles were so swollen with oedema that he was unable to wear shoes. Despite a loss of appetite his body weight had been rising with progressive accumulation of oedema fluid. On admission, Mr Anderson's serum digoxin was 2.2 nmol/l and his serum potassium 3.6 mmol/l. Over the next two days he was given large oral doses of the diuretic frusemide to remove accumulating fluids; by day three of admission this had resulted in a 12 kg fall in body weight. At this point, although Mr Anderson's body weight was now normal, he felt nauseous, retched frequently, felt very weak and complained of a headache; he became increasingly drowsy. As these are all signs of digoxin toxicity, blood was taken for serum digoxin; a urea and electrolytes request was made at the same time. The laboratory reported the following results

     serum digoxin   2.1 nmol/l
     serum potassium   2.4 mmol/l

(1) Did digoxin results either at the time of admission or 3 days later indicate that Mr Anderson might be receiving too much digoxin?
(2) Are serum potassium results normal? (See Chapter 4.)
(3) Why might Mr Anderson be suddenly suffering from digoxin toxicity despite no increase in dose for the past five years?

Discussion of case history

(1) Both digoxin results are within the therapeutic range. The deterioration in Mr Anderson's heart failure prior to hospital admission cannot be attributed to failure on his part to continue with his

digoxin medication. Results do not indicate digoxin toxicity; rather they indicate that he was receiving an appropriate digoxin dose.

(2)   The normal range for serum potassium is 3.6–5.0 mmol/l. On admission, then, Mr Anderson's serum potassium was at the low end of the normal range but after diuretic therapy on day three of admission, his potassium level was markedly reduced.

(3)   The water diuresis induced by administration of frusemide which Mr Anderson urgently required was accompanied by increased losses of potassium in urine. This is a well documented side effect of some diuretic therapies. Since before this treatment serum potassium was already at the low end of the normal range, possibly due to low dietary potassium intake because of loss of appetite, this increased loss of potassium in urine sent Mr Anderson's serum potassium plummeting; he became severely hypokalaemic. A reduced serum potassium potentiates the toxicity of digoxin so that, as in Mr Anderson's case, symptoms of toxicity appear despite the fact that serum digoxin is within the therapeutic range. Treatment of digoxin toxicity in this case is based not on withdrawal of digoxin, which might exacerbate Mr Anderson's underlying heart failure, but on restoring serum potassium to a level within the normal range by administration of potassium supplements.

Further reading

Digitalis Investigation Group (1997) The effect of digoxin on mortality and morbidity in patients with heart failure. *New Engl. J. Med.* **336**: 525–33.

Frings C. (1987) Lithium monitoring. *Clinics Lab. Med.* **7**: 545–50.

Jefferson J. (1998) Lithium. *BMJ* **316**: 1330–31.

Rowe D., Watson I., Williams J. *et al.* (1988) The clinical use and measurement of theophylline. *Ann. Clin. Biochem.* **25**: 4–26.

Sharff J. & Bayer M. (1982) Acute and chronic digitalis toxicity: presentation and treatment. *Ann. Emerg. Med.* **11**: 327–31.

Part

3

Haematology Tests

Full Blood Count (FBC) – 1: Red blood cell count, haemoglobin and red cell indices

Of all laboratory blood tests the full blood count (FBC) is the most frequently requested, reflecting the wide range of both common and less common disturbances of health which may be associated with abnormalities in FBC results. It is of course not one test but a panel of tests including a count of each of the three cellular or formed elements of blood: red cells (erythrocytes), white cells (leucocytes) and platelets (thrombocytes). In the first of two chapters which focus on the FBC we consider the red cell count and several other tests included in the FBC which all relate to red cell function. All these tests (listed in Table 14.1) are used primarily to identify those patients who are anaemic; they also help in elucidating the cause of that anaemia. In the next chapter we consider the significance of the total and differential white cell count whilst the platelet count will be dealt with in Chapter 16, which focuses on tests of blood coagulation.

Normal physiology

Red cell (erythrocyte) production

Red cells are the most abundant of the three formed elements in blood, outnumbering leucocytes (white cells) by around 1000:1 and platelets by 100:1. The process of blood cell production, called haemopoiesis, takes place within the bone marrow. During infancy the bone marrow of all bones has the capacity to manufacture blood cells but in adulthood this is limited to the bone marrow within the vertebrae, ribs, sternum, skull and pelvis as well as the ends of the long bones, femur and humeri. All blood cells are derived from the so-called pluripotent stem cells present in bone marrow which have the potential to differentiate cells which are

Table 14.1   Tests relating to red cells included in routine full blood count (FBC)

Test	What is measured	Units of measurement
Red blood cell (RBC) count	The number of red cells in blood	Number of thousand million cells, i.e. 10^9 in every litre of blood (10^9/l)
Haemoglobin (Hb)	Concentration of the protein haemoglobin in blood	Grams in every 100 ml of blood (g/dl)
Red cell indices:		
Packed cell volume (PCV)	The percentage of total blood volume occupied by red cells	Percentage (%)
Mean cell volume (MCV)	The average (mean) volume of red cells	Femtolitre (fl) (1 femtolitre = 1×10^{-15} litre)
Mean cell haemoglobin concentration (MCHC)	The average (mean) concentration of haemoglobin in red cells	Grams in every 100 ml of red cells (g/dl)

Blood film. For this test, blood is spread in a thin film on a glass microscope slide, then stained and examined under the microscope. A blood film report includes the details of any abnormalities in appearance or size of red cells. A blood film is usually only examined if results of above test indicate an abnormality.

committed to becoming either mature red cells, white cells or platelets. The most primitive of those cells within bone marrow which are destined to become mature red cells is the pro-normoblast. The pro-normoblast develops by cell division and differentiation through recognisable stages to normoblast, reticulocyte and finally the mature red cell or erythrocyte (Fig. 14.1). This development from stem cell to mature red cell is characterised by:

- gradual reduction in cell size
- loss of nucleus and therefore ability to divide
- loss of internal cell organelles.

The final stage of maturation, reticulocyte to erythrocyte, occurs both within the bone marrow and in the peripheral bloodstream; normally around 1–2% of the circulating red cell population is reticulocytes. No red cell more primitive than the reticulocyte is normally present in blood.

Red cells have a lifespan of around 120 days. Constant replacement is necessary; on average around 2.3 million red cells are produced every

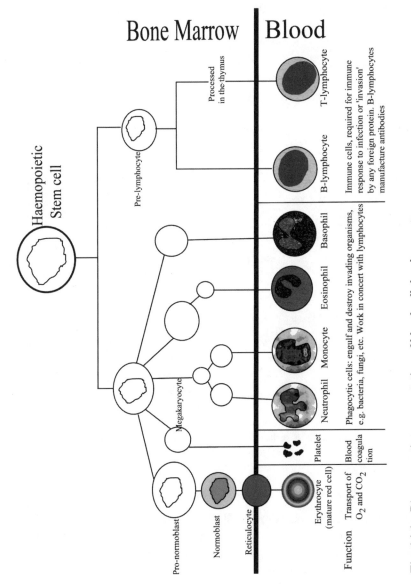
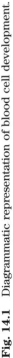

Fig. 14.1 Diagrammatic representation of blood cell development.

second by the bone marrow throughout life. This is regulated by erythropoietin, a hormone synthesised in the cells of the kidney (Fig. 14.2). In response to a falling blood oxygen level, the kidney releases erythropoietin into the bloodstream for transport to the bone marrow. Here erythropoietin stimulates red cell production. As red cell numbers increase, the oxygen content of blood rises and kidney production of erythropoietin is stepped down.

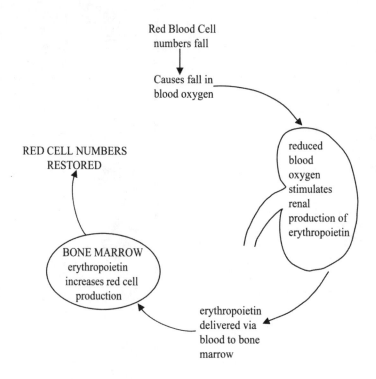

Fig. 14.2   Regulation of red cell numbers.

Structure and function of red cells

The structure of the mature red cell is well suited to its primary function: transport of oxygen from the lungs to the tissues and transport of carbon dioxide from tissues to the lungs. Central to this function is haemoglobin, the protein contained within red cells. Haemoglobin production occurs within the red cell during its early development in the bone marrow and is complete before full maturation. Each mature red cell leaves the bone marrow with its full complement of 640 million molecules of haemoglobin. Commonly described as a biconcave disc the mature red cell can be imagined as a flattened sphere with its sides pushed in. This singular shape allows the largest surface area for a given volume, providing maximum possible area for oxygen and carbon dioxide gas exchange.

The diameter of the red cell is around 8 μm, twice the diameter of the smallest blood vessels through which it must pass. The membrane is able to deform itself, altering the overall shape of the red blood cell so that it can 'squeeze' through the microvasculature within tissues and the alveoli of lungs, where gas exchange occurs. Without a nucleus and other internal organelles, the mature erythrocyte may be regarded as a deformable membranous bag stuffed full of haemoglobin.

Haemoglobin structure and function

Haemoglobin is the oxygen-carrying pigment present in red cells, which gives blood its colour. The haemoglobin molecule (Fig. 14.3) comprises four folded chains of amino acids. These together form the protein or *globin* portion of the molecule. Each of the four globin subunits has a *haem* group attached, and at the centre of each haem group is an atom of iron in the ferrous state (Fe^{2+}). Whilst the structure of the haem group is always the same, the exact sequence of amino acids in the globin sub-units varies slightly, giving rise to four possible globin chains; alpha (α), beta (β), gamma (γ) and delta (δ). Around 97% of adult haemoglobin is haemoglobin A (HbA) comprising two α and two β globin subunits. The

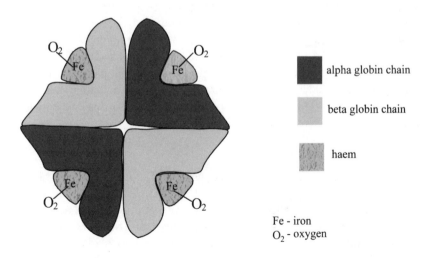

Fig. 14.3 Representation of molecular structure of oxygenated adult haemoglobin.

remaining 3% is HbA2 (two α and two δ globins). In the developing foetus and for the first few months of life, foetal haemoglobin (HbF) is the only haemoglobin produced; HbF is composed of two α and two γ globin subunits. The structure of haemoglobin is of more than passing academic interest. There are a large group of inherited disorders of haemoglobin synthesis and structure. These are collectively known as the haemoglobinopathies. Most are rare, but two, thalassaemia and sickle cell disease, warrant special attention (see separate boxes).

THE THALASSAEMIAS

These are a group of genetic (inherited) disorders characterised by deficient synthesis of α or β globin chains, with resulting low haemoglobin and anaemia. These genetic defects (more than 150 have been identified) are found most frequently in parts of Africa, the Mediterranean countries, the Middle East, the Indian subcontinent and South East Asia. All immigrants from these areas are at risk.

There are four genes which code for α globin production; if the defect lies in these genes, the condition is known as α-thalassaemia, but if the defect lies in the single gene which codes for β globin production, it is known as β-thalassaemia. The effect of these genetic defects varies greatly depending on the precise nature of the defect and whether the defect is inherited from both parents or just one.

β-THALASSAEMIA MINOR (β-THALASSAEMIA TRAIT)

This is the condition when a defective β globin gene is inherited from just one parent. Since a normal gene is inherited from the other parent, β globin is only slightly affected and patients can produce near normal amounts of HbA (two α and two β chains). Synthesis of HbA2 (two α and two δ chains) is increased (this is used to make the diagnosis), so that patients usually have normal total Hb. They are generally not anaemic and are usually fit and healthy. Affected women are, however, at high risk of anaemia during pregnancy and intercurrent illness.

β-THALASSAEMIA MAJOR

This is the much more severe homozygous form of thalassaemia, which occurs when β-thalassaemia trait is inherited from both parents. Production of β globin is severely affected. This is no problem during foetal development and the early months of life when Hb F (two α and two γ chains) is the only haemoglobin synthesised. But from around 3 to 6 months when

'cont.'

Box 1 The haemoglobinopathies – thalassaemia

'continued'

haemoglobin production switches from foetal haemoglobin (HbF) to adult haemoglobin (HbA), the deficiency of β globin chains becomes apparent, with gradual development of severe anaemia. Excessive red cell destruction leads to enlarged liver and spleen. Without regular blood transfusion every 4–6 weeks, affected children fail to develop, and die in childhood or early adolescence. Iron overload, consequent on repeated blood transfusions, is a major problem, which can be ameliorated by iron sequestering drugs. Bone marrow transplantation is a treatment option.

α-THALASSAEMIA

The genetic defect is actual deletion of α genes. The severity depends on how many of the four genes which code for α chain production are deleted. In the most severe case – known as hydrops fetalis – all four genes are deleted with complete absence of α chain synthesis. Since α chains are required for HbF, HbA and HbA2 the haemoglobin deficiency is too severe for foetal survival; death occurs *in utero*. Other forms of α-thalassaemia in which one, two or three genes are deleted result in varying degrees of anaemia.

All forms of thalassaemia, whether severe enough to cause anaemia or not, are associated with changes to red cells which are evident on FBC analysis as reduced MCV and MCH. That is, red cells are microcytic and hypochromic.

SICKLE CELL ANAEMIA

Sickle cell anaemia is caused by inheritance of a very specific genetic defect in the gene which codes for β globin synthesis. Like all proteins, β globin is composed of amino acids joined in a very precise sequence. The sixth amino acid in normal β globin is valine. The genetic defect of sickle cell anaemia results in synthesis of β globin with the amino acid glutamic acid instead of valine at position 6. This single amino acid substitution results in production of abnormal haemoglobin, HbS, composed of two normal α chains and two abnormal β chains. If the defective gene is inherited from just one parent carrier, half of the haemoglobin synthesised is normal HbA and the remainder is HbS. This heterozygous state is known as sickle cell trait. If the defective gene is inherited from both parents, no normal haemoglobin (HbA) is synthesised. Almost all the haemoglobin is abnormal HbS. This is sickle cell disease.

'cont.'

Box 2 Haemoglobinopathies – sickle cell anaemia

'continued'

HbS polymerises at low oxygen tensions causing structural changes to the red cell membrane which becomes rigid. The red cells deform into the familiar sickle shape that gives the condition its name. These deformed red cells are fragile and haemolyse easily, with development of haemolytic anaemia.

The sickle gene is most frequently found in African people and those of African descent (e.g. West Indians). It is also prevalent in some Mediterranean countries, the Middle East and parts of India.

SICKLE CELL TRAIT

Only around 30–45% of haemoglobin in those with sickle cell trait is HbS. Most of the rest is normal adult haemoglobin HbA. The condition is benign. Those affected are not generally anaemic. Tissue anoxia, which may occur in severe illnesses (e.g. clinical shock and systemic infection) may result in a sickling crises sufficient to cause anaemia. Particular care is required to maintain adequate tissue oxygenation during anaesthesia.

SICKLE CELL DISEASE

The expression of sickle cell disease varies greatly; a minority are virtually unaffected and live a normal healthy lifespan, whilst some die in early childhood. Symptoms may begin after the first six months of life when production HbF is switched to adult haemoglobin production. A chronic haemolytic anaemia is the hallmark of the disease. For most, the disease is characterised by periods of good health punctuated by extremely painful sickle cell crises. These crises may be precipitated by a variety of environmental factors including infection, violent exercise, emotional disturbance, anoxia, dehydration, etc. A sickle cell crisis is associated with increased haemolysis and sequestration of sickled cells in the microvasculature of various organs (spleen, bone, lungs, brain) and this accounts for many of the complications of sickle cell disease. Blocked vessels prevent normal blood flow, and tissue, starved of oxygen and nutrients, dies. When the microvasculature of the brain is affected, patients may suffer a stroke as a result of cerebral infarction. Occlusion of vessels in the eye causes visual impairment. Infarcts in growing bone tissue early in childhood may leave single fingers or toes permanently shorter than the rest. Sickle cell disease is associated with increased risk of infection, due partly to splenic damage. Pneumococcal septicaemia was once a significant cause of death before prophylactic antibiotics were introduced into routine care. Other treatments include regular blood transfusion to replace HbS with normal HbA.

Haemoglobin transport of oxygen

The oxygen combining property of haemoglobin depends on the single atom of iron present at the centre of each of the four haem groups. An oxygen molecule forms a weak, reversible ionic link with each of these iron atoms in turn; the product of this reaction is oxyhaemoglobin. When all four haem groups are occupied with oxygen the haemoglobin molecule is said to be saturated. The affinity of haemoglobin for oxygen, that is, the extent to which it is saturated, depends on the oxygen content of the blood. This is described graphically in the oxygen dissociation curve (Fig. 6.2). It is clear from this graph that haemoglobin becomes increasingly saturated with oxygen as the partial pressure of blood oxygen (PO_2) increases. The physiological implications of this relationship are central to the oxygen carriage and delivery function of haemoglobin. In the lungs, oxygen in inspired air passes across the alveoli to the blood so that PO_2 is high (around 95 mmHg). This high PO_2 facilitates haemoglobin affinity for oxygen and the haemoglobin quickly (within a few seconds) becomes almost 100% saturated. Conversely, in the tissues the blood PO_2 is relatively low (only around 40 mmHg) reducing affinity of haemoglobin for oxygen. As a result oxygen is released from haemoglobin and diffuses out of the red cells to tissue cells where it is required for cell metabolism.

Role of red cell and haemoglobin in the transport of CO_2

Whilst the transport of oxygen from lungs to tissues is almost entirely due to haemoglobin in red cells, the transport of carbon dioxide in the reverse direction is slightly more complex. Carbon dioxide, unlike oxygen, is soluble in blood plasma so that much CO_2 is transported simply dissolved in blood plasma. The remainder is transported in red cells. In the tissues, carbon dioxide diffuses out of tissue cells into the passing bloodstream; some remains dissolved in blood plasma and some diffuses into red cells. Within the red cell some carbon dioxide combines with deoxygenated haemoglobin to form carbamino-Hb and some combines with water in the red cell cytoplasm to form carbonic acid. This reaction is catalysed by the enzyme carbonic anhydrase. Carbonic acid dissociates to hydrogen ions (which are buffered by haemoglobin) and bicarbonate ions which diffuse out of the red cell into surrounding plasma. In the lungs these red cell reactions are reversed and the CO_2 diffuses out of red cells and passes along with CO_2 dissolved in plasma from the blood to alveoli for excretion in expired air.

Normal red cell destruction

After around 120 days, red cells are no longer viable and are removed from blood by the reticulo-endothelial system as it passes through the bone marrow, spleen and liver. In these sites the membrane of the cells breaks down, releasing haemoglobin which is split into its constituent parts: haem and globin (Fig. 10.2). The iron present in haem is recycled for production of new red cells, and globin chains are broken down to amino acids which enter the amino acid pool. What remains of haem after removal of iron is converted to the yellow pigment bilirubin, which is transported in blood to the liver for further metabolism and eventual excretion, mostly via bile in faeces; the remainder is excreted as the bilirubin metabolites, urobilin and urobilinogen, in urine.

LABORATORY MEASUREMENT OF FBC

PATIENT PREPARATION

No particular patient preparation is necessary.

TIMING OF SAMPLE

There are no special timing requirements so blood is best sampled at a time which will coinicide with routine transport to the laboratory. Blood for FBC should not be stored longer than 12 hours before transport to the laboratory. FBC is one of those tests that can be performed urgently and out of normal laboratory hours if necessary. In such circumstances it is essential to telephone the laboratory and transport the blood immediately it has been sampled.

TYPE OF SAMPLE

Venous blood is preferable, ideally collected without the use of a tourniquet (if used, a tourniquet should not be left for more than a minute or two before blood is sampled). Properly collected capillary blood can be used if venous blood collection poses difficulty (e.g. in babies and those with 'difficult' veins).

BLOOD COLLECTION BOTTLE

Blood for FBC must be collected into a special tube (usually lavender- or pink-coloured top) which contains the anticoagulant, K⁺EDTA. This prevents the blood from clotting and preserves the structure of blood cells.

'cont.'

'continued'

SAMPLE VOLUME

The sample bottles for FBC have a 'line to fill' marked on the label. This is usually 2.5 ml or 0.5 ml in the case of paediatric-sized bottles for capillary blood sampling. This volume will result in the correct ratio of blood to anticoagulant. It is vital for an accurate result that neither too much nor too little blood is added to these tubes and that anticoagulant and blood are mixed by gentle inversion as soon as the blood is sampled. Inadequate mixing can result in the formation of tiny blood clots and inaccurate results.

INTERPRETATION OF HB, RBC AND RED CELL INDICES RESULTS

APPROXIMATE REFERENCE RANGES

Red Blood cell (RBC)   Males $4.5–6.5 \times 10^{12}/l$
Females $3.9–5.6 \times 10^{12}/l$
Haemoglobin (Hb)   Males 13.5–17.5 g/dl
Females 11.5–15.5 g/dl
Packed cell volume (PCV) or haematocrit (Ht)
Males 40–52%
Females 36–48%
Mean cell volume (MCV) 80–95 fl
Mean cell haemoglobin concentration (MCHC) 20–35 g/dl

CRITICAL VALUES

Haemoglobin   < 7.0 g/dl or > 20.0 g/dl
PCV (Haematocrit)   < 20% or > 60%

TERMS USED TO DESCRIBE RED CELLS WHEN VIEWED UNDER A MICROSCOPE

Normocytosis	average size of red cell appears normal
Microcytosis	average size of red cells appears smaller than normal
Macrocytosis	average size of red cells appears larger than normal
Anisocytosis	red cells vary in size
Poikilocytosis	red cells vary in shape
Normochromasia	red cells stain normally, indicating they contain a normal amount of haemoglobin
Hypochromasia	red cells appear weakly stained indicating they contain less haemoglobin than normal

Conditions associated with reduction in RBC, Hb and PCV (Ht)

Anaemia

Anaemia (literally, without blood) is the collection of signs and symptoms that result from reduced oxygen delivery to tissues due to a decrease in the total number of red blood cells and/or reduction in haemoglobin content of blood. There are many possible causes so that anaemia is not a disease in itself, rather a sign of some underlying disease which must be identified if treatment of anaemia is to be successful. Whatever the cause, anaemia is accompanied by reduction in haemoglobin (Hb). Anaemia is defined as an Hb of less than 13.5 g/dl in adult males and less than 11.5 g/dl in adult females. In children, who normally have slightly lower levels of haemoglobin, a diagnosis of anaemia is made if Hb is less than 11.0 g/dl; the lower the result, the more severe the anaemia. A reduced red cell count and PCV is also a feature of anaemia, although the magnitude of that reduction depends not only on the severity of the anaemia but also on its cause. Delivery of oxygen to the tissues is reduced in anaemia but the extent to which this causes symptoms depends on several factors including:

- severity of the anaemia: many patients with mild anaemia, i.e. Hb greater than 10 g/dl, have no symptoms, but severe anaemia, Hb < 6 g/dl, is almost always associated with symptoms
- speed of onset: rapid onset of anaemia is more likely to result in symptoms than that which has developed slowly
- age: the elderly are less well equipped with the compensatory mechanisms for anaemia and are more likely to suffer symptoms than the young.

Signs and symptoms of anaemia

There are some generalised signs and symptoms of anaemia no matter what the cause. Most are the result of reduced oxygenation of tissues (tissue hypoxia). Some reflect the body's attempt to compensate for anaemia.

- pallor (particularly evident in the highly vascularised mucosal membranes of the eye)
- tiredness and lethargy
- shortness of breath, particularly on exertion

- dizziness, fainting
- headaches
- increased pulse rate, palpitations, increased heart rate (tachycardia).

Causes of anaemia

Whilst Hb, RBC and PCV measurement all help in identifying those patients who are anaemic, and in assessing the severity of anaemia, they provide no information about cause. Anaemia may be caused by:

- Acute blood loss (haemorrhage), e.g. trauma or surgery.
- Deficiency of iron (required for haemoglobin production), the most common cause of anaemia.
- Chronic inflammation or infection (e.g. rheumatoid arthritis, tuberculosis) and malignancy. This anaemia, called anaemia of chronic disease, is the second most common cause of anaemia.
- Deficiency of vitamin B_{12} and/or folate (required for production of red cells). So-called pernicious anaemia accounts for most anaemias in this group.
- Deficiency of erythropoietin (required for regulation of red cell production). This is the principal cause of the anaemia that occurs in chronic renal failure.
- Increased rate of red cell destruction (the haemolytic anaemias: examples include sickle cell anaemia, transfusion reactions, haemolytic disease of the newborn).
- Bone marrow stem cell failure (aplastic anaemia), usually the result of cytotoxic drug or radiation therapy for treatment of cancer.
- Malignant disease of bone marrow (e.g. the leukaemias, myeloma).

The red cell indices, MCV and MCHC, along with microscopic examination of red cells, help in identifying the cause of anaemia. Anaemias can be classified according to the average size of red cell (MCV) and the average concentration of haemoglobin in each red cell (MCHC). These two indices allow any anaemia to be classified into one of three broad groups:

- **Microcytic (low MCV), hypochromic (low MCHC) anaemia.** Iron deficiency anaemia and thalassaemia. The anaemia of chronic disease can sometimes result in microcytic, hypochromic red cells.
- **Normocytic (normal MCV), normochromic (normal MCHC) anaemia.** Most cases of anaemia associated with chronic disease are normocytic and normochromic. Other anaemias in this group include those which result from acute blood loss (haemorrhage), anaemias

which result from increased rate of red cell destruction (the haemolytic anaemias), anaemia caused by decreased erythropoietin
production (chronic renal failure), anaemia caused by damage to bone
marrow stem cells (aplastic anaemia), and anaemia which results
from malignant disease of the bone marrow (i.e. the leukaemias).

- **Macrocytic (raised MCV) anaemia.** The anaemia which results
from abnormal red cell production due to deficiency of vitamin B_{12}
and folate.

The examination of a stained blood smear under the microscope is
useful in establishing the cause of anaemia. The shape, size and staining
characteristics of the red cells from an anaemic patient may give
important clues as to the cause. For example, the red cells of patients
with sickle cell anaemia, a genetic defect of haemoglobin structure, have
a characteristic sickle shape which gives the condition its name. Relatively small red cells which stain weakly (due to abnormally low
concentration of haemoglobin) indicate possible iron deficiency,
whereas large cells, typically oval in shape, indicate anaemia is probably
due to vitamin B_{12} or folate deficiency. Many more anaemias are
associated with characteristic changes in red cell shape.

Causes of increased RBC, Hb and PCV (Ht)

Polycythaemia

Polycythaemia (literally many blood cells) is the opposite of anaemia.
Increased red cell count and haemoglobin concentration is the hallmark
of polycythaemia. Since PCV is dependent on the number of red cells,
this too is raised in polycythaemia. Polycythaemia may arise as a
response to any physiological or pathological condition in which blood
contains less oxygen than normal. In response to a low blood oxygen
level, the kidney increases erythropoietin production resulting in turn in
increased red cell production. This so called secondary polycythaemia is
a feature of

- living at high altitude (where inspired air has relatively less oxygen)
- cigarette smoking (carbon monoxide binds to haemoglobin, dis-
placing oxygen)
- chronic lung disease (passage of oxygen from lungs to blood is
compromised)
- cyanotic heart disease (blood is less well oxygenated than normal
due to structural defects in the heart).

Primary polycythaemia or polycythaemia vera is a quite separate malignant disease of the bone marrow in which bone marrow stem cell proliferation results in marked over-production of red cells (white cell and platelet numbers are also often increased). This huge increase in red cell numbers increases the viscosity (fluidity) of blood, and several of the signs and symptoms (headache, increased blood pressure) are related to this increased blood viscosity.

Effect of hydration on RBC, Hb and PCV (Ht)

It must be remembered that the red cell count and haemoglobin are measures of concentration in total plasma volume. If the volume of plasma is reduced or increased, as in dehydration and over-hydration respectively, the concentration of red cells (i.e. the measured red cell count) and haemoglobin concentration will be affected even though the absolute number of red cells and the amount of haemoglobin in blood remain normal. Dehydration is thus associated with an increased red cell count, haemoglobin and PCV and conversely a patient who has received too much fluid and is over-hydrated will have a reduced red cell count, Hb and PCV. This effect of hydration on red cell count, haemoglobin concentration and PCV must be taken into account when interpreting results from patients who are either dehydrated or over-hydrated. An increased plasma volume is a normal physiological effect of pregnancy, so that pregnancy is associated with a decrease in Hb, PCV and RBC even though absolute numbers of red cells and haemoglobin are normal. Thus a pregnant woman with a slight reduction in Hb is not necessarily anaemic.

Other causes of a raised MCV

It is worth noting that MCV may be raised in patients who are not anaemic, i.e. who have a normal Hb. The principal causes of an isolated increase in MCV are alcohol abuse and cirrhosis of the liver, although in both cases patients may also be anaemic. An isolated MCV in a patient suspected of alcohol abuse is considered sound objective evidence of such abuse. The test is widely used in conjunction with the GGT test to monitor alcoholic patients, since a normal MCV implies sustained abstinence.

Case history 13

Jane Baker, a 32-year-old solicitor, attends her GP's surgery complaining of feeling 'washed out'. Although normally an active woman, who enjoys horse riding at weekends and regular visits with her children to the local swimming pool, Jane now reports becoming increasingly tired over the past month or two. She feels unable to do much more than a normal day's work. During examination of Jane's eyes, her GP noted a slight degree of pallor in conjunctival mucous membranes, suggesting anaemia might be the cause of her tiredness. No other abnormal signs were detected. He sampled blood for a full blood count (FBC). The laboratory report, which he received two days later, contained the following results.

Hb 9.2 g/dl
RBC 3.8×10^{12}/litre
PCV 28%
MCV 73 fl
MCHC 20 g/dl

(1) What is the laboratory evidence of Jane's anaemia; is it severe?
(2) Using the red cell indices classify the anaemia to either:
   (a) microcytic anaemia
   (b) normocytic anaemia
   (c) macrocytic anaemia
(3) Suggest possible causes of the anaemia.
(4) What further test(s) is indicated?

Discussion of case history

(1) The haemoglobin concentration (Hb) is used to confirm or exclude anaemia. Jane's Hb is well below the reference range for adult females. This is sufficient evidence to make a diagnosis of anaemia. An Hb of 9.2 g/dl indicates that Jane is moderately anaemic; anaemia is usually considered severe only if Hb is less than 6.0 g/dl. Although not required to make a diagnosis, both PCV and RBC results are low, reflecting anaemia.
(2) The MCV (mean cell volume) is a measure of the average size of red cells. Jane's MCV is reduced, which means that on average her red cells are smaller than normal; her anaemia is microcytic in nature.
(3) Almost all cases of microcytic anaemia are due to either

- iron deficiency
- the anaemia of chronic disease (infection, inflammation, malignancy), or
- β-thalassaemia (an inherited disorder of haemoglobin synthesis found particularly in those of Mediterranean descent).

Of these, iron deficiency is by far the most common, and thalassaemia the least common. Since Jane has no medical history of chronic disease, iron deficiency is the most likely cause of her anaemia.

(4)   A serum iron and serum ferritin test will confirm the diagnosis of iron deficiency anaemia. (Chapter 17). As will be made clear in Chapter 17 there are many causes of iron deficiency. If iron deficiency is confirmed, Jane may require further investigation to establish the cause in her case.

Further reading

Frewin R., Henson A. & Provan D. (1997) ABC of clinical haematology: iron deficiency anaemia. *BMJ* **314**: 360–63.

Hoffbrand A. & Pettit J. (1993) Blood cell formation. In: *Essential Haematology*, 3rd edn. Blackwell Science, Oxford.

Hoffbrand A. & Provan D. (1997) ABC of clinical haematology: macrocytic anaemia. *BMJ* **314**: 430–33.

Weatherall D.J. (1997) ABC of clinical haematology: the hereditary anaemias. *BMJ* **314**: 492–96.

Full Blood Count (FBC) – 2:
White cell count and differential

In this second of two chapters devoted to the full blood count, the most commonly requested blood test, the clinical value of the white blood cell count is considered. Unlike the mature red cell population, which is homogeneous in nature, the white cell (leucocyte) population is heterogeneous, composed as it is of five morphologically and functionally distinct populations. These are: neutrophils, eosinophils, basophils, monocytes and lymphocytes. The total white cell count (WBC) is the sum of all of these white cell types, whilst the differential white cell count or 'diff' is a count of each of the five types. An increase in white cell numbers is a very common feature of disease, which can be attributed to one of several pathological processes including infection, inflammation, and malignancy. A reduced white cell count, which is much less common, implies a reduction in immunity and therefore a high risk of infectious disease.

Normal physiology

In common with all other formed elements in blood, white cells (leucocytes) are derived from the pluripotent stem cell present in bone marrow (Fig. 14.1) Mature white cells have a limited lifespan, so constant bone marrow production is necessary throughout life. An increase in bone marrow production of white cells is part of the body's normal (inflammatory) response to any insult to the body (i.e. any tissue injury, whatever the cause). The purpose of the inflammatory response is to contain and control injury, to eliminate potential pathogens (bacteria, viruses, fungi, protozoa, parasitic worms) and initiate healing and tissue repair. As key players in the inflammatory response, white cells must leave the blood and enter the tissues. Although, as we shall see, each type of white cell has a different and well defined job to do in the overall process of inflammation, they operate in concert, communicating via a range of chemical messengers called cytokines.

Neutrophils

Comprising between 40 and 70% of the total white cell population the neutrophil is the most abundant of all white cells in blood. The mature neutrophil has a multi-lobed nucleus and dark blue staining granules in the cytoplasm. It has a diameter of about 15 μm, around twice that of a red cell. The function of these cells is to enter the tissues and kill invading micro-organisms. On release from the bone marrow, mature neutrophils spend only around 8 hours in the bloodstream and the rest of their 4- to 5-day maximum lifespan in the tissues. Chemicals called chemotactic factors released from bacteria and other cells (including basophils, macrophages and lymphocytes, see below) attract neutrophils to the site of tissue infection or inflammation. In the tissues, neutrophils surround and engulf bacteria by a process called phagocytosis. Once inside the neutrophil, bacteria are killed by enzymes and highly reactive free radical chemicals produced within the darkly staining granules of the neutrophil cytoplasm. Pus, the thick yellowish fluid that oozes from an infection site, is a visible reminder of neutrophil function. It is largely composed of dead and dying neutrophils, bacterial debris and other cellular detritus produced during the fight against infection.

Eosinophils

Although many fewer in number, comprising only between 0.2 and 5% of the total white cell population, eosinophils have similarities in both appearance and function to neutrophils. The nucleus of the eosinophil, like the neutrophil, is lobed in appearance, though whereas the neutrophil nucleus is multi-lobed, the eosinophil nucleus has just two lobes. The granules of the eosinophil cytoplasm stain orange–red in contrast to the dark blue of the neutrophil, due to the presence of chemicals peculiar to the eosinophil. Like neutrophils, eosinophils are capable of phagocytosis, although it seems unlikely that they have a role in the killing of bacteria. Instead it is thought that they target foreign material too large for normal phagocytosis. For example, they bind parasitic worms and inflict damage by releasing enzymes and then phagocytose the products. Their main function, then, is protection against infection by organisms larger than bacteria and viruses. Eosinophils are present at the site of inflammation caused by allergic reactions, such as the airways of allergic asthma and hay fever sufferers. Release of chemicals from eosinophils contributes to the pathogenesis of allergic inflammatory disease.

Basophils

These are so few in number that they are only rarely seen in peripheral blood. They have a multi-lobed nucleus which is hidden by dense dark blue staining granules. Basophils migrate into tissues where they mature to mast cells. When activated, mast cells release many chemical mediators of the inflammatory response, which include a chemotactic factor that attracts neutrophils; histamine, a chemical which dilates blood vessels, increasing the blood flow to damaged areas; and heparin, an anticoagulant required to begin the process of repair to damaged blood vessels.

Monocytes

The monocyte has a non-lobed, circular or oval nucleus, with usually a clear (non-granulated) cytoplasm. After a short period of 20–40 hours circulating in the blood, these phagocytic cells migrate to the tissues where they mature to cells called macrophages. These macrophages phagocytose and kill foreign organisms in the same way that neutrophils do, but have a second important role in processing and presenting foreign proteins or antigens (derived from bacteria, etc.) to T-lymphocytes for initiation of a cell-mediated immune response (see below).

Lymphocytes

Between 20 and 40% of the circulating white cell population are lymphocytes; these are the second most abundant type of white cell in blood. Like all other blood cells they are derived from the bone marrow, but a proportion undergo further processing within the thymus; these are thymus-dependent lymphocytes or T-lymphocytes, which comprise around 70% of all circulating lymphocytes. Most of the remaining 30% are B-lymphocytes. There is an additional small population of non-B , non T-lymphocytes called natural killer (NK) lymphocytes. The routine lymphocyte count is the sum of these three types.

Like neutrophils, lymphocytes are required for immunity (protection) from infection. B-lymphocytes produce antibodies. These are proteins which bind specifically with complementary proteins called antigens. Micro-organisms (bacteria, viruses, etc.) all have specific surface proteins which act as antigens. Antibody binding of these surface antigens prevents bacteria and viruses from invading tissue cells. Furthermore, antibody-coated bacteria are much more easily phagocytosed (destroyed) by neutrophils and macrophages. Antibodies can also bind to and thereby neutralise bacterial toxins.

Although antibodies are effective in the process which leads to destruction of microbes outside cells, they cannot enter cells and therefore have no effect on the microbes harbouring within cells. The body's defence against these depends on T-lymphocytes.

T-lymphocytes can 'recognise' and destroy body cells which are infected, thereby preventing further spread. Since all viruses must infect cells in order to replicate, and many bacteria parasitise body cells, this so-called cell-mediated immunity invoked by the T-lymphocyte is a vital component of the body's defence against infection. T-lymphocytes also have the capacity to recognise and kill cancerous cells, so are part of the body's defence against cancer.

An important feature of lymphocyte-mediated immunity, whether it be B-lymphocyte (i.e. antibody) mediated or T-lymphocyte (i.e. cell) mediated, is that, unlike all other white blood cells, both classes of lymphocytes have the capacity to 'remember' an invading organism so that the response to a subsequent encounter is greater and more rapid. This so-called 'acquired' immunity explains why we seldom suffer more than once from a particular infection. First exposure provides immunity from subsequent infections with the same organism.

Laboratory measurement of full blood count is described in the previous chapter.

INTERPRETATION OF WBC AND DIFFERENTIAL RESULTS

APPROXIMATE REFERENCE RANGES

Total white blood cell (leucocyte) count		$4.0–11.0 \times 10^9/l$
Neutrophils	(40–75% of total white cells)	$2.5–7.5 \times 10^9/l$
Lymphocytes	(20–40% of total white cells)	$1.5–4.0 \times 10^9/l$
Monocytes	(2–10% of total white cells)	$0.2–0.8 \times 10^9/l$
Eosinophils	(1–5 % of total white cells)	$0.04–0.44 \times 10^9/l$
Basophils	(< 1% of total white cells)	$0.01–0.10 \times 10^9/l$

At birth the total white cell count is very high ($18.0–22.0 \times 10^9/l$). This falls sharply to around $8.0–16.0 \times 10^9/l$ during the first week of life and to normal adult levels by 6 months of age.

'cont.'

'continued'

CRITICAL VALUES

Total white blood cell count (WCC) $< 2.0 \times 10^9/l$ or $> 30.0 \times 10^9/l$

TERMS USED IN INTERPRETING RESULTS

Polymorphonuclear cells (polymorphs). Literally 'many shaped nucleus' cells, the term refers to all white blood cells with a lobed nucleus, i.e. neutrophils, eosinophils and basophils. Lymphocytes and monocytes are non-polymorphs because they have a more regularly shaped nucleus.

Granulocytes. All white cells with visibly staining granules in the cytoplasm (i.e. neutrophils, eosinophils and basophils.) Lymphocytes and monocytes are non-granulocytes.

Agranulocytosis. Complete or near absence of granulocytes in blood.

Phagocytes and non-phagocytes. Phagocytes are cells which are able to phagocytose foreign material (bacteria, etc.). Neutrophils, eosinophils, basophils and monocytes are all phagocytes. Lymphocytes do not have this ability; they are non-phagocytes.

Leucocytosis. An increase in total white cell count.

Neutrophilia, eosinophilia, basophilia. A selective increase in neutrophil, eosinophil and basophil count, respectively.

Lymphocytosis. An increase in lymphocyte count.

Leucopaenia. A reduced total white cell count.

Neutropaenia. A reduced neutrophil count.

Lymphocytopaenia. A reduced lymphocyte count.

Pancytopaenia. A reduction in all blood cells (red cells, white cells and platelets).

TERMS USED TO DESCRIBE WHITE CELLS WHEN VIEWED UNDER THE MICROSCOPE

'Increase in band forms'. Band cells are slightly immature neutrophils recognisable by the non-segmented shape of the nucleus. Normally only 3% of total neutrophils in peripheral blood are of this sort. An increase implies the bone marrow is increasing white cell production in response to infection or inflammation.

'Shift to left'. An alternative term to 'increase in band cells' denoting increase in immature neutrophils in peripheral blood.

Blast cells. Very primitive white cells never normally seen in peripheral blood. Their presence almost always indicates a haematological malignancy (e.g. acute leukaemia).

Causes of an increase in total white cell numbers

General considerations

An increase in white cell numbers (leucocytosis) occurs most commonly as a result of infection, inflammation or indeed any significant tissue damage. Since the role of white cells is to defend the body against infection, it is entirely appropriate that numbers should increase under these circumstances. This so-called benign or reactive leucocytosis must be distinguished from the much less common and entirely inappropriate leucocytosis that is a feature of leukaemia, a malignant disease of the blood.

The leukaemias are a group of bone marrow cancers characterised by the unregulated proliferation of one sort (a clone) of immature blood cell at the expense of normal blood cell production. Nearly all cases can be classified to one of four groups depending on whether the clinical course of the disease is rapid (acute) or slow (chronic) and whether the immature cells are derived from the myeloid bone marrow cells (which normally mature to either red cells, platelets, neutrophils, eosinophils, basophils or monocytes) or lymphoid bone marrow cells (which normally mature to lymphocytes). The four types of leukaemia, then, are: acute myeloid leukaemia (AML), chronic myeloid leukaemia (CML), acute lymphoblastic leukaemia (ALL) and chronic lymphocytic leukaemia (CLL). Some of the distinguishing features of the four sorts of leukaemia are outlined in Table 15.1. Since in all cases normal blood cell development is impaired, anaemia (due to deficiency of normal red cells), impaired blood coagulation with increased tendency to bleed (due to low platelet count) and high risk of infection (due to reduced numbers of normal white cells) can be features of all leukaemias.

Whether it be benign or malignant, leucocytosis is usually the result of a predominant, though not necessarily entirely selective, increase in one of the five types of white cell. The differential count thus provides clues as to the cause of an increased total white cell count. A more detailed account of the cause of increased white cell numbers follows, focusing on each type of white cell in turn.

Table 15.1 Some features of the four main types of leukaemia

Acute myeloid leukaemia	Acute lymphoblastic leukaemia	Chronic myeloid leukaemia	Chronic lymphocytic leukaemia
Most common form of acute leukaemia. Rare in childhood. Incidence increases with increasing age	Majority (80%) of cases occur in children with peak incidence at age 3–4 years	Accounts for around 15–20% of all cases of leukaemia. Occurs predominantly in those aged between 40 and 60 years but may occur at any age	Most common form of leukaemia. Accounts for around 30% of all cases. Occurs almost exclusively in those aged more than 50 years
French–American–British (FAB) classification based on appearance of abnormal blood cells allows identification of eight types (M0–M7)	French–American–British (FAB) classification based on appearance of abnormal blood cells allows identification of three types (L1–L3)	No FAB classification of type	No FAB classification of type
Rapidly fatal without treatment	Rapidly fatal without treatment	Disease typically progresses slowly over a period of several years. Later a rapidly progressive (acute) phase may occur	Disease typically progresses slowly over a period of several years
May or may not be acutely ill at the time of diagnosis. Symptoms include tiredness and lethargy due to anaemia. Fever and infection due to low numbers of mature functioning white cells. Bruising and increased tendency to bleed (low platelets)	Typically acutely ill at the time of diagnosis. Symptoms include tiredness and lethargy due to anaemia. Fever and infection due to low numbers of mature functioning white cells. Bruising and increased tendency to bleed (low platelets). Infiltration of central nervous system is common, resulting in headaches and vomiting	Not usually acutely ill at the time of diagnosis. Symptoms include tiredness and breathlessness on exertion due to slowly progressive anaemia. Bruising due to low platelets. History of weight loss. Night sweats	Around 25% of patients are symptom free at the time of diagnosis when the disease is identified by chance blood testing. This symptom-free period may last for several years. In symptomatic patients, symptoms similar to CML
Initial treatment is with chemotherapy (combination of three cytotoxic drugs) Bone marrow transplantation considered for young patients if chemotherapy fails. Although 80–90% of young patients achieve remission, only 30% are cured. Older patients fare less well	Initial treatment is with chemotherapy (a combination of three or four cytotoxic drugs). Radiation therapy for CNS disease treatment of prevention. Bone marrow transplantation considered if chemotherapy fails. Chemotherapy effects a cure in the majority of children but only around 30% of adults	Bone marrow transplantation (BMT) first line treatment of choice for younger patients (less than 40 years) otherwise single drug chemotherapy, the cytotoxic bisulphan or alpha interferon. Only BMT can effect a cure	No treatment necessary until the onset of symptoms. Control of symptoms but no cure possible with chemotherapy. Survival variable, 1–20 years. Median 3–4 years

Causes of increased neutrophil count (neutrophilia)

Neutrophilia is the most common derangement of white cell numbers.

Reactive neutrophilia

This is a feature of:

- most acute bacterial infections; particularly high (up to $50 \times 10^9/l$) in pyogenic (pus forming) infections, e.g. those caused by *Staphylococcus* and *Streptococcus* bacterial species
- non-infective acute inflammation (e.g. rheumatoid arthritis, inflammatory bowel disease, etc.)
- tissue damage (surgery, trauma, burns, myocardial infarction)
- solid tumours, e.g. lung cancer (an appropriate response to the tissue necrosis (death) which accompanies tumour growth)
- extreme physical exercise
- pregnancy and labour of pregnancy

Malignant cause of neutrophilia

In chronic myeloid leukaemia the total white cell count is very high, usually greater than $50 \times 10^9/l$ and sometimes up to $500 \times 10^9/l$. These cells are predominantly of the myeloid series with greatly increased numbers of neutrophils.

Causes of increased lymphocyte count (lymphocytosis)

Reactive lymphocytosis

This is a feature of:

- Infectious mononucleosis (glandular fever). This acute infectious disease, caused by the Epstein–Barr virus, is the most common cause of an isolated marked lymphocytosis. Most cases occur among teenagers and young adults. Symptoms include sore throat, fever, extreme tiredness, nausea and headache. Swollen and tender lymph nodes of the throat and neck are usual. Lymphocyte count rises a few days after symptoms appear and may peak very high (in the range $10–30 \times 10^9/l$) before gradually returning to normal over the following month or two.

- Other less common viral infections include cytomegalovirus, early stages of HIV infection, viral hepatitis, rubella, mumps and chicken pox.
- Chronic bacterial infection. Although bacterial infections are usually associated with neutrophilia rather than lymphocytosis, bacterial infections which are longstanding (chronic) in nature are characterised by lymphocytosis. The most common chronic bacterial infection is tuberculosis.
- Other miscellaneous infections: whooping cough (caused by the bacteria *Bordetella pertussis*), toxoplasmosis (caused by the protozoan, *Toxoplasma gondii*).

Malignant causes

- Chronic lymphatic leukaemia. The total white cell count is usually raised (often very high, in the range $50\text{--}100 \times 10^9/\text{l}$). Most of these cells are mature lymphocytes. Severe lymphocytosis (i.e. $> 50 \times 10^9/\text{l}$) in an older person is most likely due to CLL.
- Some cases of non-Hodgkin's lymphoma (a malignant tumour (cancer) of the lymph nodes).

Causes of increase in eosinophil count (eosinophilia)

Eosinophilia is much less common than either neutrophilia or lymphocytosis. Principal causes are:

- parasitic worm infections (e.g. tapeworm, hookworm, *Strongyloides*, *Schistosoma*, etc.) and
- allergic diseases (e.g. hay fever, eczema, allergic asthma, food sensitivity)
- sometimes raised in Hodgkin's (lymphoma) disease.

Causes of increase in basophils and monocyte counts

An increase in the numbers of either of these cells is rare. Basophil numbers are raised in chronic myeloid leukaemia. Monocytosis may be a feature of TB, subacute bacterial endocarditis and other chronic bacterial infections.

Causes of a reduction in white cell numbers (leucopaenia)

General considerations

A reduction in total white cell numbers is much less common than an increase; it is never 'appropriate' in the same way as an increase in white cell numbers often is. A reduced white cell count is almost always the result of a decrease in either neutrophils or lymphocytes, or both.

Low neutrophil count (neutropaenia)

■ A slight neutropaenia is a feature of some viral infections (mumps, influenza, viral hepatitis, HIV, etc.). The combination of a low neutrophil count and raised lymphocyte count (see above) explains why in some viral illnesses the total white cell count may remain normal despite a reduction in neutrophils.

■ Overwhelming bacterial infection. In rare cases of extreme infection the bone marrow is unable to replace neutrophils at a sufficiently rapid rate.

■ Aplastic anaemia, a condition of bone marrow stem cell failure which results not only in life-threatening severe neutropaenia but also in failure to produce adequate numbers of all types of blood cell (red cells, white cells and platelets). In many cases there is no identifiable cause. However, aplastic anaemia is a known although often unpredictable side effect of some drug therapies. Among these are cytotoxic drugs used to kill malignant (cancerous) cells, some antibiotics (e.g. chloramphenicol) and gold therapy for treatment of rheumatoid arthritis. Exposure to radiation (e.g. radiation therapy for cancer treatment) can also cause aplastic anaemia. The risk of aplastic anaemia is one of the reasons for the policy of restricting the use of diagnostic X-rays whenever possible.

■ Acute leukaemia. Malignant blood cells proliferate at the expense of normal blood cell development, with resulting neutropaenia.

■ Many solid malignant tumours spread (metastasise) to the bone where they infiltrate and suppress normal bone marrow blood cell production. Neutropaenia may therefore be a feature of advanced cancer.

Causes of reduced lymphocyte count

■ AIDS. Human immunodeficiency virus (HIV-1) which causes AIDS exerts its devastating effects by specifically infecting T-lymphocytes.

The virus replicates within the T-lymphocytes causing cell death, so AIDS is characterised by progressive T-lymphocyte destruction with severe, progressive lymphocytopaenia.

■ Autoimmune destruction of lymphocytes is the cause of the lymphocytopaenia which is a common feature of systemic lupus erythematosus (SLE).

■ A slight decrease in lymphocyte numbers often accompanies some acute inflammatory conditions; examples include pancreatitis, appendicitis and Crohn's disease.

■ Influenza virus infection.

■ Burns, surgery and severe trauma.

■ A profound deficiency of lymphocytes is a feature of several very rare congenital disorders discovered at birth. These include DiGeorge's syndrome in which, due to failure of thymus development, babies are born with no T-lymphocytes. A lack of both B- and T-lymphocytes is a feature of severe combined immunodeficiency syndrome (SCID).

Clinical consequences of abnormal white cell numbers

An increase in white cell numbers is a protective response to injury, infection and inflammation. An increase in white cell numbers is therefore physiological and usually has no deleterious consequences. In some cases of leukaemia, however, the white cell count rises so high ($> 100 \times 10^9$/l) that the sheer numbers of white cells reduce the fluidity of blood, making it more viscous. This increased viscosity of blood increases blood pressure causing headaches, confusion, visual disturbances and in the long term congestive heart failure.

A reduction in white cell numbers leaves affected patients at risk of infection. This becomes clinically evident as neutrophil count drops below 1.0×10^9/l, particularly when bacterial infections of the mouth and throat occur. Without adequate numbers of protective neutrophils these infections fail to resolve, causing ulceration. Those with neutrophil counts of less than 0.5×10^9/l are at high risk of death from uncontrolled bacterial infection. Even normally harmless bacteria which are present on the skin pose a serious threat to life for these patients; such patients require careful barrier nursing to minimise the risk of infection.

A severe reduction in lymphocyte numbers compromises the immune response leaving affected patients also at high risk of infection from bacterial, viral and fungal infection. The life-threatening opportunistic infections suffered by AIDS patients are a result of reduction in T-lymphocyte numbers.

Case history 14

James Herron, a 14-year-old boy, was admitted to the local hospital A&E department via his GP, with severe central abdominal pain. James had been vomiting before admission and was slightly pyrexial (temperature 38°C) on admission. Physical examination and symptoms suggested that James was suffering acute appendicitis. The admitting doctor sampled blood for urgent urea and electrolytes and full blood count (FBC).

The following FBC results were telephoned to A&E, 30 minutes later.

Hb 13.1 g/l
PCV 42%
RBC 5.1×10^{12}/l
WBC (total) 15.1×10^{9}/l
Neutrophils 10.8×10^{9}/l
Lymphocytes 2.0×10^{9}/l
Monocytes 0.7×10^{9}/l
Eosinophils 0.2×10^{9}/l
Basophils $<0.1 \times 10^{9}$/l

(1) Are there any abnormalities in these results?
(2) Would you expect abnormalities in FBC results in a patient with acute appendicitis?

Discussion of case history

(1) Yes. There are two abnormal results. James has a slightly raised total white cell count due to an increase in neutrophil numbers (neutrophilia).
(2) Yes. Appendicitis is an acute inflammation of the appendix. Any active inflammatory disease process is likely to result in an increase in neutrophil numbers. Such an increase is found in the vast majority of cases of acute appendicitis and therefore provides further evidence to support the provisional diagnosis made on the basis of physical examination, reported history and symptoms. A slight decrease in lymphocyte numbers is also sometimes a feature of acute appendicitis.

Further reading

Cranfield T. & Bunch C. (1995) Acute leukaemias. *Medicine*: 503–9.

Gawlikowski J. (1992) White cells at war. *Am. J. Nursing* **92**: 45–51.

Moss P. (1995) Chronic leukaemias. *Medicine*: 509–13.

Peterson L. & Hrinkso M. (1993) Benign lymphocytosis and reactive neutrophilia. *Clin. Lab. Med.* **13**: 863–75.

Shapiro M. & Greenfield S. (1987) The complete blood count and leukocyte differential count. *Annals Int. Med.* **106**: 65–74.

Shoentag R. & Cangliarella J. (1992) The nuances of lymphocytopaenia. *Clinics in Lab. Med.* **13**: 923–34.

16 Tests of Haemostasis: Platelet count, prothrombin time (PT), activated partial thromboplastin time (APPT) and thrombin time (TT)

In health, blood loss following tissue injury is minimised by the ability of the blood to coagulate or clot. Normal haemostasis is the name given to the complex process by which blood retains its ability to quickly form a plug at the site of vessel injury, preventing undue blood loss, whilst remaining fluid and free from coagulated blood within undamaged vessels. Disturbance of this fine balance, a feature of many disease processes, can result either in an increased tendency to bleed if the coagulability of blood is less than normal or to form small blood clots within blood vessels (thrombi) reducing blood flow, if coagulability of blood is abnormally increased. The four blood tests described in this chapter are the most commonly used tests in the first-line investigation of patients who are suspected of suffering disease which results in an increased tendency to bleed. Two of the tests, prothrombin time (PT) and activated partial thromboplastin time (APPT), are also used to monitor anticoagulation drug therapy, prescribed for those who are at risk of thrombi formation.

Normal physiology

The sequence of events which leads to the formation of a stable fibrin plug and cessation of bleeding following blood vessel injury is described in Fig. 16.1.

Reduced blood flow to the injured site minimises blood loss. Vessel injury also initiates two vital physiological responses. The first is platelet

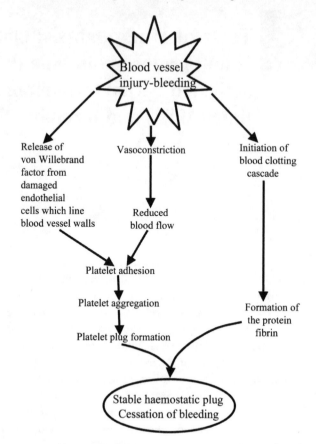

Fig. 16.1 Overview of normal haemostasis.

adhesion and aggregation, with formation of a physical plug of platelets, and the second is initiation of the so-called clotting cascade which results in production of the protein, fibrin. Fibrin strands form around and between the aggregated platelets, stabilising the somewhat fragile platelet plug.

Normal haemostasis is crucially dependent, then, on two factors:

■ adequate numbers of normally functioning platelets, and
■ a normally functioning blood clotting cascade.

In order to understand the defects of haemostasis which are associated with disease and the use of laboratory testing in those diseases, it is necessary to examine these two factors in a little detail.

Platelet production, structure and function

Like the other two formed elements (red cells and white cells), which circulate in blood, platelets (alternative name thrombocytes) are derived from the stem cells of the bone marrow (Fig. 14.1). A proportion of stem cells differentiate by stages within the bone marrow to megakaryocytes. Platelets are produced within the cytoplasm of these cells. Still within the bone marrow, platelets are released from mature megakaryocytes and pass from bone marrow to the blood. Each megakaryocyte produces around 4000 platelets. Platelets have a lifespan of only around 10 days in blood so that constant bone marrow production is necessary.

Having a diameter of between 1 and 2 μm, platelets are far smaller than either red cells or white cells. Like mature red cells, they have no nucleus. The principal function of the platelet is to plug 'holes' in vessel walls caused during injury. The first stage in this process is adhesion of platelets to the wall of the damaged vessel. This adhesion is facilitated in part by a protein called von Willebrand factor, which is released from injured vessel wall cells (endothelial cells). Adhesion proteins present on the surface of passing platelets bind to von Willebrand factor which itself is bound to proteins present on the surface of damaged endothelial cells. Following adhesion, platelets secrete many substances which modulate both the clotting cascade (see below) and further platelet function. Among these are substances (e.g. ADP and thromboxane A_2), which both induce platelets to stick to each other and swell in size. This process, called aggregation, continues until the mass of aggregated swollen platelets is sufficiently large to plug the damaged vessel.

Blood clotting cascade

As platelets are aggregating at the site of vessel injury, fibrin is being produced locally by the blood-clotting cascade. This is a series of reactions in which proteins present in blood plasma, called *factors*, are activated in sequence. Each activated factor promotes activation of the next and so on down the cascade; the final product being fibrin. These reactions are enzymic in nature; in their inactive state factors are proenzymes (i.e. have no enzymic activity). Enzymic action converts proenzymes (unactivated factors) to active enzymes (activated factors). Whilst most factors are proenzymes/enzymes, some are not actually enzymes but substances which are required for enzymic action to occur. Thirteen factors have been identified, numbered by convention in Roman numerals in the order in which they were first discovered (Table 16.1). The once postulated Factor VI is no longer thought to exist.

A simplified account of current understanding of the blood clotting

Table 16.1   Blood clotting factors

Factor	Alternative name(s)	Notes
Factor I	Fibrinogen	Glycoprotein precursor of fibrin synthesised in liver
Factor II	Prothrombin	Proenzyme synthesised in liver
Factor III	Tissue factor, thromboplastin	Protein present in most tissues initiates extrinsic pathway
Factor IV	Calcium	Inorganic ion cofactor
Factor V	Labile factor	Protein, cofactor synthesised in liver
Factor VI	Once proposed but no longer thought to exist	
Factor VII	Proconvertin Stable factor	Proenzyme synthesised in liver
Factor VIII	Antihaemophilic factor	Protein, cofactor
Factor IX	Christmas factor	Proenzyme synthesised in liver
Factor X	Stuart factor	Proenzyme synthesised in liver
Factor XI	Plasma thromboplastin antecedent	Proenzyme
Factor XII	Hagemann factor contact factor	Proenzyme
Factor XIII	Fibrin stabilising factor	Proenzyme

cascade is described in Fig. 16.2. The cascade comprises the intrinsic and extrinsic pathways, which both result in activation of Factor X. The route from activated Factor X to fibrin production is referred to as the common pathway.

The intrinsic pathway is initiated when Factor XII is activated by contact with a structural protein called collagen, exposed as a result of vessel wall injury. Activated Factor XII then activates Factor XI, which in turn activates Factor X. Co factors, Factor VIII (antihaemophilic factor) and Factor IV (calcium), are required for this last reaction.

The extrinsic pathway is initiated by Factor III. This is a substance called thromboplastin, found in most tissues and released to the blood during tissue injury. Factor III activates Factor VII, which in turn activates Factor IX. In the final common pathway, activated Factor X activates Factor II (prothrombin) to the active thrombin, which in turn converts Fibrinogen (Factor I) to fibrin. Factor V is a cofactor required for conversion of prothrombin to thrombin.

Most of the factors of the blood clotting cascade, including Factor I (fibrinogen), Factor II (prothrombin) and Factors V, VII, IX, X, XI and XII

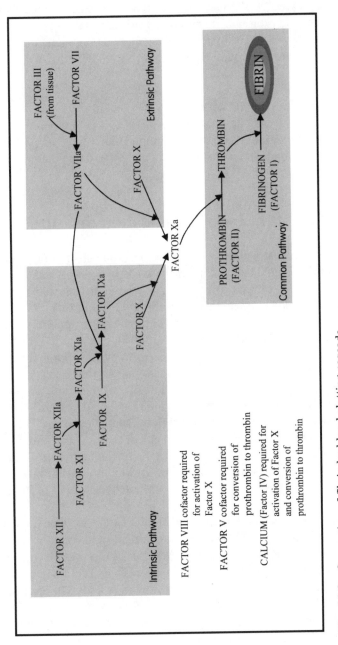

Fig. 16.2   Generation of fibrin by blood clotting cascade.

are synthesised and released to the blood in their inactive form by the liver. The synthesis of Factors II (prothrombin), VII, IX and X is crucially dependent on Vitamin K. The later is derived from two sources, diet and vitamin-K-synthesising bacteria normally present in the gut.

The formation of fibrin by the clotting cascade depends, then, on an adequate concentration of all clotting factors which in turn is dependent on:

- a normally functioning liver
- an adequate dietary source of Vitamin K
- a normal bacterial flora in the gastrointestinal tract
- normal gastrointestinal absorption of dietary and non-dietary vitamin K.

What do tests of blood coagulation measure?

Whilst it is clear that a platelet count is simply a measure of the number of platelets present in blood, it might be less obvious what is being measured by the other three tests considered in this chapter. Pro-thrombin time (PT), activated partial thromboplastin time (APPT) and thrombin time (TT) all test the ability of the blood to generate fibrin by the blood clotting cascade. In essence, they all measure the time taken for a sample of patient's blood plasma to form a fibrin clot in a test tube after addition of a reagent which initiates the clotting cascade. Results are expressed in time (seconds). In the case of the prothrombin test, commercially produced thromboplastin (Factor III) is added to the plasma. This is the clotting factor which initiates the extrinsic pathway. Prothrombin time is thus a test specifically of the extrinsic pathway and common pathways; a deficiency of any factor or factors of these two pathways (i.e. Factors VII, X and V, prothrombin and fibrinogen) will result in an abnormally long time for a fibrin clot to form (i.e. PT will be raised).

In a similar way, by adding only an initiator of the intrinsic pathway to patient's plasma, the APPT tests only the intrinsic and common pathway. In this case, an abnormally prolonged result indicates a deficiency of one or more of those factors required by the intrinsic and common pathways.

Finally, in the thrombin time test, thrombin is added to the patient's plasma. This is a test specifically of the final stages of the common pathway: fibrinogen to fibrin. An abnormally prolonged thrombin test indicates a deficiency of Factor I (fibrinogen).

If PT, APPT and TT are all normal, the blood clotting cascade is working normally.

LABORATORY MEASUREMENT OF PLATELET COUNT, PT, APPT AND TT

A platelet count is one of the tests included in a full blood count. Laboratory measurement and sample requirements for full blood count are discussed in Chapter 14. This section is concerned only with PT, APPT and TT.

PATIENT PREPARATION

No particular patient preparation is necessary.

TIMING OF SAMPLE

Blood for PT, APPT and TT may be sampled at any time. However, the proteins of the clotting cascade are not well preserved in a blood sample and falsely abnormal results can occur if blood is not tested within 4–6 hours of sampling. This period can be extended to 15 hours if sample is stored in a refrigerator at 4°C. Samples more than 15 hours old are not suitable for analysis.

SAMPLE REQUIREMENTS

The tests are performed on plasma, the fluid that remains when all cellular elements are removed from anticoagulated blood. The blood must be collected into a tube containing the anticoagulant sodium citrate (usually a light blue top), which also preserves blood clotting proteins. The volume required (usually 5 ml) is indicated on the bottle; it is important that neither more nor less than the volume indicated is added to the bottle. Gentle inversion to mix blood with the anticoagulant is essential. It is inadvisable to sample blood for these tests via an indwelling catheter, since heparin flushes are often used to keep these lines patent. Falsely abnormal results will be obtained if blood samples are contaminated with heparin.

INTERPRETATION OF RESULTS

APPROXIMATE REFERENCE RANGES

Platelet count	$150–400 \times 10^9/l$
Prothrombin time (PT)	10–14 seconds
Activated partial thromboplastin time (APPT)	30–40 seconds
Thrombin time (TT)	14–16 seconds

'cont.'

'continued'

CRITICAL VALUES

Platelet count	$< 40 \times 10^9/l$ or $> 1000 \times 10^9/l$
Prothrombin time	> 30 seconds
Activated partial thromboplastin time	> 78 seconds

TERMS USED IN INTERPRETATION

Thrombocytes – Alternative name for platelets.
Thrombocytopaenia – Reduced platelet count, i.e. $< 150 \times 10^9/l$
Thrombocytosis – Increased platelet count, i.e. $> 400 \times 10^9/l$

Causes of decreased platelet count

A reduction in platelet numbers, which is more common than an increase, can be caused by either reduced bone marrow production or an increased rate of platelet destruction or consumption. Reduced bone marrow production of platelets, with resulting severe decrease in platelet numbers (may be less than $50 \times 10^9/l$) is a feature of aplastic anaemia, acute leukaemia, cytotoxic drug therapy and radiotherapy. Megaloblastic anaemia, that is, anaemia caused invariably by deficiency of vitamin B_{12} or folate (Chapter 16), is also associated with decreased bone marrow production of platelets, although not usually severe. Secondary spread of primary cancer to the bone marrow can result in reduced platelet production so that a reduced platelet count is sometimes a feature of advanced cancer.

Immune thrombocytopaenic purpura (ITP) is the most common cause of increased platelet destruction. This relatively common disorder, affecting usually young to middle aged women, results from production of autoantibodies against the patient's platelets. The cause of this autoantibody production is not known. In most cases the condition arises in otherwise well women, but it can arise as a secondary complication of some other primary disorder; these include systemic lupus erythematosus (SLE), infection with HIV and chronic lymphatic leukaemia. The antibodies bind to the platelets, resulting in their premature removal and destruction within the reticuloendothelial system. In this condition, platelet lifespan is reduced from a normal 10 days to just a few hours. Bone marrow production cannot keep pace with this rate of destruction and the reduction in platelet numbers is severe, in the range

10–50×10^9/l. A similar disorder may complicate recovery from vaccination and some viral infections (e.g. chicken pox and measles) in childhood.

Increased platelet consumption is a feature of disseminated intravascular coagulation (DIC), a complication of many serious illnesses including severe infections of the blood (septicaemia), malignant disease, severe tissue damage during major surgery or trauma, some obstetric disorders and incompatible blood transfusion. DIC is characterised by abnormal coagulation, and platelet aggregation within blood vessels. The result is depletion of both platelets and clotting factors.

Many commonly used drugs sometimes induce production of antibodies directed at platelets with resulting increased platelet destruction. Drugs which may result in a reduction in platelet numbers include some anti-inflammatories, antibiotics (penicillin, sulphonamide) and some diuretics (frusemide, acetazolamide).

Causes of increased platelet count

A severe increase in platelet numbers is a feature of those malignant disorders of the bone marrow that are characterised by abnormal proliferation of myeloid stem cells. An increase in platelet numbers in these so-called myeloproliferative disorders is due to the fact that it is the myeloid stem cells which normally give rise to platelet-producing megakaryocytes. The myeloproliferative disorders in which an increase in platelet numbers can be expected include chronic myeloid leukaemia (around a third of all cases), polycythaemia vera (around a half of all cases) and essential thrombocythaemia (all cases).

A mild to moderate increase in platelet numbers (usually between 400 and 1000×10^9/l) is a relatively common phenomenon and may be seen in severe stress caused by surgery or trauma, severe infectious illness (e.g. septicaemia), chronic inflammatory conditions (e.g. rheumatoid arthritis), non-haematological malignancy, and following severe blood loss (haemorrhage). Surgical removal of the spleen results in particularly high values.

Consequences of abnormality in platelet numbers

Since platelets are required for normal haemostasis, patients with a reduced platelet count are at increased risk of excessive bleeding.

Spontaneous bleeding occurs if platelet count falls below $50 \times 10^9/l$. Fatal haemorrhage almost inevitably occurs if count falls to $5 \times 10^9/l$. An increased tendency to bleed due to platelet deficiency has several clinical manifestations, including increased menstrual blood loss (menorrhagia), easy or even spontaneous bruising, bleeding gums, nose bleeds (epistaxis), petechial (tiny pinpoint) haemorrhages into the skin giving a red rash-like appearance and purpura. Widespread purple/ brown discoloration of skin (ecchymosis) occurs following massive haemorrhage into tissues.

An increase in platelet numbers carries with it the risk of increased coagulability of blood and resulting thrombosis. In practice this risk of thrombosis is not real until count rises in excess of $1000 \times 10^9/l$.

Causes and consequences of increased PT, APPT and TT

An increase in any of these tests indicates a deficiency of one or more clotting factors. Deficiency may be congenital (i.e. inherited) or, much more commonly, acquired as a result of disease. Haemophilia A, which accounts for around 85% of all known inherited blood clotting defects, is the most common congenital defect of blood clotting. The defect is in the gene which codes for production of Factor VIII (also called anti-haemophilia factor). This is the cofactor required for activation of Factor X by Factor IXa (Fig. 16.2). The result of the genetic defect is a marked deficiency or complete absence of Factor VIII and severely impaired blood clotting. Without Factor VIII replacement therapy, affected patients are at risk of life-threatening haemorrhage. The extrinsic and common pathways are intact in the patient with haemophilia A so that PT and TT are normal. However, APPT (a test of the intrinsic pathway) is abnormally increased. Haemophilia B (Christmas disease) is a less common but equally devastating inherited defect of the clotting cascade in which the deficiency is of Factor IX rather than Factor VIII, and also causes raised APPT.

Since many clotting factors are synthesised in the liver, multiple factor deficiency is a feature of liver disease (acute and chronic hepatitis, cirrhosis, etc). PT, APPT and TT may all be increased in severe liver disease, although a raised TT is less usual. Of the three, PT is the most sensitive marker of liver disease and is routinely used as a test of liver function, both in its detection and to monitor progress.

The production of several factors of both the intrinsic and extrinsic pathway are dependent on vitamin K, so that deficiency of vitamin K is associated with an increase in both PT and APPT. Newborn babies who are often deficient of vitamin K and are therefore at risk of haemorrhage are often given prophylactic vitamin K at the time of birth. In adults vitamin K deficiency usually arises as a result of impaired absorption from the gastrointestinal tract. Diseases which may be associated with poor absorption of vitamin K include those that result in obstruction of the bile tract (e.g. gallstones, cancer of the head of the pancreas) and pancreatitis.

Dietary deficiency of vitamin K may occur in malnourished adults. Antibiotic use can be associated with deficiency because it affects the balance of normal gut flora, and therefore bacterial production of vitamin K. Whatever the cause, vitamin K deficiency is associated with an increase in PT and APPT; TT is normal.

Consumption and resulting deficiency of several clotting factors is a feature of the abnormal coagulation within blood vessels which characterises DIC (see above). PT, APPT and TT are all raised in DIC. The increase in TT is particularly marked.

Clotting factors are not well preserved in stored blood, so those patients who receive massive blood transfusion (i.e. total blood volume replaced) are paradoxically at increased risk of haemorrhage because the blood that is being transfused is relatively deficient of clotting factors. Increased PT, APPT and TT may all be evident in the patient who has received massive blood transfusion.

An increase in any or all of these tests implies a deficiency of clotting factors and therefore an increased tendency to bleed.

Anticoagulation therapy

One of the major uses of the prothombin time (PT) and activated partial thromboplastin time (APPT) tests is to monitor anticoagulation therapy. The anticoagulant drugs warfarin and heparin are widely used in the treatment and prevention of deep vein thrombosis (DVT) and its life-threatening complication, pulmonary (thrombo) embolism. DVT is characterised by formation of thrombi (plugs of coagulated blood and platelets) within veins, usually of the legs. Patients most at risk are those recovering from surgery, particularly of the hip and pelvis, and those who are immobile or obese. Old age and pregnancy also carry an increased risk of DVT. Some people inherit defects of blood coagulation which predispose to DVT.

The aim of anticoagulation therapy is to dissolve existing thrombi and prevent further thrombus formation by artificially reducing the coagulability of blood. Heparin, which is administered intravenously or sub-cutaneously, functions in this regard by inhibiting the action of several activated factors of the extrinsic pathway; it also impairs platelet function. Warfarin is an oral anticoagulant which operates by inhibiting the action of vitamin K in production of vitamin K dependent factors. Of course reducing the coagulability of blood carries with it the risk of increased bleeding, so anticoagulation therapy must be carefully monitored to ensure a maximum level of anticoagulation consistent with minimum risk of excessive bleeding. Heparin is monitored using APPT, and warfarin is monitored using the PT test. In the case of heparin use, dose is adjusted so that APPT is between 1.5 and 2 times the normal value.

Warfarin, prothrombin and INR

As we have seen, when PT is used to investigate a suspected coagulation defect, results are expressed in time (seconds). This is not the case when PT is used to monitor warfarin therapy. Instead, the internationalised normalised ratio (INR) is used. The INR provides a way of expressing PT results to take account of the differing activity of commercially prepared tissue thromboplastin used in the test. This ensures that prothrombin results are more directly comparable and provides a more accurate control of warfarin therapy. The INR is defined as the patient's PT in seconds, divided by the mean of the PT reference range, raised to the power of the international sensitivity index (ISI) of the particular thromboplastin being used:

$$\text{Patient's INR} = \left(\frac{\text{Patient's prothrombin time (seconds)}}{\text{Mean normal prothrombin time (seconds)}} \right)^{\text{ISI}}$$

Warfarin dose is adjusted so that the INR is maintained within a therapeutic range which depends on the precise clinical reason for prescribing warfarin. For most patients the INR must be maintained within the range 2.0–3.0. In some circumstances an increased level of anticoagulation is required in which case the therapeutic INR range is 3.0–4.5. If INR rises above the prescribed range (i.e. 2.0–3.0 or 3.0–4.5), dose must be adjusted downwards. All patients on long-term warfarin therapy should have their INR checked at regular (2- to 3-week) intervals.

Advances in technology have allowed the development of portable analysers for monitoring warfarin therapy. These have been designed to allow monitoring outside the laboratory, in either clinics or primary care centres. Several studies have demonstrated that using these analysers nursing staff can perform the INR test as well as experienced laboratory staff.[1] In some centres, specialist trained nurses are not only performing the test but also interpreting results and adjusting patient dose. At least one study has demonstrated that a nurse specialist anticoagluant service is as good as a haematology-consultant-run service in maintaining therapeutic control among patients receiving warfarin.[2]

Some studies[3,4] have demonstrated the feasibility of patients themselves taking control of their own blood testing and dose management. Just as diabetic patients monitor their own blood glucose and adjust insulin dose accordingly, so too patients can successfully self-manage their long-term anticoagulation therapy, thereby avoiding the inconvenience of frequent hospital appointments.

Case history 15

Amy Waters, now aged 68 years, had to retire 10 years prematurely from her physically demanding work because of rheumatoid arthritis. Two months ago she was given a hip replacement to increase her mobility. Her postoperative recovery was complicated by an infection and on the tenth day following surgery she suddenly became extremely breathless. Understandably panicked, Amy also reported chest pain. During physical examination, the orthopaedic senior house officer noted some swelling of the left calf which Amy described as slightly tender when touched. A diagnosis of pulmonary embolus secondary to deep vein thrombosis in her left leg was eventually made. For the next few days Amy was given a continuous intravenous infusion of heparin and then daily warfarin tablets. Gradually the breathlessness resolved and she was eventually discharged home feeling well, and delighted with her new hip. She was given a prescription to continue her daily dose of warfarin and asked to attend the haematology outpatients' clinic every three weeks for a blood test.

(1) What blood test does Mrs Waters need?
(2) Why does she need this test?
(3) How long will she have to continue to attend outpatients for this test?

Discussion of case history

(1) The blood test required is prothrombin time (PT).
(2) Mrs Waters is receiving long-term anticoagulation therapy in the

form of warfarin tablets to prevent recurrence of the deep vein thrombosis (DVT) she suffered during postoperative recovery. This drug decreases the tendency of the blood to coagulate by inhibiting the production of several clotting factors (proteins) required for blood coagulation; in lay terms, it 'thins the blood'. The drug carries with it the risk of increased bleeding (haemorrhage) and so must be carefully monitored to ensure that the dose given continues to give the maximum protection against thrombus formation consistent with minimum risk of haemorrhage.

(3)   Mrs Waters must continue to have her prothrombin time checked at regular intervals for the duration of time she is receiving warfarin. This may be for up to six months, after which time it may be considered not necessary. If she has a recurrence of DVT, then warfarin and regular testing would be resumed, most likely for a much longer period.

References
(1)   Hobbs F.D., Fitzmaurice D., Murray E. *et al.* (1999) Is the internal normalised ratio (INR) reliable? A trial of comparative measurement in hospital laboratory and primary care settings. *J. Clin. Pathol.* **52**: 494–7.
(2)   Taylor F.C., Gaminara E., Cohen H. *et al.* (1997) Evaluation of a nurse specialist anticoagulant service. *Clin. Lab. Haem.* **19**: 267–72.
(3)   Ansell J., Patel N., Ostrovsky D. *et al.* (1995) Long term patient self management of oral anticoagulation. *Arch. Intern. Med.* **155**: 2185–89.
(4)   Sawacki P. (1999) A structured teaching and self-management program for patients receiving oral anticoagulation. A randomised controlled trial. *JAMA* **281**: 145–50.

Further reading
Griesshammer M., Bangerter M. & Sauer T. (1999) Aetiology and clinical significance of thrombocytosis: analysis of 732 patients with an elevated platelet count. *J. Int. Med.* **245**: 295–300.
Hickey A. (1994) Catching deep vein thrombosis in time. *Nursing* **94** October: 34–40.
Hoyer L. (1994) Haemophilia A. *New Engl. J. Med.* **330**: 38–46.
Tritshler I. (1994) Anticoagulation therapy. *Nursing Standard* **8**: 54–55.

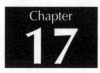
Laboratory Investigation of Anaemia: Serum iron, total iron binding capacity, serum ferritin, serum B_{12} and folate

The means by which full blood count (FBC) results identify those patients who are anaemic was discussed in Chapter 14. It was emphasised that anaemia is not a disease but rather a symptom of disease with many possible causes. Successful treatment of anaemia depends crucially on identifying its cause. It will be remembered that tests included in the full blood count (most notably the MCV) suggest possible likely causes of anaemia, but further testing is necessary. The principal use of the five tests described in this chapter is to confirm the cause of anaemia. Deficiency of iron is the most common cause of anaemia worldwide, affecting an estimated 500 million.[1] Measurement of the concentration of serum iron, total iron binding capacity (TIBC) and serum ferritin concentration together provide a means of making the diagnosis of iron deficiency anaemia. Similarly measurement of the concentration of vitamin B_{12} and folate in serum or plasma and folate in red cells provides a means of identifying those patients who are suffering so-called megaloblastic anaemia which is caused by a deficiency of these vitamins. As we shall see, anaemia is not the only condition in which abnormalities in results of these five tests can be expected.

Normal physiology

Function of iron and iron metabolism

The oxygen carrying capability of haemoglobin contained within red cells is dependent on the presence of iron in the haem part of haemoglobin (Fig. 14.3). Oxygen forms a reversible weak link with the single atom of iron in the haem molecule. Iron is thus essential for haemoglobin production and function. The muscle protein myoglobin and the function of some enzymes are also dependent on iron, although compared with the role of iron in haemoglobin production and function these are of much less clinical significance.

Around 70% of the approximately 4–5 g of iron present in the body is contained in the haemoglobin in circulating red cells (Fig. 17.1). Most of the rest is stored in tissues (principally the liver but also the spleen and bone marrow). In these storage 'compartments' iron is contained within the proteins ferritin and haemosiderin. Some ferritin is present in the plasma part of blood, and the concentration of ferritin in plasma is a reliable indicator of the body's total iron tissue stores. Just 3 to 4 mg (i.e. 0.1% of total body iron) circulates in the liquid (plasma) part of blood; this is bound to the transport protein transferrin. It is the concentration of this transferrin-bound fraction of total body iron which is measured in the serum iron test.

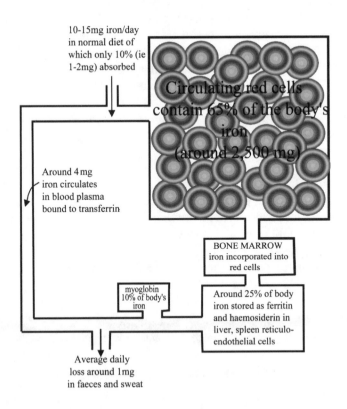

Fig. 17.1 Daily intake and loss of iron and distribution of iron in the body; circulating red cells contain 65% of the body's iron (approximately 2500 mg).

Iron is well conserved by the body. When red cells die at the end of their 120-day lifespan, iron is returned to the body stores for bone marrow production of new red cells. Since iron is protein bound and therefore cannot be filtered out of blood at the glomerulus, very little iron is excreted in urine; the only significant loss is that contained in surface epithelial cells constantly shed from the skin surface. Just 1 mg/day is lost from the body. Since most of the body's iron is contained within red cells, blood loss represents a potential route for significant iron deple-tion. For example, normal menstruation is associated with a loss of around 15 mg of iron every month. When this is taken into account, healthy menstruating women lose on average 1.5–2 mg of iron a day. To replace these minimal losses and maintain normal iron stores, at least 1 mg of iron in the case of healthy children, males and non-menstruating females and up to double this in the case of menstruating females must be absorbed every day from the diet. In fact a normal well balanced diet contains approximately 10 to 15 mg of iron per day. The principal sources of dietary iron are meat (particularly red meat) and fish, green-leafed vegetables and breakfast cereals. Vitamin C increases the availability for absorption of the iron present in vegetables and cereals. Absorption of dietary iron occurs in the upper small intestine. Just 10% of available dietary iron is normally absorbed, sufficient to replace daily loss. It is vital for good health that iron stores remain replete but are not over-loaded with iron. Too much iron can be at least as damaging to health as too little iron. Since there is no control of the iron lost from the body, control of iron body stores depends crucially upon the control mechanisms of absorption of dietary iron. Absorption of available diet-ary iron is adjusted to meet the body's requirements and increased if:

- iron stores are depleted, and/or
- anaemia (whatever its cause) is present.

Since anaemia, whatever its cause, increases iron absorption, dangerous iron overload may occur if anaemic patients who are not iron deficient are given iron supplements.

Function and metabolism of vitamin B_{12} and folate

Vitamins are a group of organic substances of widely differing chemical structure which are essential, albeit in tiny amounts, for life. They cannot be synthesised by the human body and our only source is the food we eat. Most vitamins of the B group, which includes both B_{12} (alternative name cobalamin) and folate (alternative name folic acid), function as essential coenzymes or cofactors in the enzymic reactions of cellular metabolism. Specifically B_{12} and folate are both required for the action of key enzymes in the synthesis of deoxyribonucleic acid (DNA) during cell division. Tissues characterised by rapid cell turnover and consequent unremitting cell division are particularly dependent on intact DNA synthesis and therefore vitamins B_{12} and folate. Bone marrow is one such tissue; blood cell production by the bone marrow continues minute by minute throughout life and an adequate supply of B_{12} and folate is essential for the continuing normal production of blood cells. Although essential for several other cellular enzyme reactions, the role of B_{12} and folate in the cell division required for normal production of blood cells is the one which is of prime clinical significance.

Both B_{12} and folate are synthesised in nature by bacteria and we obtain them by eating animal and plant foods that are naturally contaminated with these bacteria. The principal dietary source of vitamin B_{12} is meat (animal liver is a particularly rich source), fish and dairy products. Vegetables do not contain B_{12}. Folic acid is present in green leafy vegetables; liver is a rich source. Most breakfast cereals are fortified with both B_{12} and folate. The minimum daily requirement for B_{12} is 1–2 mg and for folate 150 µg. A normal healthy diet provides well in excess of the minimum requirement of B_{12} but only just twice the amount of folate required.

Absorption of B_{12} (Fig. 17.2)

The acid medium of the stomach is important for release of B_{12} from foods prior to absorption from the gastrointestinal tract. B_{12} is absorbed at the ileum, but for this to occur the vitamin must first be bound to so-called intrinsic factor, a peptide produced by the gastric parietal cells of the stomach. Absorbed B_{12} is transported in blood to bone marrow and other cells, bound to the transport protein transcobalamin.

Normal production of red cells in the bone marrow is dependent, then, on:

■ a healthy diet containing sufficient B_{12}
■ production of acid and intrinsic factor by the stomach
■ normal absorption at the ileum (i.e. functioning gastrointestinal tract) and
■ adequate production of transcobalamin.

The body has considerable capacity to store large reserves of vitamin B_{12} in the liver, sufficient in fact to remain in normal health for several years on an entirely B_{12}-free diet.

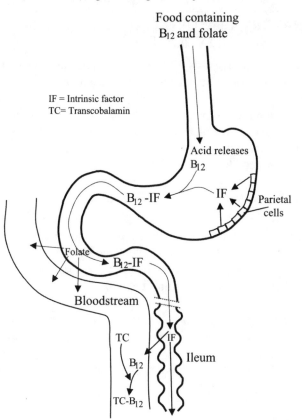

Fig. 17.2 Absorption of vitamin B_{12} and folate.

Absorption of folate

Absorption of folate is less complex. It is absorbed at the upper small intestine and is transported in blood to bone marrow and other folate-requiring tissues either in its free form or bound to albumin.

Normal blood cell production is dependent on:

- a diet containing adequate folate
- a normally functioning small intestine for absorption of folate.

Like B_{12}, folate is stored principally in the liver. However, folate stores are sufficient to last only a few months on a folate-free diet.

LABORATORY MEASUREMENT OF IRON, TIBC, FERRITIN, B_{12} AND FOLATE

With few exceptions the tests described in this chapter should be reserved for those patients in whom anaemia has been demonstrated by FBC (Chapter 14). The results of mean cell volume (MCV) indicate which of these tests are most appropriate. A reduced MCV indicates possible iron deficiency anaemia, in which case serum iron, total iron binding capacity and serum ferritin are appropriate. If MCV is raised, then B_{12} and folate should be measured first.

WHAT IS BEING MEASURED

Serum/plasma iron. This is the concentration of the small proportion of total body iron which circulates in the plasma part of blood; it does not include the iron contained in red cells or that contained in ferritin.

Total iron binding capacity (TIBC). This is a test performed on plasma or serum and is essentially a measure of plasma transferrin concentration. Transferrin is the protein to which iron in plasma is bound.

Serum ferritin. The concentration of ferritin in serum. Ferritin is a protein in which iron is stored in tissues. The concentration of ferritin in serum reflects total iron stores.

Serum B_{12} and Folate. The concentration of vitamin B_{12} and folate in serum. A low result indicates deficiency.

Red cell folate. The concentration of folate in red cells. A low result indicates deficiency.

PATIENT PREPARATION

No particular patient preparation is necessary.

TIMING OF SAMPLE

No particular timing is required. It is best practice to collect blood at a time to coincide with routine transport to the laboratory.

SAMPLE REQUIREMENTS

Around 5 ml of venous blood is sufficient for iron, TIBC and ferritin. Most commonly serum is used, in which case blood should be collected into a plain tube containing no anticoagulant. Blood for red cell folate must be collected into a tube containing the anticoagulant EDTA (lavender-coloured top). A further 5 ml of venous blood is required for serum B_{12} and folate (collected into a plain tube containing no additives).

'cont.'

'continued'

INTERPRETATION OF RESULTS

APPROXIMATE REFERENCE RANGE

Serum Iron	10–30 µmol/l
Serum TIBC	40–75 µmol/l
Serum ferritin	10–300 µg/l
Serum B$_{12}$	Of the order 150–1000 ng/l but values vary – consult local laboratory
Red cell folate	Of the order 150–700 µg/l but values vary – consult local laboratory

Conditions associated with abnormal results of serum iron, TIBC and ferritin

These are

- iron deficiency anaemia
- chronic infection, inflammation
- iron overload.

Iron deficiency anaemia

Causes

Iron deficiency is caused by either:

- insufficient iron in the diet
- poor absorption of iron due to gastrointestinal disease
- increased loss of iron (in blood) from the body
- increased demand for iron (e.g. during pregnancy or periods of growth).

It is unusual for poor diet to be the sole cause of iron deficiency in developed countries, although a diet relatively deficient of iron (e.g. a high proportion of 'junk food') may be a contributory factor in some cases. Poor nutrition is, however, a major cause of iron deficiency in some areas of the developing world. Gastrointestinal diseases in which defective absorption of iron can predipose and even cause iron deficiency include coeliac disease and tropical sprue, but these are relatively rare causes of iron deficiency.

Since red cells contain 70% of the body's iron, blood loss is a significant potential cause of iron deficiency. So long as iron tissue stores are replete, a single acute episode of even severe blood loss will not cause iron deficiency. However, chronic blood loss, that is, the continuous or regular loss of small amounts of blood over a prolonged period, will slowly exhaust iron stores. Chronic blood loss is the most common cause of iron deficiency anaemia in adults. For pre-menopausal women, excessive menstrual blood loss (menorrhagia) is a frequent cause of iron deficiency. Chronic bleeding into the gastrointestinal tract is a feature of many quite common diseases including ulcerative colitis, duodenal and gastric ulcer, liver failure (oesophageal varices), and cancer of the stomach, colon or rectum. Long-term use of non-steroidal anti-inflammatory drugs such as aspirin is associated with an increased risk of chronic blood loss via the stomach wall. In most cases of gastrointestinal bleeding, blood is lost imperceptibly to the patient, in faeces.

Increased physiological demand for iron for the growing foetus is the usual cause of the iron deficiency that can occur during pregnancy.

In all cases of iron deficiency anaemia, a cause should be sought; it may be a presenting symptom of serious underlying gastrointestinal or gynaecological disease.

Symptoms

There are no early symptoms of iron deficiency, and symptoms of anaemia appear only after iron stores are depleted. In addition to the general symptoms of anaemia listed on p. 216, patients with iron deficiency anaemia may exhibit some other specific symptoms which include:

■ glossitis (inflammation of the tongue)
■ angular cheilosis (ulceration of lips at the corners of the mouth)
■ changes to nails (unusually brittle; may become ridged or spoon shaped (koilonychia).

Blood test results

Ferritin concentration reflects iron stores so a reduction in serum ferritin is evident before symptoms develop, during the period of progressive iron store depletion. By the time that iron stores are totally depleted, when signs and symptoms of iron deficiency occur, serum ferritin concentration is extremely low or undetectable. Serum iron is usually reduced, but may remain at the low end of the reference range. Serum total iron binding capacity is always raised.

Typical blood results in iron deficiency anaemia are:

- serum iron usually reduced, in the range 5–10 μmol/l (may be at the low end of the reference range)
- serum TIBC raised (i.e. greater than 75 μmol/l)
- serum ferritin greatly reduced (usually undetectable, i.e. < 5 μg/l).

Chronic inflammation and infection

As outlined in Chapter 14, many patients with chronic infectious or inflammatory disease may become mildly to moderately anaemic (it is unusual for Hb to fall lower than 9 g/dl in such cases). Although the anaemia of chronic disease is not the result of iron deficiency (iron stores are not depleted), it is associated with poorly understood abnormalities in iron metabolism. These abnormalities are reflected in blood test results. Serum iron is usually reduced as it is in iron deficiency anaemia. However, in contrast to iron deficiency anaemia, serum TIBC is reduced and serum ferritin is either normal or in some cases increased. Since a deficiency of iron is not the problem, iron supplements are of no use to these patients. Indeed such treatment may be harmful by putting them at risk of iron overload. Instead treatment is directed at the underlying condition; as this resolves, anaemia disappears.

To summarise, patients with chronic infections (e.g. TB, bacterial endocarditis, pneumonia, etc.) and chronic inflammation (e.g. rheumatoid arthritis, SLE, Crohn's disease, etc.) as well as some patients with malignant disease may be anaemic. The severity of anaemia reflects the severity of the underlying disorder. This anaemia is associated with:

- reduced serum iron concentration
- reduced serum TIBC
- normal or raised serum ferritin concentration.

Iron overload

In the physiological state all iron is bound to a protein (haemoglobin in red cells, ferritin in storage compartments and transferrin in blood plasma). In this state it is non-toxic. However, free (unbound) iron is toxic. There is a finite amount of each of the 'protective' proteins and once they are saturated with iron, any additional iron in cells exists in its toxic free (unbound to protein) state. Free iron is toxic because it promotes production of highly reactive free radicals which disrupt normal cell structure and function. Unchecked this can lead to tissue damage. Tissues affected in disease caused by chronic iron overload include:

Pancreas – fibrosis of pancreas leading to diabetes
Liver – cirrhosis and eventual liver failure, liver cancer
Heart – arrhythmias, heart failure
Gonads – impotence
Joints – severe joint pain (similar to arthritis)

Causes

Hereditary haemachromatosis. Those with this genetically determined disease absorb increased amounts of available iron in diet, 3–4 mg per day instead of the normal 1–2 mg. There is no physiological means of increasing iron excretion so iron accumulates at the rate of 0.5–1.0 g per year. In late middle age when the first clinical effects of iron overload occur, total body iron may be in the range 20–40 g rather than the normal 4–5 g. The condition was once thought to be rare but renewed interest in recent years, including the discovery of the precise genetic defect, has revealed that the condition is probably underdiagnosed. Around 1 in 10 of us carry a single copy of the defective gene (it is the most common inherited genetic defect). Only inheritance of the defective gene from both parents (i.e. two copies of the defective gene) results in the most severe form of haemachromatosis which leads to diabetes, cirrhosis, etc.

Other causes of iron overload include repeated blood transfusion and inappropriate iron therapy. One unit of blood contains around 250 mg of iron in red cells, 100 times the daily requirement. Patients whose treatment includes repeated blood transfusion over a prolonged period (e.g. those suffering thalassaemia and sickle cell anaemia) are particularly at risk of iron overload.

Anaemic patients who are not in fact iron deficient may be given iron supplements inappropriately. Since anaemia, whatever the cause, increases iron absorption, such patients are also at risk of iron overload.

Blood test results

The blood test results of those with iron overload are, as might be expected, the opposite of those associated with iron deficiency. No matter what the cause, iron overload is associated with:

- raised serum iron
- reduced serum TIBC
- raised serum ferritin.

Conditions associated with reduced vitamin B_{12} and folate

Megaloblastic anaemia

Megaloblastic anaemia is a term applied to all those anaemias in which, due to impaired DNA synthesis, there is abnormal development of blood cells in the bone marrow. Impaired DNA synthesis results in production of large (mega) immature (blast) red cells, many of which do not develop to maturity and die within the bone marrow. There is thus a marked reduction in the number of circulating red cells, hence the anaemia. Those red cells that do survive and appear in peripheral blood are larger than normal, often characteristically oval in shape. Large red cells in peripheral blood are called macrocytes, so the term macrocytic anaemia is sometimes used as an alternative name for megaloblastic anaemia, although the terms are not strictly speaking synonymous. The effect of impaired DNA synthesis is not confined to red cells; numbers of both white cells and platelets may be reduced in those with severe megaloblastic anaemia. With a few, very rare exceptions, the cause of the impaired DNA synthesis which leads to megaloblastic anaemia is either vitamin B_{12} or folate deficiency.

Causes of vitamin B_{12} and/or folate deficiency

These are:

- dietary deficiency
- failure to absorb B_{12} due to inadequate production of intrinsic factor
- failure to absorb either B_{12} or folate due to gastrointestinal disease
- increased demand for B_{12} and folate during pregnancy.

Dietary deficiency of B_{12} is rare except among strict vegetarians (vegans) who eat no dairy products. Dietary deficiency of folate is more common; in fact it is the most common cause of folate deficiency. Folate in foods can be destroyed by cooking and the normal dietary intake is close to the minimum required. Dietary deficiency of folate is quite common among chronic alcoholics. This, combined with the effects of alcohol on folate metabolism, render this group particularly susceptible to folate deficiency. Old people living alone often have a diet relatively deficient in folate and must be considered at risk.

The most common cause of vitamin B_{12} deficiency is failure to absorb the vitamin due to lack of intrinsic factor. This specific type of megaloblastic anaemia is known as pernicious anaemia. Those with pernicious anaemia (most often late middle aged and elderly women) are unable to produce intrinsic factor because of damage (autoimmune in nature) to the cells of the stomach, where intrinsic factor is produced. The condition tends to run in families and is often associated with other autoimmune disease (e.g. thyroid disease and Addison's disease). Absorption of folate is not affected in pernicious anaemia. Patients with pernicious anaemia must be given B_{12} by injection, as that given by the oral route cannot be absorbed.

Partial and total gastrectomy can of course also result in reduced production of intrinsic factor.

Various gastrointestinal diseases associated with inflammatory or other damage to the areas where B_{12} and folate are normally absorbed can result in poor absorption and eventually vitamin deficiency. These include Crohn's disease, coeliac disease and tropical sprue. Surgical removal of areas of the gastrointestinal tract (e.g. jejunal or ileal resection) can lead to either B_{12} or folate deficiency. Patients receiving such surgery may be given regular injections of B_{12} and folate to prevent anaemia developing.

Symptoms of megaloblastic anaemia

Whether it be caused by dietary deficiency or poor absorprtion of B_{12} or folate, the resulting symptoms include:

- generalised symptoms of all anaemias (p. 216), plus
- mild jaundice
- glossitis (inflamed tongue)
- angular cheilosis (sores at the corner of the mouth).

Patients with B_{12} deficiency but only extremely rarely those with folate deficiency may also suffer neuropathy. Neurological symptoms include:

- paraesthesia (abnormal sensation, e.g. tingling in fingers and toes)
- gait ataxia resulting in difficulty in walking
- increased irritability
- memory loss
- rarely personality changes and obvious psychiatric problems.

The neurological symptoms of B_{12} deficiency may be present without any signs or symptoms of anaemia.

Blood test results

Serum B_{12} is usually reduced in pernicious anaemia and all other cases of megaloblastic anaemia and neuropathy caused by deficency of B_{12}. In some cases the serum level remains at the low end of the reference range, causing some diagnostic difficulty. Serum folate is usually normal but may be slightly raised. Red cell folate by contrast is either normal or low in cases of B_{12} deficiency.

In cases of megaloblastic anaemia caused solely by folate deficiency, serum B_{12} is normal, but as might be expected both serum and red cell folate are reduced. Red cell folate is considered a more reliable test of folate status because serum folate may be low in some illnesses (e.g. severe liver and kidney disease) despite normal folate status.

Case history 16

Jane Baker is a 32-year-old solicitor who is being investigated by her GP because of increasing tiredness of several months' duration (Case history 13). The results of an FBC demonstrate that she is anaemic and that the anaemia may be due to iron deficiency. Jane's GP takes a further sample of blood for iron studies and sends it to the laboratory. Four days later the following report is received at the GP's surgery:

Serum Iron	$9\,\mu mol/l$
Serum TIBC	$113\,\mu mol/l$
Serum Ferritin	$<5\,\mu g/l$

(1) Are the results normal?
(2) What is ferritin, and why is its concentration in blood serum measured in patients who are suspected of being iron deficient?
(3) What do the results indicate?
(4) Why might further investigation be necessary?

Discussion of case history

(1) No. Serum iron and ferritin are abnormally reduced and serum TIBC is raised.

(2) Ferritin is a water-soluble molecule composed of an outer protein shell enclosing an iron core. Each molecule contains 4000–5000 atoms of iron and this iron constitutes around 20% of its weight. Most of the body's ferritin is in tissue cells (liver, spleen, bone marrow) where its function is iron storage. A small fraction circulates in blood plasma where its concentration reflects total iron body stores. A reduction in serum ferritin as iron stores become progressively depleted is the first objective evidence of iron deficiency. A reduction in serum ferritin occurs before iron is sufficiently depleted to affect haemoglobin production and therefore occurs before symptoms of iron deficiency anaemia occur. Serum ferritin remains low or undetectable until iron stores are replete.

(3) Reduced serum iron and increased serum TIBC in association with undetectable levels of ferritin in blood serum are the typical pattern of results expected in iron deficiency. There can be no doubt that Mrs Bishop is iron deficient and requires iron supplements.

(4) A diagnosis of iron deficiency should be followed by investigation of its cause. Why has Mrs Bishop become iron deficient? In a woman of reproductive age like Mrs Bishop, the most common cause is menorrhagia (increased loss of iron due to excessive menstrual bleeding) but this is by no means the only cause of iron deficiency.

References

(1) DeMaeyer E. & Adiels-Tegman M. (1985) The prevalence of anaemia in the world. *World Health Stat. Q.* **38**: 302.

Further reading

Burke W., Thomson E., Khoury M. *et al.* (1998) Hereditary haemochromatosis. *JAMA* **280**: 172–8.

Guyatt G. *et al.* (1992) Laboratory diagnosis of iron deficiency: an overview. *J. Gen. Intern. Med.* **7**: 145–55.

Hoffbrand A. & Pettit J. (1993) Megaloblastic anaemias and other macrocytic anaemias. In *Essential Haematology*, pp. 53–73. Blackwell Science, Oxford.

Kent S., Weinberg, E. & Stuart-Macadam P. (1994) The etiology of the anaemia of chronic disease and infection. *J. Clin. Epidemiol.* **47**: 22–33.

Lucas C., Logan E. & Logan, R. (1996) Audit of the investigation and outcome of iron deficiency anaemia in one health district. *J. Roy. Coll. Physicians London* **30**: 33–5.

Pheeko K., Williams Y., Shey S. *et al.* (1997) Folate assays: serum or red cells? *J. Roy. Coll. Physicians London* **31**: 291–5.

18 Erythrocyte Sedimentation Rate (ESR)

The ESR test is one of the oldest and simplest tests still performed in clinical laboratories, and is based on a very visible phenomenon familiar to all those who have collected blood. If a blood sample collected into a tube containing an anticoagulant is left undisturbed, the red cells (erythrocytes) gradually fall or sediment to the bottom of the container, leaving the clear, straw-coloured plasma fluid above. At the end of the last century, physicians investigated this phenomenon and discovered that the red cells in a blood sample taken from healthy volunteers sediment slowly, but that the cells in a blood sample taken from those suffering a range of diseases sediment much faster. From these observations the erythrocyte sedimentation rate (ESR) test was born.

Despite minor modifications, measurement of ESR has remained essentially unchanged since its introduction nearly 80 years ago. A narrow-bore tube of standard length is filled with anticoagulated blood and placed in a vertical position. The tube is left undisturbed for a defined time (usually 1 hour). During that time the erythrocytes sediment leaving an increasingly large column of clear plasma above. After 1 hour has elapsed, the distance from the top of the tube to the interface between clear plasma and red cells is measured. This distance is the ESR expressed in mm/hour. In other words the ESR is the distance in millimetres which red cells fall in one hour.

Normal physiology: what affects red cell sedimentation?

Although apparently simple, the rate at which erythrocytes sediment is a complex phenomenon which even now is not entirely understood. Clearly red cells fall because they have a greater density than the plasma in which they are suspended. Red cells have a net negative charge due to the presence of membrane-bound proteins on their surface. This electrostatic force tends to make red cells repel each other. This is the situation in health; red cells are for the most part separate and fall individually. If, for any reason, this tendency of cells to repel each other is overcome, then they aggregate together to form 'rouleaux' (red cells stacked together rather like a pile of coins). Since an aggregation of red cells has greater density than single cells, aggregated cells sediment faster. It is this abnormal tendency for cells to overcome their natural repulsion for each other and aggregate which explains the increased ESR found in disease. The crucial question is: what makes red cells aggregate? Part of the answer lies in the plasma in which red cells are suspended. Certain proteins in plasma, most notably fibrinogen and immunoglobulins, act as molecular bridges between red cells. When present in high concentration, the effect of these proteins is a marked increase in the aggregation of red cells. As will become clear, it is disease states which are associated with abnormally high concentration of these proteins in plasma which most commonly result in a raised ESR.

In addition to the composition of the plasma in which they are suspended the rate at which red cells sediment is also affected by both numbers and shape of red cells themselves. So, for example, a significant decrease in the number of red cells as occurs in some forms of anaemia is associated with an increase in ESR whilst an abnormal increase in red cell numbers (polycythaemia) reduces ESR. The shape of red cells of those suffering sickle cell anaemia is abnormal; these so-called sickle cells sediment slower than normal red cells.

LABORATORY MEASUREMENT OF ESR

PATIENT PREPARATION

No particular patient preparation is necessary.

SAMPLE TIMING

Depending on the method being used a delay of more than a few hours in processing samples can affect results. Samples stored overnight may be unsuitable for analysis. It is therefore best practice to take samples at a time which coincides with routine transport to the laboratory.

'cont.'

'continued'

SAMPLE REQUIREMENTS

A sample of venous blood is required. Most laboratories provide a specific tube for ESR only (black top) which contains the anticoagulant sodium citrate. The required volume is printed on the label. It is essential that anticoagulant in the bottle be mixed with the blood by gentle inversion.

INTERPRETATION OF RESULTS

APPROXIMATE REFERENCE RANGE

Males	1–10 mm/hour
Females	5–20 mm/hour

Causes of a raised ESR

General considerations

ESR increases gradually with age, rising at the rate of around 0.8 mm/hour every 5 years. From the fourth month of pregnancy ESR usually rises to a peak of 40 to 50 mm/hour, returning to normal after parturition. ESR is one of the least specific of all laboratory tests. In other words, like a raised temperature or pulse, a raised ESR occurs in many different sorts of illness. The changes in plasma proteins which give rise to increased red cell aggregation and raised ESR are a feature of any illness associated with significant tissue injury, inflammation, infection or malignancy. Unfortunately, from a diagnostic point of view in most of these disease states it is possible for the ESR to be normal. Furthermore it is clear that ESR is occasionally raised in normal healthy individuals. Despite these awkward anomalies which tend to confound interpretation of an ESR result, the ESR continues to be used in clinical practice. In general the higher the ESR the greater is the likelihood of a significant inflammatory, infectious or malignant disease.

Inflammatory disease

The inflammatory response to tissue injury results in an abnormal increase in the synthesis of plasma proteins including fibrinogen which tend to promote rouleaux formation and raise ESR. Potentially, then, any disease with an acute or chronic inflammatory component may be associated with an increase in ESR. In clinical practice the test is used as supportive evidence of inflammation in the diagnosis of disease associated with chronic inflammation such as rheumatoid arthritis, Crohn's disease and ulcerative colitis. It is frequently used to monitor disease activity in these conditions. A rising ESR in a patient with a known chronic inflammatory condition such as rheumatoid arthritis implies that disease activity is continuing or increasing and therefore not responding to current therapy. Conversely a falling ESR indicates reduced inflammation and therefore response to therapy.

Although the ESR has a limited diagnostic role for most diseases with an inflammatory component, because there are other more reliable and specific tests available there are two related conditions in which ESR is the only investigation which is abnormal. These are temporal arteritis (sometimes called giant cell artertitis) and polymyalgia rheumatica. The first is an inflammatory disease of arteries, usually in the head and neck. The condition is relatively common in the elderly causing general feeling of malaise and tiredness along with severe headaches; sudden blindness may occur if the optic artery is affected. The second is an inflammatory condition affecting muscles causing severe muscle pain and stiffness, particularly after resting. The two conditions often appear together in the same patient and both are associated with very high ESR, usually greater than 75 mm/hour and often higher. The ESR gradually returns to normal during treatment with steroids and the test is used to monitor response to therapy. These are the only conditions in which diagnosis depends on the ESR test.

Infectious disease

All infections are associated with an immune response with increased production of immunoglobulins (antibodies). These immunoglobulins increase the tendency to rouleaux formation, so all infections may be associated with an increased ESR. In general, bacterial infections tend to result in an increased ESR more frequently than those caused by viruses. Particularly high ESR (i.e. greater than 75 mm/hour) is most frequently found in those suffering chronic infections, e.g. TB and subacute bacterial endocarditis (infection of valves of the heart), but any bacterial infection, if sufficiently severe, may be associated with very high ESR. The ESR may be used to monitor the effectiveness of therapy among those suffering chronic infection and for early detection of postoperative infection following surgery. Orthopaedic surgery is associated with high risk of postoperative infection, so it is in this setting that this particular use of the ESR test has been exploited in some centres.

Malignant disease

Many patients suffering cancer of all types have a raised ESR. However, since a significant proportion of cancer patients do not have a raised ESR, the test has no place in cancer diagnosis. In the absence of infectious or inflammatory disease a significant increase in ESR (i.e. greater than 75 mm/hour) might suggest that further tests to detect cancer are warranted. Some authorities believe that a particularly raised ESR (i.e. greater than 100 mm/hour) in a patient with cancer is reliable evidence of tumour spread beyond the primary site (metastasis).

The only widely accepted use of the ESR so far as malignant disease is concerned is in the diagnosis of multiple myeloma, a malignant disease of bone marrow in which uncontrolled proliferation of plasma cells within the bone marrow causes bone pain and bone destruction. These malignant plasma cells synthesise huge quantities of abnormal immunoglobulin at the expense of normal immunoglobulin (antibody) production. Since immunoglobulin is one of those proteins which increase rouleaux formation and thereby the ESR, multiple myeloma is almost always associated with an increase in ESR (often greater than 100 mm/hour). So consistent is this finding that a raised ESR is among the criteria required for diagnosis of multiple myeloma.

Finally ESR is almost always raised in patients with Hodgkin's disease (malignant tumour of lymph nodes). The ESR is not used to make a diagnosis but is frequently used to monitor disease progress and therapeutic effectiveness.

Other common causes of raised ESR

Myocardial infarction (heart attack) involves tissue injury to heart muscle (myocardium). The consequent inflammatory response to this injury includes increased synthesis of plasma proteins (fibrinogen) which causes increased red cell aggregation and therefore raised ESR. Thus myocardial infarction is a common cause of raised ESR. Typically ESR rises after an infarct, peaking 1 week later. A gradual return to normal is usual over the next few weeks. A raised ESR is also common in patients suffering renal disease and those anaemic patients whose red cells are significantly depleted.

Causes of a reduced ESR

A reduced ESR is far less common than an increased ESR and is actually of little clinical significance. An abnormally high red cell count (polycythaemia) is the most frequent cause. Rare causes include sickle cell anaemia and hereditary spherocytosis; both conditions are associated with abnormally shaped red cells which slow the rate at which they sediment.

Alternative tests to ESR

In recent years there has been increasing interest in alternative tests to the ESR and some laboratories offer instead either plasma viscosity or plasma C-reactive protein (CRP) measurement. Viscosity is a measure of the fluidity of a liquid; a 'thick' liquid like oil has high viscosity compared with that of a 'thin' liquid like water. An abnormal increase in the viscosity of plasma results from an increase in the concentration in plasma of the same proteins which give rise to a raised ESR.

C-reactive protein is present in low concentration in the plasma of healthy individuals. It is one of the proteins which rises during inflammation, infection and malignancy. Broadly speaking, then, both plasma viscosity and plasma CRP are raised in the same pathological conditions which give rise to a raised ESR. The two newer tests, unlike ESR, are unaffected by abnormalities in red cell numbers so remain normal in anaemia and polycythaemia.

Case history 17

Alex Manson was a cheerful healthy 5-year-old until he first became acutely ill just over six months ago. His first complaint was a sore throat. Over the next two weeks he had a spiking fever almost every day and a recurring rash on his trunk. His knee joints became painful, making him uncharacteristically tearful. He was often tired and spent long periods just lying on the couch. After a course of antibiotics prescribed by his GP failed to have any effect and during a particularly severe fever, Alex was admitted for investigation to his local hospital nearly three weeks after the first sign of illness. Among the blood tests performed was an ESR, which was reported as 89 mm/hour. A diagnosis of Still's disease (a form of juvenile chronic arthritis) was eventually made and the intensity of symptoms resolved with administration of the anti-inflammatory drug, naprosyn. After three weeks in hospital Alex was discharged home with prescription for naprosyn and methotrexate. At his most recent rheumatology outpatients clinic, blood was collected from Alex for ESR. The result on this occasion was 18 mm/hour.

(1) Was Alex's ESR normal at the time of admission to hospital?
(2) Was this ESR result consistent with a diagnosis of Still's disease?
(3) What is the significance of the ESR result at Alex's recent outpatient appointment?
(4) What is meant when ESR is described as a non-specific test?

Discussion of case history

(1) No. Alex's ESR was grossly elevated.
(2) Yes. Like many other forms of arthritis, Still's disease is a chronic condition characterised by inflammation of the joints. A raised ESR is almost always a feature of active inflammatory disease.
(3) The most recent ESR shows a marked reduction, reflecting a reduction in disease activity. The result provides objective evidence that the prescribed drug regime (naprosyn and methotrexate) is, for the moment at least, keeping this chronic disease under control.
(4) A non-specific test like ESR is one which is abnormal in a wide range of pathological conditions. By contrast a specific test is one which is abnormal in one or a few related conditions. There are few tests which are absolutely specific for a single disease but nearly all are more specific than ESR. In the context of this case history the non-specificity of the ESR means that although ESR is usually raised in patients with Still's disease it is not useful to make the diagnosis: there are many other conditions in which a raised ESR is equally likely.

Further reading

Bedell S. & Bush B. (1985) Erythrocyte sedimentation rate. From folklore to facts. *Amer. J. Med.* **78**: 1001–8.

Dinant G., Knottnerus J., Van Wersch J. (1991) Discriminating ability of the erythrocyte sedimentation rate: a prospective study in general practice. *Br. J. Gen. Practice* **41**: 365–70.

Fincher R. & Page M. (1986) Clinical significance of extreme elevation of the erythrocyte sedimentation rate. *Arch. Intern. Med.* **146**: 1581–3.

Kanfer E. & Nicol B. (1997) Haemoglobin concentration and erythrocyte sedimentation rate in primary care patients. *J. Roy. Soc. Med.* **90**: 16–18.

Lowe G. (1994) Should plasma viscosity replace the ESR? *Br. J. Haematology* **86**: 6–11.

Part

4 Blood Transfusion Testing

19 Blood Transfusion Testing: Blood grouping, antibody screen and crossmatch

Blood transfusion is such a commonplace procedure that it is perhaps easy to underestimate the dangers involved. Although often of life-saving benefit, transfusion of donated blood is associated with considerable potential risk to the recipient patient. The two most significant risks are transmission of serious blood-borne infections, and the potentially fatal haemolytic transfusion reaction which can occur if patients receive incompatible blood. The risk of infection is virtually eliminated[1,2] by careful donor selection and rigorous screening of all blood donations for evidence of infection (Table 19.1). An additional measure, leucopletion (the removal of white cells from all units of donated blood), was introduced in late 1999 to prevent transmission of new variant Creutzfeldt–Jacob disease (vCJD). These measures, which ensure a supply of the safest possible blood to local hospital blood transfusion laboratories, are the responsibility of the four national blood transfusion services in the UK.

Prevention of the second major risk associated with blood transfusion, i.e. incompatible transfusion reaction, begins with the pre-transfusion tests of donor and recipient blood conducted in local hospital blood transfusion laboratories. Of crucial importance are the three tests which are the subject of this chapter: determination of blood group, antibody screen and crossmatch. In order to understand what is meant by an incompatible blood transfusion and the significance of these tests for its prevention, a little background immunology is required.

Background immunology

What are antigens and antibodies?

Our ability to withstand attack from invading micro-organisms such as bacteria and viruses depends in large part on antibody-producing white

Table 19.1   Selection criteria for blood donors and mandatory blood tests to prevent transmission of infectious disease

---

Blood donors must:

- be aged between 18 and 56 years
- be in good health
- have a haemoglobin (Hb) greater than 13.1 g/dl (men) or 12.5 g/dl (women).

Blood donors must not:

- be pregnant or have been pregnant during previous 12 months
- ever have suffered from cancer, syphilis or brucellosis
- have a recent history of malaria, hepatitis, jaundice, or glandular fever
- be in a high-risk group for HIV infection
- donate blood more than twice in one year.

All donated blood units tested for the presence of:

- hepatitis B surface antigen
- antibody to hepatitis C antibody } To prevent transmission of viral hepatitis

- antibody to *Trepanema pallidum*   To prevent transmission of syphilis

- antibody to HIV-1
- antibody to HIV-2 } To prevent transmission of HIV

---

blood cells called B-lymphocytes. Antibodies are immunoglobulin proteins which bind to and neutralise bacteria and viruses. Each antibody is very specific in its action so that an antibody which binds and neutralises one sort of bacteria will have no effect on another. This specificity is due to the specific nature of the molecular target on the surface of each sort of bacteria. This molecular target is called the antigen. Recognition by B-lymphocytes of specific bacterial or viral antigens induces specific antibody production.

This ability of the body to produce destructive antibodies to 'foreign' antigens is not confined to those antigens present on the surface of bacteria or viruses. Proteins and other molecular substances present on the surface of any foreign (i.e. non-self) cell are 'seen' as antigens and provoke a similarly destructive specific antibody response. It is, for example, this same antibody response to foreign antigens which accounts in part for the tissue rejection that occurs following organ transplantation.

To summarise then:

- An *antigen* is any substance (most commonly a protein, but it may be a carbohydrate) which causes production of antibodies by lymphocytes. Antigens are found usually, although not exclusively, on the surface of cells.

■ An *antibody* is a protein (immunoglobulin) which circulates in blood plasma and binds only with the antigen which provoked its production.

When an antibody binds with an antigen present on the surface of a cell, be it a bacterium, a virus or a tissue cell, a sequence of events follows which invariably leads to that cell's disruption or destruction.

One of the characteristics of the immune system is its ability to remember. On the first occasion lymphocytes 'meet' a foreign antigen, antibody production is low and therefore not very effective. However, the immune system is now primed. Specialised B-lymphocytes (called memory lymphocytes) 'remember' the antigen so that when it is encountered on subsequent occasions, both speed and intensity of antibody production are greatly increased. This is the basis of the concept of acquired immunity; we have little protection (immunity) against a particular bacteria or virus until our immune system has been primed by an initial infection.

Clearly it is vital for health that we do not produce antibodies to our own antigens, and the immune system has a means of preventing this occurring. However, it is worth mentioning in passing that there are a large group of pathological conditions, collectively known as the auto-immune diseases, in which this ability to distinguish self from non-self antigens is lost. These diseases are characterised by the production of antibodies directed at self antigens. Such antibodies (known as auto-antibodies) bind to antigens present on the surface of the body's own cells. The result is cellular damage or destruction. Common diseases with an autoimmune component include rheumatoid arthritis, Type 1 diabetes, most thyroid diseases and systemic lupus erythematosus (SLE); there are many others.

Notwithstanding these pathological exceptions, it is important to remember that it is normally not possible to produce antibodies to one's own antigens.

Red cell antigens and the blood group

The surface of red cells like that of all other cells is covered with inherited antigens. These red cell antigens (or the lack of them) determine an individual's blood group. More than 400 different red cell antigens (most very rare) have been identified, and make up the 24 blood group systems so far described. Fortunately, only a tiny minority of these are of significance in transfusion medicine. Of those that do have significance, the antigens of the ABO and Rh blood group system are of prime importance.

ABO blood group system

We all belong to one of four groups of the ABO blood group system determined by the inheritance or non-inheritance of two red cell antigens A and B. Those who inherit neither A nor B red cell antigens belong to group O; those who inherit the A red cell antigen belong to group A, those who inherit the B red cell antigen belong to group B and those who inherit both the A and the B red cell antigen belong to group AB. Most (88%) of the UK population belong to either group O or group A.

Rh blood group system

The Rh blood group system, so called because much of the early research was conducted on rhesus (Rh) monkeys, is the only other blood group system of major significance to blood transfusion. There are five red cell antigens in the Rh system: C, c, D, E, and e but only the D antigen is of major significance. Around 85% of the UK population have the D antigen on their red cells and are said to be Rh D positive; the remaining 15% do not have the D antigen and are Rh D negative.

Other less significant red cell antigens

A routine blood group means determination of the ABO group and Rh D typing (either positive or negative). Of the remaining nearly 400 red cell antigens which may or may not be present on the surface of an individual's red cells, a few have occasional significance for transfusion medicine. Among these are the remaining antigens of the Rh blood group system (i.e. the c, C, e and E antigens) and the antigens of the Kell (K), Duffy (Fy), Kidd (Jk) and Lewis (Le) blood group systems. These antigens are rare causes of transfusion reaction either because they are themselves rare, or because they are relatively weakly immunogenic.

Antibodies to red cell antigens: incompatible blood transfusion

The significance of red cell antigens for blood transfusion medicine lies in the specific antibodies to these red cell antigens, which may or may not be present in the recipient's plasma. An incompatible transfusion reaction occurs when antibodies present in the patient's (recipient's) plasma binds to its complementary antigen present on the red cells of donated blood. Such antibody–antigen binding can result in the destruction of the donated red cells; this destruction is called haemolysis, so the term immune haemolytic transfusion reaction is used to describe this complication of blood transfusion. So long as the patient's plasma contains no significant antibodies to the antigens present on the red cells of donated blood, the patient and donor blood are said to be compatible and donor blood can be safely transfused.

Production of red cell antibodies

It was stated above that antibodies are only produced when lymphocytes come into contact with the relevant 'foreign' antigen. There are two situations in which an individual's antibody-producing lymphocytes may come into contact with 'foreign' red cell antigens. The first of course is blood transfusion, and the second is pregnancy. During pregnancy, foetal blood leaks to maternal circulation. If foetal blood red cells bear antigens inherited from the father which are not present on the mother's red cells, they are 'seen' as foreign by the mother's lymphocytes, which then proceed to manufacture antibody.

As with any other immune response, initial antibody production during the first immunising blood transfusion or pregnancy is low and usually has no effect. But the immune system is now primed to synthesise large quantities of antibody the next time the 'foreign' red cell antigen is encountered. Antibodies produced in this way are called immune red cell antibodies. The clinically most significant immune red cell antibody is anti-D, the antibody to the Rh D antigen. Of course only those who lack the Rh D antigen (i.e. the 15% of the population who are Rh D negative) can be immunised to produce anti-D in this way. In fact around 1% of the population have anti-D in their plasma as the result of previous immunising transfusion or pregnancy. If such people were transfused with Rh D positive blood, the anti-D in their plasma would bind to the D antigen on the surface of donated red cells, resulting in a haemolytic transfusion reaction.

If immune red cell antibodies were the only red cell antibodies present in plasma, then only those who have a history of previous immunising blood transfusion or pregnancy would be at risk of incompatible blood transfusion; this is not the case.

The overriding clinical significance of the ABO blood group system lies in the fact that antibodies to these antigens are naturally occurring, that is they do not arise as a result of previous immunisation by foreign red cells. All of us have antibodies to the A or B antigen that we lack. Thus all those who belong to group O and lack both the A and B antigen have antibodies to both antigens (i.e. anti-A and anti-B) in their plasma; all those who belong to group A and have the A antigen on their red cells have antibodies to the B antigen (i.e. anti-B) in their plasma and all those of group B have the antibody to the A antigen (i.e. anti-A) in their plasma. Only the 3% of the population belonging to group AB who have both the A and B antigen on their red cells have no naturally occurring anti-A or anti-B in their plasma. The antigens and antibodies associated with the four groups of the ABO blood group system are summarised in Table 19.2.

Table 19.2   The ABO blood group system and Rh D type

ABO blood group	Antigen present on red cells	Naturally occurring antibody in plasma	Relative frequency in UK population (%)
O	O	anti-A and anti-B	47
A	A	anti-B	42
B	B	anti-A	8
AB	A and B	None	3

Notes:
Rh D antigen present on the red cells of 85% of UK population; these are Rh D positive.
Rh D antigen not present on the red cells of 15%; these are Rh D negative.
For a routine blood group only ABO group and Rh D status (i.e. negative or positive) are determined.

It is the relative ubiquity and potency of naturally occurring anti-A and anti-B which determine the prime clinical importance of the ABO blood group system. Like anti-D, all other clinically significant red cell antibodies are immune antibodies so they cannot be present in the plasma of a person who has not been immunised by a previous transfusion or pregnancy. Thus the only significant red cell antibodies present in a patient who has never received a blood transfusion or been pregnant is naturally occurring anti-A or anti-B. It has been estimated that if only ABO compatibility is ensured, and no other tests are performed, blood transfusion would be immunologically safe in 97% of cases.

Immune haemolytic transfusion reaction – ABO incompatibility

The consequences of transfusing ABO-incompatible blood are described in Fig. 19.1. Such a reaction can occur after only a few millilitres of blood have been transfused. In this example, blood from a donor who is blood group A is given to a patient who is blood group B. Anti-A present in the patient's plasma binds to the A antigen on the surface of donated red

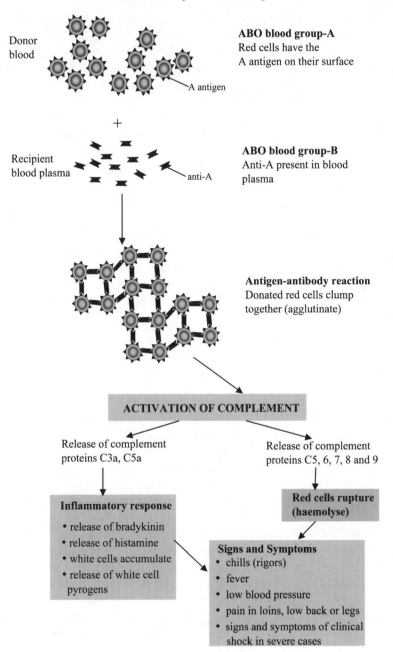

Fig. 19.1 Incompatible transfusion reaction.

cells. The red cells clump together (agglutinate). Antigen–antibody binding activates the so-called complement pathway; it is the complement proteins (by convention denoted by the letter C followed by a number) produced as a result of this activation that accounts for many of the signs and symptoms of a haemolytic transfusion reaction. Complement proteins C5, C6, C7, C8 and C9 are all involved in the process of red cell destruction (haemolysis), in which holes are made through the red cell membrane. By this complement-mediated haemolysis, all donated red cells are destroyed in the most severe cases of ABO incompatibility. Complement proteins C3a and C5a initiate an inflammatory response which includes release from activated mast cells of various potent chemicals (e.g. histamine, bradykinin) which result in a sudden fall in blood pressure (hypotension) and other very visible symptoms. The fall in blood pressure leads to symptoms of clinical shock and reduced flow of blood to the kidneys with the onset of acute renal failure in the most severe cases. Other complications of severe haemolytic transfusion reaction include disseminated intravascular coagulation (DIC), and jaundice as haemoglobin released from damaged red cells is metabolised to bilirubin.

Other immune haemolytic transfusion reactions

Even if donated blood is ABO compatible with the recipient's blood, there remains a risk of haemolytic transfusion reaction if there are other significant red cell antibodies present in the patient's plasma. Since these are all immune antibodies, they can only be present in the plasma of those patients who have been immunised by previous blood transfusion or pregnancy. The most important of these is anti-D. Others include anti-C, anti-c, anti-E, and anti-e (i.e. remaining antibodies to Rh blood group antigens); anti-K (antibody to the Kell (K) blood group antigen); anti-Fy^a and anti-Fy^b (antibodies to two of the Duffy (Fy) blood group antigens); and anti-Jk^a and anti-Jk^b (antibodies to two of the Kidd (Jk) blood group antigens). Symptoms of haemolytic transfusion reaction which result from these antibodies are generally speaking less severe than those associated with ABO incompatibility. The reaction may be delayed for up to ten days after the transfusion, when chills and fever develop. Red cell destruction may cause anaemia and mild jaundice.

LABORATORY TESTING OF BLOOD GROUP, ANTIBODY SCREEN AND CROSSMATCH

SAMPLE COLLECTION

When a patient requires a blood transfusion, 10 ml of venous blood must be collected into a plain tube containing no additives; this is sufficient for all three tests. Most blood transfusion laboratories supply designated tubes (usually pink top) that are to be used only for these tests.

Because of the potentially fatal consequences of giving donated blood to the 'wrong' patient, scrupulous attention to the detail of patient identification and documentation is vital when collecting blood for any of these tests. Before taking blood ensure beyond any doubt the identification of the patient, preferably by asking his or her name and cross-checking with the identification armband.

The following minimum information must be written legibly on the sample label and accompanying request card.

- patient's first and last name (taken from the patient's armband)
- patient's unique identification number, gender and date of birth
- patient's ward or department
- date and time of collection
- initials of person taking the blood.

The request card should include the following additional details:

- the nature of donated blood required (whole blood, packed red cells, etc.)
- the number of units required
- when the blood is required – level of urgency
- why the blood is required (acute blood loss, chronic anaemia, elective surgery, etc.)
- ABO and rhesus blood group (if known)
- any relevant transfusion or obstetric history (if known)
- signature of the medical officer making the request.

These are guidelines only; healthcare workers involved in the collection of blood for pre-transfusion testing should adhere to locally agreed protocols. These local protocols must now reflect best practice as defined by the British Committee for Standards in Haematology (BSCH) in collaboration with the Royal College of Nursing and the Royal College of Surgeons.[3,4] If in doubt, consult your local blood bank for acceptable practice in this area. Blood-bank staff will reject specimens which are inadequately labelled or if

'cont.'

'continued'

sample label does not match information recorded on accompanying request card.

PRINCIPLES OF THE THREE TESTS

The purpose of the three tests is to prevent haemolytic transfusion reaction by issuing only donated blood which is immunologically compatible with the blood of the patient who is to receive the transfusion. In essence this means first determining which antibodies to red cell antigens are present in the patient's plasma and then selecting donated blood which has none of the relevant red cell antigens. The only significant antibodies that can be expected with certainty to be present in most patients' plasma are the naturally occurring antibodies to the red cell antigens of the ABO group system, so determination of the patient's ABO blood group is the prime test. At the same time as the ABO group is determined, the Rh D status (either negative or positive) is also determined. Together these comprise the blood group.

The binding of red cell antibody to its complementary antigen results in agglutination (clumping together) of cells. This visible phenomenon is exploited in all blood banking tests and is reflected in the alternative name for red cell antibodies and antigens. In many texts red cell antibodies are referred to as agglutinins and antigens as agglutinogens.

BLOOD GROUPING

Patient's ABO blood group is determined by simply mixing a sample of patient's red cells with sera containing anti-A and sera containing anti-B. The red cells either agglutinate or stay separate in suspension (Fig. 19.2). As an additional check a reverse group is performed in which the patient's serum is added to red cells of known ABO group. Rh D type is determined by mixing the patient's cells with a solution of anti-D. Agglutination indicates the presence of the D antigen on the patient's cells (Rh D positive). No agglutination indicates the patient's blood is Rh D negative.

ANTIBODY SCREEN

By performing an ABO blood grouping we know that the patient's plasma contains either anti-A or anti-B or both of these or neither of these. In around 97% of cases no further antibody is present. With a few rare exceptions all other significant red cell antibodies, including antibody to the Rh D antigen, are immunogenic in nature and present in the patient's

'cont.'

'continued'

serum only as a result of previous immunising blood transfusion or pregnancy. However, the presence of these red cell immune antibodies may potentially provoke a haemolytic reaction, if red cells to be transfused bear the relevant antigen. Therefore, a search for the presence of any significant atypical antibodies is performed on the serum of all patients who are to receive donated blood. This is the antibody screening test.

Essentially the antibody screening test is performed by adding a drop of the patient's serum to a panel of different group O red cells each bearing a different and known combination of the most common red cell antigens known to cause immune reactions. Since group O red cells do not have the A or B antigen on their surface, any agglutination when the patient's serum is added to this panel of red cells must be due to the presence of an atypical antibody in the patient's serum. No agglutination indicates no atypical antibodies, and the result antibody screen negative is reported. The antibodies tested for in the antibody screening test usually include at least all of the following:

- anti-D, anti-C, anti-c, anti-E, and anti-e (antibodies to Rh blood group antigens)
- anti-K (antibody to the Kell (K) blood group antigen)
- anti-Fy^a and anti-Fy^b (antibodies to two of the Duffy (Fy) blood group antigens) and
- anti-Jk^a and anti-Jk^b (antibodies to two of the Kidd (Jk) blood group antigens).

If the screen is positive, the identity of the antibody causing the positive result can usually be deduced from the pattern of reactions displayed by the panel of O red cells.

SELECTION OF DONOR BLOOD

Having established what significant red cell antibodies are present in the patient's plasma, the next step is selection of suitable donor unit. What is required is blood whose red cells do not bear any of the antigens which react with any significant antibodies present in the patient's (recipient's) serum. For those patients whose antibody screen is negative, the only consideration is ABO and Rh D compatibility. In most instances this simply means selecting blood which has the same ABO and Rh D blood group as the patient. However, if ABO or Rh D identical blood is not available, there is some room for manoeuvre:

'cont.'

'continued'

- A patient whose blood group is AB has no ABO antibodies in his or her plasma so can receive red cells of any ABO group. Under these circumstances consideration must be given to the naturally occurring antibodies (i.e. anti-A and anti-B) present in the plasma of donated blood. These would bind to A and B antigens present on the surface of the patient's AB red cells and cause patient red cell destruction. This can be avoided by removing the plasma containing the antibody from donor blood before transfusion. If group O, A or B blood is to be transfused to a patient of blood group AB, only packed red cells can be selected.
- The red cells of blood group O have no A or B antigens on their surface so can be safely transfused to all patients. However, the plasma of group O blood contains anti-A and anti-B which will react with the A and B antigens present on the surface of patients' red cells if they are of blood group A, B or AB. To minimise the risk of this reaction, if group O blood is to be given to patients who are not group O, then plasma should be removed from the unit; only packed red cells should be transfused.
- Patients who are Rh D positive cannot have antibodies to the D antigen and can therefore be given blood which is either Rh D positive or negative.
- Patients who are Rh D negative may or may not have antibodies to the D antigen but whether they do or not, transfusion of Rh D positive blood almost invariably invokes anti-D production. For this reason only Rh D negative blood should be selected for transfusion to Rh D negative patients.

Table 19.3 summarises the criteria for selection of donor unit for transfusion, based on the ABO group and Rh D type of the patient. It will be noted that O Rh D negative red cells can be safely transfused to all patients; for this reason, those with this particular blood group are known as 'universal donors'. In the very rare event of life-threatening haemorrhage, where the clinical need for a blood transfusion is so urgent that it does not allow time for laboratory testing, O Rh D negative blood is transfused. It will also be noted from Table 19.3 that patients with the blood group AB Rh D positive can be safely transfused with red cells of any blood group. Those with this blood group are known as 'universal recipients'.

For those patients whose antibody screen is positive, a further step is required. First ABO Rh D identical or compatible donated blood units are selected as described above. The red cells of these are tested for the

'cont.'

'continued'

presence of red cell antigens that react with the atypical antibody found in the patient's serum. So, for example, suppose the antibody screen revealed that the patient had the antibody which reacts with the Rh C antigen (i.e. anti-C): the red cells of donated blood must be tested for the presence of the C antigen. Only blood which is negative for the C antigen can be transfused.

CROSSMATCH

Having selected a unit of donated blood whose red cells have no antigens which could react with antibodies present in the patient's plasma, one final checking test must be performed to ensure compatibility. This is the crossmatch in which transfusion is simulated in a test tube. Essentially a sample of donor red cells is mixed with a sample of the patient's (recipient's) serum and inspected for agglutination. No agglutination indicates there is no red cell antigen/antibody reaction and that the donor's red cells are compatible with the patient's plasma and can be safely transfused.

Pre-transfusion checks on the ward

Severe acute immune haemolytic reactions (invariably caused by ABO incompatibility) are rare events but when they do occur the cause is usually transfusion of blood to the 'wrong' patient due to clerical error or error in patient identification.[2] Strict adherence to the agreed local protocol for pre-transfusion checks at the bedside is vital. Local policy must now reflect best practice as defined by the BSCH in collaboration with the Royal College of Nursing and the Royal College of Surgeons.[3,4]

Pre-transfusion checks at the bedside should include:

- confirmation of patient's identity, preferably by asking him or her and crosschecking with identity armband
- confirmation that the patient details on the blood compatibility report match in every detail the identity of the patient to be given blood
- confirmation that the identifying unit number printed on the unit of blood to be transfused matches the unit number on the compatibility report

Solution of anti-A or anti-B added to a few drops of a suspension of patient's red cells

	Patient 1	Patient 2	Patient 3	Patient 4
Anti-A	●	◌	●	◌
Anti-B	●	●	◌	◌
Result	No agglutination when either anti-A or anti-B is added.	Agglutination only when anti-A added	Agglutination only when anti-B added	Agglutination when both anti-A and anti-B are added.
Interpretation of result	**Group O**	**Group A**	**Group B**	**Group AB**
% Frequency in UK population	47	42	8	3

 agglutination - cells clumped together

● no agglutination

Fig. 19.2   Determination of ABO blood group.

- confirmation that the ABO blood group and Rh D type printed on the blood unit is the same as the patient's ABO and Rh D blood group or compatible with it
- confirmation that the unit of blood to be transfused has not passed its expiry date and that no more than 30 minutes have elapsed since the unit was removed from the blood bank refrigerator
- baseline measurement of patient's blood pressure, temperature, pulse and respiration rate must be recorded immediately before the start of blood transfusion.

Other transfusion reactions

The laboratory tests discussed in this chapter are designed solely to prevent immune haemolytic transfusion reactions but these are not the only adverse reactions that a patient can suffer during a blood transfusion.

Table 19.3 Selecting blood for transfusion

Donor blood group	Recipient (patient) blood group							
	O RhD Pos	O RhD Neg	A RhD Pos	A RhD Neg	B RhD Pos	B RhD Neg	AB RhD Pos	AB RhD Neg
O RhD Pos	✓	X	✓R	X	✓R	X	✓R	X
O RhD Neg	✓	✓	✓R	✓R	✓R	✓R	✓R	✓R
A RhD Pos	X	X	✓	X	X	X	✓R	X
A RhD Neg	X	X	✓	✓	X	X	✓R	✓R
B RhD Pos	X	X	X	X	✓	X	✓R	X
B RhD Neg	X	X	X	X	✓	✓	✓R	✓R
AB RhD Pos	X	X	X	X	X	X	✓	X
AB RhD Neg	X	X	X	X	X	X	✓	✓

Key:

✓   ABO compatible. No risk of Rh D sensitisation. Safe to transfuse if patient antibody screen is negative.

X   ABO incompatible or risk of Rh D sensitisation. Not safe to transfuse.

✓R ABO compatible. No risk of Rh D sensitisation. Safe to transfuse packed red cells if patient antibody screen negative.

Non-haemolytic febrile transfusion reactions (NHFTR)

Patients who have received previous blood transfusions may have developed antibodies to antigens present on the surface of white cells. If blood whose white cells bear these antigens is transfused to such patients, a febrile reaction characterised by shivering and fever may develop. The symptoms are due to potent chemicals (cytokines) released from damaged white cells. Although quite common among patients who have previously received multiple transfusions, febrile reactions are usually mild and self-limiting. It is likely that the incidence of these febrile reactions will be greatly reduced by the new policy of leucopletion.

Allergic reaction

Some people suffer allergic reactions to one or more of the many proteins in the plasma of transfused blood. These are the most frequently observed adverse effects of blood transfusion. They are usually mild in nature and evidenced by urticaria (appearance of extremely itchy weals on the skin). Very rarely, allergy can result in severe anaphylactic shock, a clinical emergency characterised by hypotension, chest pain and breathlessness. Such severe reactions, like the haemolytic reactions caused by ABO incompatibility, are of life-threatening significance.

Bacterial infection

Scrupulous aseptic technique during donor blood collection and care that donated blood is stored at a temperature ($+4°C$) which minimises bacterial growth ensure that donated blood is free from bacteria at the time of transfusion. Additional safeguards include the disposal of blood which has passed its expiry date and protocols which ensure that donated blood is not left at room temperature for longer than absolutely necessary before it is transfused. Although rare, reactions due to transfusion of bacterially contaminated blood can occur. Depending on the nature of the contaminating bacteria, symptoms vary. In the most severe cases symptoms of life-threatening septicaemia can develop within a few minutes of starting the transfusion. These include fever, sudden chills and shivering (rigors), nausea and vomiting. A severe fall in blood pressure can herald clinical shock and acute renal failure.

Patient monitoring during transfusion

The vast majority of blood transfusions are uneventful, but because of the potentially serious adverse effects, careful observation of the patient is necessary during blood transfusion. Locally agreed protocol for the monitoring of patients receiving a blood transfusion must reflect best practice as defined by the BCSH in collaboration with the Royal College of Surgeons.[3,4] Some general points are made here. Monitoring is particularly important during the early stages, when most severe reactions develop. Temperature, pulse, respiration and blood pressure should be recorded at 15 minutes after the start of the transfusion; further measurements may be considered, particularly for patients who are unconscious. Patients should be observed for signs and symptoms of all adverse reactions. In the event of a suspected reaction, the transfusion should be stopped immediately and medical staff summoned. The management of a patient suffering a transfusion reaction depends on its cause and severity. Mild febrile reactions may require only the administration of an anti-pyretic drug (e.g. aspirin) to control temperature. The transfusion can be restarted, only at a slower rate. Mild allergic reactions may be treated with antihistamine drugs. For severe reactions, that is, immune haemolytic reactions, severe allergic reactions and those caused by bacterial infection, the principal first objective is to maintain blood pressure in order to preserve blood flow to the kidneys. Adrenalin and steroids may be administered to control allergy and shock. Diuretics may be administered to increase urine flow. In the case of suspected bacterial infection, broad spectrum antibiotics are administered.

Laboratory investigations of transfusion reaction

In all cases of severe reaction, the laboratory must be informed as soon as possible, so that the cause of the reaction can be investigated. Along with the donor blood pack a fresh sample of the patient's blood collected into a plain tube must be sent to the laboratory for this purpose. Blood group, antibody screen and crossmatch will be repeated. Because of the risk of disseminated intravascular coagulation (DIC) and resulting excessive bleeding, associated with severe immune haemolytic reaction and reaction due to transfusion of bacterially contaminated blood, a sample of blood for haemoglobin estimation and a further sample of blood for coagulation studies should also be sent to the laboratory. Finally blood from the donor pack and blood from the patient must be cultured for the detection of bacteria.

Post-transfusion reactions

For the vast majority of patients, blood transfusion passes uneventfully. There remains a small risk of a delayed immune haemolytic reaction (usually mild) during the hours and days which follow a blood transfusion. The sudden onset of chills, a rise in temperature, and the occurrence of anaemia and jaundice at any time during the ten-day period following a transfusion may signal such a reaction.

Haemolytic disease of the newborn (HDN)

Both determination of blood group and the antibody screening test are important not only for the prevention of immune haemolytic transfusion reactions but also for the diagnosis and prevention of haemolytic disease of the newborn (HDN). As part of their antenatal care, pregnant women have a sample of blood taken, usually at their first antenatal appointment, for blood group determination and antibody screen. The purpose of this testing is to identify those women whose developing baby is at risk of this potentially fatal condition.

What is HDN?

Some red cell antibodies (most notably antibodies to the antigens of the Rh blood group system, e.g. anti-D) can pass from the mother's blood across the placenta to the foetal circulation. If the baby has inherited red cell antigens from the father which these maternal antibodies react with, an immune haemolytic reaction occurs and foetal red cells are destroyed.

Pregnancies most at risk are those in which the mother is group O Rh D negative and the father is group O Rh D positive. There is a one in four chance that the baby of such a union will be Rh D positive. If the baby is in fact Rh D positive, then when foetal red cells pass from foetal circulation to the mother's blood, as they do in all pregnancies, the mother's lymphocytes 'see' the D antigen as foreign and produce anti-D. During the first such pregnancy the titre (amount) of anti-D in the mother's plasma is usually insufficient to have any effect. But the mother's immune system is now primed to produce massive quantities of anti-D the next time it encounters Rh D positive red cells. In subsequent pregnancies, if the baby is once again Rh D positive, large amounts of anti-D pass from the mother to foetal circulation and bind to the D antigen on foetal red cells, provoking a massive haemolytic reaction, with destruction of the developing baby's red cells.

In the most severe cases, the anaemia that results from red cell destruction can lead to death *in utero*. More often babies are born anaemic and jaundiced. The jaundice is due to increased production of bilirubin from haemoglobin released from haemolysed (destroyed) red cells. There is a risk of permanent brain damage if excess bilirubin is deposited in the cells of the brain, a condition called kernicterus. An affected baby may need exchange transfusion, in which O Rh D negative blood (which because it lacks the Rh D antigen cannot be destroyed by any anti-D present) is transfused as the baby's O Rh D positive blood, containing the damaging antibody, is removed. This transfusion corrects the anaemia and prevents further red cell damage; the severe jaundice resolves. If the developing foetus is severely affected, consideration may be given to intrauterine transfusion from as early as 18 weeks into the pregnancy.

Prevention of Rh D HDN

To prevent HDN caused by Rh D incompatibility, all Rh D negative women carrying a Rh D positive baby for the first time are given an injection of anti-D at the time of birth or at any time during the pregnancy when there is good evidence to suppose that foetal red cells have passed to the mother's circulation. This administered anti-D destroys any foetal cells before the mother can mount an immune response, thus preventing maternal production of anti-D which could jeopardise subsequent pregnancies.

HDN can be caused by other red cell antibodies

Although Rh D incompatibility between mother and baby is the most significant cause of HDN, other red cell antibodies which may or may not be present in the mother's serum can cause HDN. It is rare for ABO incompatibility to cause HDN because anti-A and anti-B cannot normally cross the placenta so therefore do not come into contact with foetal red cells. When HDN is caused by ABO incompatibility, it is usually mild and of much less clinical significance than that due to Rh D incompatibility. Other antibodies of significance are the antibodies to other rhesus group antigens (i.e. anti-C, anti-E and anti-e), anti-K (antibody to Kell blood group antigens) and anti-Dfy (antibody to Duffy blood group antigens). An antibody screen performed early in pregnancy is designed to detect if any antibodies capable of causing HDN are present in the mother's blood plasma.

Case history 18

Mrs Greenwood, a 24-year-old mother, attends surgical outpatients to have blood taken for various tests prior to surgery scheduled later in the week. Among the blood tests requested is 'group, screen and save'.

(1)   What sample is required?
(2)   What is the purpose of the tests?

Mrs Greenwood's blood group is found to be AB Rh D negative. During surgery Mrs Greenwood suffers a significant haemorrhage and a request for 3 units of crossmatched packed red cells is sent urgently to the laboratory. During the pre-transfusion checks in the recovery room prior to administration of the first unit, it is noted that the blood to be transfused is A Rh D negative.

(3)   In view of the ABO blood group discrepancy between donor and Mrs Greenwood, is it safe to go ahead with the transfusion?
(4)   Why is it important that Mrs Greeenwood does not receive Rh D positive blood?

Discussion of case history

(1)   A 10 ml sample of venous blood collected into a plain bottle specially designated for blood transfusion tests.
(2)   These tests are performed to reduce the delay should Mrs Greenwood require a blood transfusion during surgery. Her ABO group and Rh D type will be determined. The term 'screen' refers to the antibody screening test in which her plasma is tested for the presence of any atypical red cell antibodies which may complicate the selection of a suitable donor unit. 'Save' simply means store the sample. Should a blood transfusion become necessary, the only remaining test to be performed is the crossmatch test in which Mrs Greenwood's stored sample of plasma is mixed with the red cells of a selected ABO and Rh compatible donor unit. If Mrs Greenwood were scheduled for major surgery in which excessive bleeding were a routine and expected complication, blood would be crossmatched prior to surgery.
(3)   Although the ABO blood group of the donated unit is not identical, it is compatible with Mrs Greenwood's group. The cells of the donated blood group bear the A antigen; it is imperative that this

blood is not given to a patient whose serum contains anti-A. Mrs Greenwood is group AB and her serum therefore contains no anti-A or anti-B, so she can be given group A red cells. The donor plasma contains anti-B which can react with the B antigen present on Mrs Greenwood's red cells. This is not a problem, however, because the unit requested is packed red cells, that is a donor unit from which most of the plasma (and therefore most of the anti-B) has been removed. Any anti-B remaining in the small volume of plasma will be diluted in the patient's own plasma and have no adverse effect. Only 3% of the population belong, like Mrs Greenwood, to group AB so that it is often difficult to find ABO identical blood for such patients; Group A or Group B packed red cells is a suitable alternative.

(4) Mrs Greenwood belongs to the 15% of the population whose red cells do not bear the Rh D antigen. She is Rh D negative. If she were given blood whose red cells did bear the antigen (i.e. Rh D positive blood), she would 'see' these cells as foreign and invoke an immune response with production of anti-D. This would be significant for future transfusions. If, in any subsequent transfusion, she were given Rh D positive blood, her primed immune system would produce large quantities of anti-D which would bind to the D antigen on transfused red cells and initiate an acute immune haemolytic reaction. There is also a greatly increased risk that if Mrs Greenwood became pregnant, her pregnancy would be complicated by severe Rh D haemolytic disease of the newborn. For these reasons it is vital that patients who are Rh D negative, particularly women of child-bearing age, are only given Rh D negative blood.

References

(1) Regan F., Hewitt P., Barabara J. & Contreras M. (2000) Prospective investigation of transfusion transmitted infection in respect of over 20 000 units of blood. *BMJ* **320**: 403–6.
(2) Williamson L., Lowe S., Love S. *et al.* (1999) Serious hazards of transfusion (SHOT) initiative: analysis of first two annual reports. *BMJ* **319**: 16–19.
(3) NHS Executive (1998) Better blood transfusion. *Health Services Circular 1998/224*. HMSO, London.
(4) British Committee for Standards in Haematology (1999) Guidelines for the adminstration of blood and blood components and the management of the transfused patient. *Transfusion Medicine* **9**: 227–38.

Further reading

Contreras M. (1992) *ABC of Transfusion*. BMJ Publishing Group, London.
Fitzpatrick L. & Fitzpatrick T. (1997) Blood transfusion: keeping your patient safe. *Nursing* 97 August: 34–41.

Glover G. & Powell F. (1996) Blood transfusion. *Nursing Standard* **10**: 49–54.

Mackenzie I.Z., Bowell P., Gregory H. *et al.* (1999) Routine antenatal Rhesus D immunoglobulin prophylaxis: the results of a prospective 10 year study *Br. J. Obstet. Gynaecology* **106**: 492–97.

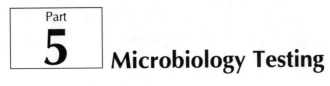

Part 5 Microbiology Testing

20 Urine Microscopy Culture and Sensitivity (M, C & S)

In this chapter and the next, attention is focused on the work of the clinical microbiology laboratory. Of all microbiological tests conducted in clinical laboratories, urine culture and sensitivity is the most frequently requested. The test is used to help make or exclude a diagnosis of urinary tract infection (UTI) among patients who exhibit signs and symptoms of UTI, and among patients who are asymptomatic but at high risk of UTI. After the respiratory tract, the urinary tract is the most frequent site of infection.

Normal physiology

The urinary tract

The urinary tract (Fig. 20.1) comprises the kidneys (the upper urinary tract), and the ureters, bladder and urethra (which together constitute the lower urinary tract). Urine formation occurs in the kidney. The functional unit of the kidney is a microscopically small tube called a nephron (Fig. 5.2); there are around 1 million nephrons in each kidney. Urine formation begins when blood delivered to the kidney via the renal artery is filtered at the glomerulus of each nephron. The fluid which passes through the glomerular filter is called the ultrafiltrate and is essentially blood from which all cells and large protein molecules have been removed. During its passage through the nephron, the volume and composition of this ultrafiltrate is adjusted. By the time the ultrafiltrate has passed to the end of the nephron, only waste products of the body's metabolic processes dissolved in a little water are left; this is urine. The urine from each nephron flows into a system of collecting ducts. These ducts join at the pelvis of the kidney, where urine leaves the kidney.

Urine is conducted from the pelvis of each kidney to the bladder, via

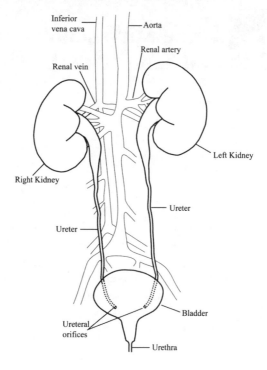

Fig. 20.1   Urinary tract.

tubes called ureters. The walls of the ureters contain smooth muscle. Peristaltic contractions of this muscle wall, occurring around three times per minute, propel urine towards the bladder. The ureters are joined obliquely to the bladder at its base, and urine enters the bladder in continuous spurts due to the peristaltic action of the ureters. The oblique entry of the ureters to the bladder ensures that the opening to the bladder is kept closed except during peristaltic contraction when urine enters. This effectively prevents urine passing from the bladder in the reverse direction up the ureters.

The bladder is an innervated muscular bag whose function is to store urine prior to urination (micturition) and expel all the urine it contains at the time of micturition. The volume of the bladder increases as it fills with urine. Between 150 and 400 ml of urine are collected in the adult bladder before the desire to urinate arises. When 700 ml of urine are present, the desire to urinate becomes urgent and painful. A sphincter muscle (the external urethral sphincter), situated where the urethra joins the bladder, prevents accumulating urine from leaving the bladder. At the time of micturition this sphincter is relaxed; the detrusor muscle in the wall of the bladder contracts, forcing urine out of the bladder, and urine flows from the bladder down the urethra.

The urethra is the tubular structure through which urine flows on the final part of its journey from the bladder out of the body. In the female the opening of the urethra (called the meatus) is in front of the vaginal orifice; in the male it is at the tip of the penis. The male urethra is thus significantly longer than the female urethra.

Bacteria in the urinary tract

The urinary tract from the kidney to the final distal third of the urethra normally contains no bacteria so in health the urine present in the bladder is sterile. Bacteria normally present on the skin of the perineum and in faeces can find their way up the urethra. Bacteria may therefore be present without any untoward effect in the lower third of the urethra. The normal flushing effect of urine as it passes down the urethra, and other non-immune and immune defences against bacterial invasion, serve to keep this bacterial contamination of the urethra under control. In health, normally voided urine is either sterile (contains no bacteria) or contains low numbers of bacteria flushed from the urethra during micturition.

Urinary tract infection

Route of infection

Urinary tract infection (UTI, Fig. 20.2) most often results from ascending infection by bacteria which constitute part of the normal bacterial flora of either the gastrointestinal tract or the skin. Bacteria normally present in the gastrointestinal tract are present in faeces. These bacteria find their way from the perianal region via the perineum to the urethra and up into the bladder. The skin of the perineum is also a source of urinary tract pathogens. Bacteria which are normally present specifically in the female genital tract are a less common cause of UTI.

Infection and resulting inflammation of the bladder are called cystitis. This is the most common form of UTI. In a minority of individuals, infection spreads on up the urinary tract, infecting the kidney. Although far less common than infection of the lower urinary tract, infection of the kidney (pyelonephritis) is more serious than cystitis. Scarring of kidney tissue can in the long term reduce kidney function. Chronic infection of the kidney may result in renal failure. Pyelonephritis is associated with

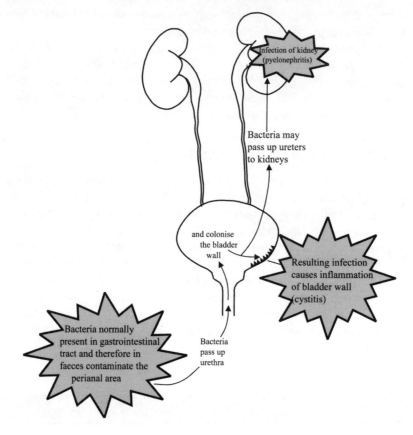

Fig. 20.2   Ascending route of urinary tract infection.

increased of risk of infection spreading to the blood causing septicaemia.

Although the ascending route of infection is the most usual, urinary tract infection may be caused by septicaemia. In this case bacteria present in blood may initiate descending infection of the urinary tract affecting first the kidneys and then the lower urinary tract.

Predisposing factors

Gender

The relatively short female urethra is considered one of the principal reasons for the particular susceptibility of women to ascending UTI. Around a third of all women have a UTI before the age of 65,[1] whilst for men under the age of 50, UTI is relatively rare. The incidence of UTI infection among men increases significantly with age past 50 years, so that there is no gender difference in UTI among elderly patients[1]. Among children, girls are more prone to UTI than boys.

Sexual activity

Women who are sexually active are more likely to suffer UTI than those who are not.

Pregnancy

Changes in the urinary tract early in pregnancy increase the risk of UTI spreading up the urinary tract with resulting pyelonephritis. For this reason all pregnant women are screened for UTI at least once during the first half of pregnancy.

Urine stasis

One of the principal physiological processes which prevent UTI is the flushing effect of sterile bladder urine through the lower urinary tract. Any disease process which inhibits urine flow or complete bladder emptying increases the risk of UTI. Obstruction of the urinary tract by stones (urinary calculi) or tumour and disease of the prostate, all of which may impair urine flow, contribute to the increased incidence of UTI in older men compared with younger men.

Immunosuppression

A suppressed immune system reduces host defence against bacterial invasion of the urinary tract. This explains the increased incidence of UTI among HIV patients and those who have been given immunosuppressive drugs (e.g. transplant patients).

Diabetes mellitus

Diabetics are more likely to suffer infections than non-diabetics. Urinary tract infection is a particular complication of longstanding diabetes.

Vesico-ureteral reflux

Anatomy of the normal urinary tract prevents urine from passing from the bladder back into the ureters. Vesico-ureteral reflux is a pathological condition in which reflux of infected urine from bladder to ureters greatly predisposes to ascending infection with resulting pyelonephritis. This is a particular problem among children and is a major cause of pyelonephritis among this age group. Other congenital abnormalities of the urinary tract cause UTI in babies and young children. If not identified and treated, these anomalies and associated recurrent UTI can lead to renal failure later in life. For this reason UTI in childhood warrants intensive urological investigation.

Hospitalisation

Illness which necessitates a stay in hospital is quite commonly associated with a temporary state of reduced immune defence against infectious disease. Furthermore the hospital environment is one in which the risk of coming into contact with infectious organisms is high. It is perhaps not surprising, then, that many patients acquire an infection as a direct result of being admitted to hospital. Around half of all patients in hospital who are suffering an infection, acquired the infection after admission. The principal site of hospital-acquired (nosocomial) infection is the urinary tract; around a third of all nosocomial infections are UTIs.[2] Patients at high risk of nosocomial UTI are those who require urine catheterisation or cystoscopy (endoscopic examination of the urinary tract). Urological surgery is also associated with an increased risk of UTI. All patients who require long-term catheterisation, i.e. for more than a month, whether in hospital or the community, almost inevitably contract a urinary tract infection, though many are asymptomatic (i.e. they have significant bacteriuria but do not feel unwell).

Signs and symptoms

Lower urinary tract infection (cystitis)

The principal signs and symptoms of cystitis are

- frequent urge to urinate even when there is not much urine in the bladder (frequency and urgency)
- burning pain during and immediately after urination (dysuria)
- fever may occasionally be a feature.

Upper urinary tract infection (acute pyelonephritis)

Those with upper urinary tract infections are usually significantly more unwell than those with uncomplicated cystitis. Principal signs and symptoms include:

- fever and rigors (fits of shivering)
- general malaise with nausea and vomiting
- renal (i.e. low back) pain
- symptoms of lower urinary tract infection may also be present.

MICROBIOLOGICAL EXAMINATION OF URINE

SPECIMEN COLLECTION (MSU)

The sample required is a 'clean catch' midstream specimen of urine (Table 20.1). It is important that the sample be taken before antibiotics are given, as these can quickly reduce the numbers of any bacteria present, possibly resulting in a falsely negative result. If antibiotics have been given, then this should be stated on the accompanying request card.

SPECIMEN COLLECTION (CSU)

The once widely adopted practice of catheterising patients simply to obtain a specimen of bladder urine for microbiological testing was abandoned when it was realised that the process of catheterisation itself increases the risk of UTI. However, the collection of a catheter specimen of urine (CSU) is necessary for the investigation of catheterised patients. Any bacteria present in bladder urine will quickly multiply as it stands in a catheter drainage bag. Urine should not therefore be sampled from the drainage bag; it will give a false impression of the bacterial content of bladder urine. Urine should instead be sampled using scrupulous aseptic technique by syringe and needle from the self-sealing sleeve of the drainage tube. Aseptic technique is important for three reasons:

- it reduces the risk of infecting the catheterised patient
- it reduces the risk of cross-infection from the catheterised patient to staff and other patients, and
- it reduces the risk of the specimen being contaminated with bacteria in the environment.

SPECIMEN COLLECTION BOTTLE

Urine (either MSU or CSU) must be collected into a sterile bottle. It is not necessary to fill the bottle; 5–10 ml is all that is required.

'cont.'

'continued'

TRANSPORT TO THE LABORATORY

Urine is a good medium for bacterial growth. Any bacteria present in the urine at collection will continue to multiply in the specimen bottle, giving falsely positive results. It is important, then, that the urine be examined within a few hours of collection. The time of sample collection should be recorded on the accompanying request card. If there is to be any delay in transportation to the laboratory, urine is best stored in a designated refrigerator as low temperature slows bacterial growth. Some laboratories provide sterile universal bottles which contain boric acid, a chemical which inhibits bacterial growth. The dip-slide culture method is designed for immediate culture of urine the moment the sample is voided. The slide which is covered with a culture medium, is dipped into freshly voided urine, drained and then sent to the laboratory.

IN THE LABORATORY

As with any specimen submitted for microbiological examination, urine is:

- examined macroscopically
- examined microscopically
- cultured to detect and identify any bacteria present
- and any potential pathogenic bacteria discovered, tested for sensitivity or resistance to a range of anti-microbial drugs.

Macroscopic examination. Normal urine is a clear straw-coloured or yellow fluid. Although by no means diagnostic, the appearance of urine can sometimes provide suggestive evidence of UTI. Like any other bacterial infection, UTI is associated with recruitment of white blood cells (WBC) to the site of infection in order to 'fight' bacteria. Dead and dying white cells are removed from the site of any infection in an inflammatory exudate called pus. Pus in urine (pyuria) turns clear urine turbid (cloudy). However, the absence of cloudiness does not rule out an infection and a cloudy urine does not necessarily mean the urine is infected; there are other causes of turbid urine. Infection with some bacteria can make urine foul smelling.

Microscopical examination. A measured volume of urine is examined under the microscope, principally for the presence of white and red blood cells. Urine normally contains a few white and red blood cells but a significant increase in white cell numbers is strong evidence of an infective process (see above). However, an increased white cell count is occasionally seen in urine which when cultured is found to contain no bacteria.

'cont.'

'continued'

Conversely a small minority of urines from patients suffering UTI contain no increase in the number of white cells. Infection is sometimes associated with an increase in red cell numbers (haematuria). There are other pathological causes (mostly renal disease) for an increase in urine red cell numbers.[3] Epithelial (skin) cells naturally shed from the surface of the female genital tract may be seen in urine; these have no pathological significance but rather indicate that the urine was not collected properly and may contain contaminating bacteria from the genital tract. Bacteria if present in large enough numbers may be seen during microscopical examination of urine.

Culture. The only sure way of confirming the presence or absence of bacteria and identifying the species is to culture the urine. Culture in this context means grow. A measured volume of urine is placed on a sterile solid culture medium in a petri dish. The culture medium contains all the nutrients necessary for bacterial growth. The petri dish is then covered and placed in an incubator at 37°C (optimum temperature for bacterial growth) and left for 24 hours. Any bacterial growth is seen as visible colonies on the surface of the solid medium. Each colony contains many thousands of bacteria, all derived from a single bacterium present in the urine sample. The number of these visible colonies is directly related to the number of organisms in the urine sample. If the urine were sterile (i.e. contained no bacteria), there would be no visible colonies: the culture medium would appear unchanged.

As previously stated it is quite normal for urine to contain small numbers of bacteria, mostly derived from the distal third of the urethra, so that the mere presence of bacteria in urine (bacteriuria) is not sufficient to make a diagnosis of UTI. The term 'significant bacteriuria' was first used in 1956 by Kass & Finland to diagnose UTI. They determined that, with some provisos, a bacterial count of more than 10^5 (i.e. 100 000) organisms per millilitre of urine was diagnostic of UTI. Although it has been demonstrated since that symptoms of UTI can occasionally occur when bacterial count drops as low as 10^3/ml and that some patients have no symptoms when their bacterial count is above 10^5/ml, Kass's dictum is still widely applied and a bacterial count of greater than 10^5/ml remains a working definition of urinary tract infection. By counting the number of colonies in culture grown from a known volume of urine, it is possible to deduce the original concentration of bacteria in the urine specimen.

Each colony is the product of division of a single bacterium, so each colony is pure (i.e. contains only one sort of bacterium). The macroscopic

'cont.'

'continued'

appearance of the colony provides some evidence of the sort of bacterium it contains but further testing is required for positive identification.

Although several types of bacteria are known to cause UTI, the commonest being *E. coli* (Table 20.2), it is very rare for the infected urinary tract of any one patient (except catheterised patients) to be colonised by more than one sort of bacterium. Thus the finding of many sorts of bacteria and no single one predominating (called a mixed bacterial growth), tends to indicate not that the urine tract is infected but rather that the urine has been contaminated with the mixture of bacteria normally present in the lower third of the urethra or genito-anal area. In other words the sample was not collected properly. A pure growth (i.e. growth of one type of bacteria) with a bacterial count of greater than 10^5 organisms/ml or urine is virtually diagnostic of urine tract infection.

Sensitivity. The results of this final test inform the decision about which antibiotic is to be prescribed in cases of bacterial infection. It is therefore a test which would not be performed if the results of urine culture revealed that the urine was sterile or contained insignificant numbers of bacteria. The object of the test is to determine the resistance or sensitivity to a range of antibiotics of the particular strain of bacteria causing the UTI. A bacterium is said to be resistant to an antibiotic if that antibiotic fails to kill it in culture. If prescribed, that particular antibiotic would not be effective in eradicating the infection. Conversely a strain of bacterium which is sensitive to a particular antibiotic will be killed by that antibiotic.

Essentially the test is performed by taking colonies of bacteria previously grown by culture of the urine specimen and re-inoculating these colonies on culture medium as before, but this time in the presence of a range of antibiotics. After a period of incubation the culture medium is inspected. If the strain is resistant to the antibiotic being tested, then no effect on bacterial growth is seen; the culture appears as it would if the antibiotic were not present. If, however, the bacteria are sensitive to the antibiotic being tested, there is no evidence of bacterial growth; the bacteria are killed and the culture medium appears as if no bacteria had been applied.

Since sensitivity testing involves a further period of incubation, there is an inevitable delay of up to 24 hours before the final report can be issued. If there is strong evidence of UTI at microscopy, that is, there is a high white cell count and bacteria are visible, some laboratories perform sensitivity tests on urine directly without waiting for the bacteria to grow in culture.

'cont.'

'continued'

INTERPRETATION OF RESULTS

- Pure growth of bacteria with a bacterial count of $> 10^5$ organisms/ml urine indicates *urinary tract infection*. Increase in the number of white cells (i.e. > 10 per mm^3 urine) provides supportive evidence.

- Pure growth of bacteria and a bacterial count of between 10^3 and 10^5 organisms/ml urine indicates an equivocal result: there may or may not be UTI. The presence of increased numbers of white cells (i.e. greater than 10 per mm^3 urine) supports a diagnosis of UTI. The higher the white cell count the stronger is the possibility of infection.

- Mixed bacterial growth indicates *probable contamination*, especially if epithelial cells are present. However, this mixed growth may be masking urinary tract infection caused by one type of bacterium within the mixed growth, particularly if the bacterial count is high (i.e. $> 10^5$ organisms/ml urine). A carefully collected repeat sample may be indicated. A normal white cell count tends to suggest there is no UTI, whereas a raised white cell count suggests there might be.

- Sterile urine (no bacteria detected) or a bacterial count of $< 10^3$/ml urine indicates *no evidence of UTI*. A white cell count of < 10 per mm^3 urine also indicates no evidence of UTI.

POST-TREATMENT TESTING

Symptoms of UTI may disappear within a few days of beginning a course of antibiotic therapy, but the only sure way of ensuring that a cure has been elicited is laboratory examination of urine. An MSU should be examined at around 1 week and 4 weeks after the course of antibiotics has been completed. If the bacteria which caused the infection cannot be isolated from urine by culture at these times, a cure can be assumed.

DIPSTICK TESTING FOR UTI

Rapid dipstick tests to screen for UTI are commercially available. These dipstick methods are widely used in the GP's surgery and side room by nursing and medical staff; they provide almost instant results. They are used for the rapid detection of bacteria and white cells in urine.

All of the common bacteria which cause UTI convert nitrate present in urine to nitrite, so an increase in nitrite concentration of urine indicates bacterial infection. This is the basis of the dipstick method for detection of bacteria in urine. The enzyme leucocyte esterase is present only in white

'cont.'

'continued'

cells. Detection of this enzyme in urine indicates the presence of white cells. The chemicals necessary for nitrite and leucocyte esterase detection are packaged on two pads on the dipstick. The dipstick is merely dipped in a freshly voided urine and the two pads are inspected for a colour change, indicating the presence of bacteria, white cells or both.

Although extremely convenient, these rapid dipstick methods have limitations. The number of false positive results associated with their use are unacceptably high to make a definitive diagnosis of UTI.[5] In any case, without culture of the urine it is not possible to identify the bacteria and perform sensitivity studies. All urines found to be positive with the dipstick test should be submitted to the laboratory for full urine culture and sensitivity.

Many studies have, however, concluded that a negative result using the dipstick method is reliable.[5,6] So long as the manufacturer's instructions are followed to the letter, the finding of no bacteria or white cells in urine by the rapid dipstick test (i.e. the absence of a colour change) is strong evidence that the patient is not suffering a UTI. Unless there is strong clinical evidence suggestive of UTI, most authorities agree that such negative urines need not normally be submitted for full microbiological examination.

CASE HISTORY 19

Hayley Smith is a 24-year-old mother of two who is 16 weeks pregnant. At her most recent routine antenatal care appointment she was asked to provide a midstream urine (MSU) specimen for microscopy, culture and sensitivity (M, C & S).

A few days later the laboratory report of this test is received. The report includes the following results:

WBC: < 5 /mm3
RBC: < 5/mm3
Urine culture: $< 10^3$ bacteria/ml 'mixed coliform growth'

(1) Why is an examination of MSU a routine part of antenatal care?
(2) Do the results suggest Hayley is suffering a urinary tract infection?

Table 20.1   Collection of a 'clean-catch' midstream urine (MSU) specimen

Object: To collect a specimen of bladder urine uncontaminated by bacteria which may be present

- on skin
- in external genital tract
- on peri-anal region
- in distal third of urethra
- and in the environment (on surfaces, outside of collection bottle, etc.)

Principle: Any bacteria present in the urethra are washed away in the first portion of urine voided. This is not collected. All other potential contamination is avoided by thorough cleansing and good clean aseptic technique

Protocol for women:

(1)   Wash hands thoroughly with soap and water and dry.
(2)   With one hand spread the labia.
(3)   Area around the urinary meatus must be cleansed from front to back with soap and water and dried.
(4)   Still with labia separated, the patient voids the first 20 ml or so of urine into the toilet bowl and then collects a portion of the remaining urine into a *sterile* universal container.
(5)   Screw on cap of urine bottle immediately, taking care not to touch either the rim of the bottle or the inside of the bottle cap.

Protocol for men:

(1)   Wash hands thoroughly with soap and water and dry.
(2)   Retract foreskin and clean around the urinary meatus with soap and water.
(3)   Patient passes the first 20 ml or so into the toilet bowl and collects a portion of the remaining urine into a *sterile* universal container.
(4)   Screw on cap of bottle immediately, taking care not to touch either the inside rim of the bottle or the inside of the cap.

Discussion of case history

(1)   Pregnancy is normally associated with changes in the gross structure of the urinary tract, in part caused by compression of the
growing uterus on the kidneys and lower urinary tract. The ureters
are elongated, widen and become more curved. One effect of these
changes is a relative urine stasis (urine flow is not as efficient as
usual) and a higher than normal risk of infection of the lower
urinary tract spreading upwards to the kidneys with resulting
infection of the kidney (pyelonephritis). An estimated 20–40% of
pregnant women with significant bacteriuria, early in pregnancy,
even if asymptomatic, will go on to develop pyelonephritis later in
pregnancy if the bacteria are not quickly eliminated with antibiotic

Table 20.2   Most common causes of urinary tract infection

Bacteria	Normally present in	% of UTI acquired in community	% of UTI acquired in hospital
Escherichia coli (*E. coli*)	GI tract: faeces	75–80	50–60
Staphylococcus epidermis (*S. epidermis*)	Skin External genital tract	5–10	< 5
Staphylococcus saprophyticus (*S. saprophyticus*)	GI tract: faeces	5–10	< 5
Proteus species	GI tract: faeces; hospital environment	< 5	10–15
Klebsiella species	GI tract: faeces; external genital tract	< 5	10–15
Pseudomonas aeruginosa (*P. aeruginosa*)	GI tract: faeces (rarely) hospital environment	<5	5–10
Other (many species)		< 5	5–10

therapy. Pyelonephritis is a serious infection which may lead to renal failure. Babies of mothers suffering pyelonephritis during pregnancy may be born prematurely or have a low birth weight. To prevent pyelonephritis, all pregnant women are screened for evidence of urinary tract infection. Since significant bacteriuria may occur without any symptoms, testing in this context should not be confined to those who have symptomatic UTI.

(2)   Despite the finding of bacteria in Hayley's urine, there is no evidence of infection. The numbers of bacteria are not significant and those discovered are a mixed growth of many sorts of bacteria suggesting contamination of the specimen with bacteria normally present in the lower part of the urethra or the perianal region. There is also no increase in the number of white blood cells in Hayley's urine, providing further evidence that her urinary tract is not infected.

References

(1) Neu H. (1992) Urinary tract infections *Amer. J. Med.* **92** (suppl. 4A): 63–9.

(2) Turk M. & Stamm W. (1981) Nosocomial urine infection. *Amer. J. Med.* **70**: 651–4.

(3) Shroder F. (1994) Microscopic haematuria: requires investigation. *BMJ* **309**: 70–72.

(4) Kass E.H. & Finland M. (1956) Asymptomatic infection of the urinary tract. *Trans. Assoc. Am. Physicians* **69**: 56–64.

(5) Fowlis G., Waters J. & Williams G. (1994) The cost effectiveness of combined rapid tests (Multistix) in screening for urine tract infections. *J. Roy. Soc. Med.* **87**: 681–82.

(6) Hiscoke C., Yoxall H. *et al.* (1990) Validation of a method for the rapid diagnosis of urinary tract infection suitable for use in general practice. *Br. J. Gen. Pract.* **40**: 403–5.

Further reading

DeGroot-Kosolcharoen (1996) Culture and sensitivity testing. *Nursing 96* **9**: 33–8.

Saint S. & Lipsky B. (1999) Preventing catheter-related bacteriuria. *Arch. Int. Med.* **159**: 800–8.

Shanson D. (1989) Infections of the urinary tract. In: *Microbiology in Clinical Practice*, 2nd edn, pp. 430–51. Butterworth, London.

Stickle V. (1993) *Microbiology for Nurses*, 7th edn. Baillière-Tindall, London.

Winn W. (1993) Diagnosis of urine tract infection – a modern Procrustean bed. *Amer. J. Clin. Pathol.* **99**: 117–19.

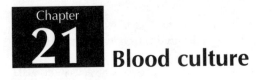

21 Blood culture

In this second of two chapters devoted to the work of the clinical microbiology laboratory, attention is focused on blood culture, a test used to confirm or exclude the presence of bacteria in blood (bacteraemia). Blood culture is useful in three broad clinical contexts. The first is among patients who are suspected of suffering septicaemia (overwhelming bacterial infection of the bloodstream). Secondly there are several infectious diseases that are caused by spread of bacteria via the bloodstream. These diseases, which include endocarditis (infection of the valves of the heart), osteomyelitis (infection of bone), and infective arthritis (infection of joints), are characterised not necessarily by septicaemia but by low grade bacteraemia. A positive blood culture provides supportive evidence for diagnosis of these conditions. The third group of patients who are likely to have their blood cultured are those with PUO (pyrexia of unknown origin). This is usually defined as a raised body temperature for more than ten days, with no immediate explanation. The clinical investigation of a patient with PUO routinely includes a blood culture in the search for an infective cause of pyrexia.

Normal physiology

Blood is normally sterile (contains no bacteria). However, normal life is associated with the risk of circulating blood coming into contact with bacteria, and transient bacteraemia may occur from time to time without ill effect. For example, the bacteria normally present in the mouth have access to the bloodstream during dental surgery; transient bacteraemia invariably follows dental surgery. Even vigorous chewing has been shown to facilitate entry to the bloodstream of bacteria normally present in the mouth. Likewise a 'dirty' cut allows access to the bloodstream of environmental bacteria and bacteria normally present on the skin. Small numbers of bacteria may enter the bloodstream from an existing infection site (e.g. the urinary tract, the respiratory tract, a wound infection, etc.). Despite scrupulous aseptic technique, any surgical procedure may be associated with passage of small numbers of bacteria from sites (e.g. the skin), where bacteria are normally present in abundance, to the bloodstream. It is the innate and acquired immune defences of the blood that maintain its sterility and prevent transient bacteraemia, which inevitably occurs from time to time, from developing into infection of the blood (septicaemia).

Innate immune defences in blood

Innate immunity is the sum of the protective mechanisms against infection with which we are born. One of the principal functions of the skin, for example, is to act as a physical barrier to invading organisms; in this way skin contributes to the body's innate immune defence. The most significant innate immune defence within blood is the neutrophils, phagocytic white blood cells. These cells engulf invading bacteria by the process of phagocytosis. Once phagocytosed, bacteria are killed by enzymes and highly reactive 'free radical' chemicals produced within the neutrophil. The process of phagocytosis is greatly enhanced by the so-called complement proteins, which also make a significant contribution to innate immunity. The production of these blood proteins is activated by some species of invading bacteria. One of the complement proteins, known as C3b, binds to bacteria. Bacteria which are coated with C3b are much more easily phagocytosed by neutrophils. Other complement proteins (C6, C7, C8 and C9), kill or damage some species of bacteria directly by insertion in bacterial membranes, and some (e.g. C5a) act by attracting neutrophils towards bacteria, thus enhancing phagocytosis.

Acquired immune defences in blood

Acquired immunity is very specific and can only arise after initial infection; we are not born with this form of immune defence. Acquired immunity against bacterial invasion of blood depends on lymphocytes, another type of white blood cell. Bacterial invasion results in production of specific antibodies (immunoglobulins) to the bacteria by B-lymphocytes. Antibody binds to the bacteria which induced its B-lymphocyte production. This antibody binding of bacteria has two effects: it enhances neutrophil phagocytosis of bacteria, and in some cases antibody binding is required for complement-mediated killing of the bacteria. Many bacteria produce chemical toxins; antibody acts to neutralise these toxins. Antibody also activates the production of the protective complement proteins by an alternative pathway to that of complement activation by bacteria.

Thus, by a synergy of innate and acquired immune effects, bacteria present in blood are destroyed and blood remains essentially sterile.

Septicaemia

Predisposing factors

If bacteria invade the bloodstream and the normal defences against invasion are overwhelmed, bacteria multiply and infection of the bloodstream (septicaemia) occurs. Contributory factors to development of septicaemia include

■ reduced host defence
■ an existing focus of infection
■ the virulence of the invasive organism
■ hospital procedures which facilitate entry of bacteria to the bloodstream.

Reduced host defences

Any condition associated with reduced immune (either innate or acquired) defence against bacterial infection predisposes to septicaemia. Severe immunosuppression associated with conditions such as AIDS and the use of immunosuppressive and cytotoxic drugs (which result in a marked reduction in production of white blood cells by the bone marrow) greatly predispose to bacterial infection of the blood by opportunistic bacteria (i.e. bacteria of low virulence which in healthy individuals would cause no problem). In fact any severe debilitating illness (e.g. cancer, renal failure, heart failure, etc.) or major trauma including surgery is associated with some degree of reduction in the normal immune response to infection. Premature babies have an underdeveloped immune system and are particularly prone to infection during the first few months of life. Response to infection is less effective in the very elderly. Finally diabetic patients are more at risk of some bacterial infections spreading to the bloodstream than non-diabetics.

Existing focus of infection

In most cases of septicaemia, there is a pre-existing infection at some site (called the focus of infection) in the body. Bacteria from this primary site invade the blood. If the organisms are not susceptible to the bactericidal (bacteria-killing) action of blood, or the numbers of organisms are overwhelming, bacteria multiply within the bloodstream with resulting septicaemia. The most common foci of infection in patients suffering septicaemia are the lower respiratory tract and the urinary tract, but bacteria may enter the blood from any site of infection and, if the conditions are 'right', multiply within the bloodstream.

Virulence of invading organism

The vulnerability of bacteria to blood defences varies between species so that, for example, gram-positive bacteria are generally speaking resistant to the bactericidal properties of antibody and complement, although they are vulnerable to phagocytosis. This variation determines that invasion by some strains of bacteria (highly virulent bacteria) are more likely to result in septicaemia than others of low virulence. However, if there is an established focus of infection in the body and/or the patient's defences are severely impaired, any species of bacteria, no matter what its virulence, can cause septicaemia. In fact although only a few species of bacteria cause most cases of septicaemia, all species of pathogenic (disease causing) bacteria and even some normally non-pathogenic species can cause septicaemia if present in large enough numbers and if host (patient) immune defences are sufficiently debilitated.

Hospital procedures that facilitate entry of bacteria to the bloodstream

Around 60% of all patients with septicaemia acquire the infection whilst in hospital.[1] Patients at greatest risk of hospital-acquired (nosocomial) septicaemia are those who are subjected to surgical procedures, intravenous and urinary catheterisation, cystoscopy and other operative invasive interventions. An infected intravenous catheter is the focus of infection in around 20% of all patients suffering hospital-acquired septicaemia, and most of those patients with hospital-acquired septicaemia, whose focus of infection is the urinary tract have been catheterised or have had their urinary tract investigated using a cystoscope. Surgery of areas which are normally heavily contaminated with bacteria (e.g. the mouth, the colon and the genital area) carry the highest risk of post-operative septicaemia.

Causative bacteria

In each case of septicaemia a single species of bacteria is invariably the cause; only rarely (less than 8% of all cases) is more than one species causative. All pathogenic (disease causing) bacteria and, rarely, some usually non-pathogenic bacteria, have been implicated as the cause of septicaemia in particular cases. There are, however, a few species of bacteria which account for the majority of cases.

The commonest cause of septicaemia is the gram-negative organism *Escherichia coli (E. coli)*.[1] Infection with this organism accounts for 20–25% of all cases of septicaemia. *E. coli* is normally present in the gut and is responsible for most cases of urinary tract infection. The focus of infection in cases of *E. coli* septicaemia is usually the urinary tract, or urinary catheter.

Staphylococcus aureus and *Streptococcus pneumoniae* are the two most common gram-positive bacteria to cause septicaemia. *Staphylococcus aureus*, a gram-positive coccus, is present without ill effect in the nose of between 20 and 30% of the population; it may also be found on the moist skin of 5–10% of healthy individuals. It is, however, also a common pathogen of the skin, being responsible for superficial skin infections such as boils and carbuncles. Surgical and trauma-induced wound infections are frequently caused by *Staph. aureus*, and this organism is responsible for most (> 80%) cases of bone infection (osteomyelitis) and joint infection (septic arthritis). In between 15 and 20% of cases, septicaemia is caused by infection with *Staph aureus*; the most common foci of infection are infected wounds and infected intravenous catheters.

Streptococcus pneumoniae, also a gram-positive coccus, is present in the mouth and nose of normally healthy people but is the most significant bacterial cause of the common lower respiratory tract infection, pneumonia. It is the causative organism in around 10% of all cases of septicaemia; almost all of these are the result of spread of the organism to blood from infected respiratory tract in patients suffering pneumonia. Together, then, these three organisms (*E. coli. Staph. aureus* and *Strep. pneumoniae*) account for just over half of all cases of septicaemia. In excess of 150 different species of bacteria are the cause in the remainder of cases. Of these the most significant are:

- *Klebsiella* and *Proteus* species which, like *E. coli*, are both gram-negative bacilli, normally present in the gut and a frequent cause of urinary tract infection.
- *Staph. epidermis*, a gram-positive coccus found in abundance on the skin and inside the nose of normal healthy individuals, is the

organism most often implicated in cases of septicaemia caused by infection of intravenous catheters.

■ *Pseudomonas aeruginosa*, a gram-negative bacillus, is an environmental pathogen which thrives on moist surfaces; this organism is frequently found contaminating the hospital environment, surfaces, equipment, etc. Most cases of septicaemia caused by this organism are related to infected venous or urinary catheters.

■ *Neisseria meningitidis* is a gram-negative diplococcus, present without harmful effect in the nose and throat of up to a fifth of the population. However, it is the most common cause of bacterial meningitis (infection of the central nervous system). If the causative organism is *N. menigitidis* the condition is known as meningococcal meningitis. In most cases of meningococcal meningitis, the organism spreads via the bloodstream from nose and throat to meninges. Meningococcal septicaemia is a life-threatening complication of meningococcal meningitis.

■ *Haemophillus influenzae* is a gram-negative bacillus normally present in the upper respiratory tract. This organism is a common cause of lower respiratory tract infection (bronchitis and pneumonia). Spread to the bloodstream it causes septicaemia. In young children this is one of the most common bacteria to cause septicaemia; in such blood-infected children the organism can spread via the blood to meninges causing meningitis. Among adults the most common focus of infection in cases of *H. influenzae* septicaemia is the lower respiratory tract and in young children there are two main foci of infection; the lower respiratory tract and the meninges.

■ *Strep. 'viridans'* is not one but a group of several bacterial species (all gram-positive cocci) which are present in abundance in the mouth of healthy individuals. They are the most significant causative organisms in bacterial endocarditis, an infection of the heart valves which is caused by spread of bacteria via the bloodstream from mouth to heart. The isolation of this organism from blood culture provides supportive evidence for a diagnosis of bacterial endocarditis.

Symptoms of septicaemia

Symptoms mostly result from the release of chemical mediators of the inflammatory response by phagocytic cells recruited to fight the infection. The cardinal symptoms of septicaemia are:

■ fever (body temperature $> 38°C$)
■ rigors (shivering chills)

- tachycardia (heart rate > 95 beats/min)
- alteration of mental state (confusion, apprehension).

If not checked with immediate antibiotic therapy, septicaemia may develop quickly to septic shock.

Septic shock

Although progression from septicaemia to septic shock is not inevitable, (it occurs in around 20% of cases), such progression is associated with a marked increase in mortality. In one study, gram-negative septicaemia uncomplicated by shock resulted in only 7% mortality compared with 47% among patients whose septicaemia developed to septic shock.[2] As a rough guide around half of all patients who suffer septic shock, die. In the intensive care setting, where most patients with septicaemia are cared for, septic shock is a major if not the most common cause of death.[3] Although more common in patients infected with gram-negative organisms, septic shock may also complicate gram-positive septicaemia. Whilst antibiotic therapy is effective in combating the underlying infection and preventing septic shock arising, it has little or no effect in combating septic shock. This is because shock is caused not directly by the bacteria themselves, but largely by the body's response to bacterial infection. A destructive cascade of chemical release by the body's own cells (monocytes, macrophages, etc.) recruited to fight the infection, accompanies release of toxins from invading bacteria. Among the many chemicals released from the body's own cells is tumour necrosis factor (TNF) and interleukin 1 (IL-1). Recent research[4] has implicated these two proteins and endotoxin (released from the walls of dying gram-negative bacteria) as particularly significant in the pathogenesis of septic shock. Damage, mediated by these chemicals, to the cells which line the internal surface of blood vessels (the vascular endothelium) results in disruption of the microvascular circulation. The tiny vessels of the microvasculature become dilated and leaky. The combination of hypovolaemia (low blood volume due to leaky vessels) and vessel dilatation causes a reduction in blood pressure (hypotension), the most significant clinical sign of septic shock. The resulting reduced blood supply to all tissue cells leads to hypoxia (relative oxygen deficiency) and tissue death. All organs may be affected, and without successful treatment multiple organ dysfunction progresses to multiple organ failure and death.

Damage to vascular endothelium not only results in hypotension but also triggers the clotting cascade, leading to inappropriate coagulation of blood within blood vessels, a condition known as disseminated intravascular coagulation (DIC). This exhausts available clotting factors and platelets, resulting in an increased tendency to bleed and a high risk of fatal haemorrhage. The immediate cause of death for many patients with septic shock is intracerebral haemorrhage.

Clinical signs and symptoms of septic shock

A patient in septic shock will usually display all the signs and symptoms of septicaemia plus, most crucially:

- hypotension (systolic pressure < 90 mmHg, diastolic < 60 mmHg).

Consequent impaired blood flow to all parts of the body may result in:

- low urine output – indicating renal failure
- cyanosis – indicating respiratory failure
- jaundice – indicating liver failure.

Disseminated intravascular coagulation results in:

- reduced platelets and clotting proteins
- increased tendency to bleed.

PRINCIPLES OF MICROBIOLOGICAL EXAMINATION OF BLOOD

The primary objective of the laboratory is to determine if a patient's blood contains bacteria. It is not possible to confirm or exclude the presence of bacteria in blood by simply examining a sample under the microscope; there simply are not sufficient bacteria present. Instead bacteria must first be grown (cultured) in a liquid (called the culture medium) which contains the nutrients necessary for bacteria to grow and multiply. The culture medium containing the blood sample is incubated at 37°C, the optimum temperature for bacterial growth, until there is evidence of such growth. This usually takes between 12 and 24 hours but may take days or even, very rarely, weeks for particularly slow growing species. In practice, if there is no evidence of bacterial growth after 3 days' incubation, it is highly unlikely that the culture (and therefore the blood sample added to the culture

'cont.'

'continued'

medium) contains any bacteria. However, the culture continues to be inspected for longer to allow for the possibility that rare, slow growing species were present in the blood sample.

As soon as there is evidence of bacterial growth, a sample of the culture, now rich in bacteria, is stained and examined under the microscope. This provides the first evidence of the identity of the species of bacteria present (e.g. whether gram-positive or negative, cocci or bacilli, etc.). More precise identification may require that the liquid culture be further grown (sub-cultured) on a solid culture medium in a petri dish. This allows the growth of visible, pure colonies of bacteria, each colony being the product of multiplication of a single bacterium. A sample of the visible colony is then subjected to a range of chemical tests which finally determine the identity of the bacteria it contains.

Having isolated and identified the bacteria present in the culture, the final step is sensitivity testing. This involves testing the bacteria isolated in culture for reaction with a range of antibiotics to establish which antibiotic is likely to be most effective in combating this particular infection.

Septicaemia is a life-threatening condition which requires immediate antibiotic treatment. It is not practicable therefore to wait for the results of laboratory tests before starting treatment, and initial antibiotic therapy must be based on the clinical history, which provides important clues as to the likely nature of the invading bacterial species. However, when the results of laboratory tests, particularly sensitivity testing, become available (usually within two to three days) antibiotic therapy can be altered if necessary.

SAMPLE COLLECTION

The objective: to introduce a sample of the patient's blood into culture bottles without *any* bacterial contamination (e.g. from environment, or from operators' or patient's skin, etc.).

TIMING OF SAMPLING

Blood for culture should be sampled before administration of antibiotic therapy as antibiotics may delay or prevent bacterial growth causing falsely negative results. For patients with intermittent fever, blood should ideally be taken while temperature is rising, or as soon after the spike of temperature as is possible, when the bacteria are present in blood at highest con-centration. Many laboratories recommend taking a second sample not less than one hour after the first to increase the chances of recovering bacteria and to distinguish true bacteraemia (which would be present in both culture sets) from bacterial contamination.

'cont.'

'continued'

BLOOD CULTURE BOTTLES

Blood must be collected into specially designated blood culture bottles. There are several commercially available blood culture systems, but they all contain a sterile liquid mixture of nutrients (called the culture medium) necessary for bacterial growth. Most laboratories supply two blood culture bottles per blood culture set. The first has oxygen in the space above the culture medium to allow growth of those species of bacteria which require oxygen. The second bottle has a mixture of gases without oxygen. This bottle is required for culture of anaerobic bacteria (i.e. bacteria which only grow best in an oxygen-free environment). A sample of blood must be introduced into both bottles.

VOLUME OF BLOOD REQUIRED

In a patient with bacteraemia there may be as few as one bacterium per millilitre of blood so a falsely negative result can occur if insufficient blood is introduced into the culture bottle. Paradoxically, a false negative result can also occur if too much blood is introduced. This is because blood continues to have a bactericidal effect in culture. This effect is diluted out in the liquid culture medium. A compromise must be sought between too small a volume of blood, which might well contain insufficient bacteria, and too large a volume, which would remove the dilution effect of the culture medium on the bactericidal property of blood. An approximate 1:10 dilution of blood in culture medium is optimal but the actual volume required (usually between 5 and 10 ml) depends on the blood culture system being used. It is vital that no less than the local laboratory recommended minimum volume of blood be sampled for each culture bottle.

TECHNIQUE

Aseptic technique is essential throughout the procedure to ensure that no bacterial contamination of the culture occurs. If successful, the only bacteria (if any) in the culture bottle will be those originally present in the patient's blood.

- Blood should be sampled from a peripheral vein, never via an indwelling catheter, which might itself be contaminated with bacteria.
- With sterile gloved or well washed hands, the venepuncture site must be cleansed with 2% tincture of iodine or some other suitable disinfectant. The iodine should be removed after a minute or two with 70% alcohol, ensuring that the site is dry. The top of both blood culture

'cont.'

'continued'

bottles through which the sample is introduced must be similarly disinfected.

■ Taking care not to touch the venepuncture site, blood is collected using a sterile syringe and needle.

■ The needle on the syringe must be changed before injecting the required volume of blood into the blood culture bottle via the rubber septum in the blood culture top. This minimises the risk of bacteria present on the needle as a result of contact with the patient's skin being transferred to the culture. Never remove the top of a blood culture bottle. This would expose the culture to environmental bacteria.

■ If blood is being collected for other tests, always inoculate blood culture bottles first to prevent bacteria present in other specimen bottles being transferred to the culture.

■ Blood culture bottles must be carefully labelled with patient details and sent along with the appropriate request card to the laboratory without delay. If blood is collected out of normal laboratory hours blood cultures must be placed in a specially designated 37°C incubator so that bacterial growth can begin. It is important to record on the request card outline clinical details and any antibiotic therapy if given before blood sampling.

BLOOD CULTURE REPORTS

Interim reports of progress in examination of a blood culture are usually issued daily. A final report will include the identity of any bacteria recovered from the culture, along with a report of the sensitivity or resistance of that particular strain to a range of antibiotics.

Results of blood culture fall into one of three main groups:

■ blood culture negative – no bacterial growth
■ blood culture positive – pure growth
■ blood culture positive – mixed bacterial growth

Blood culture negative. This is a normal result, that is, one which would be obtained from a person whose blood was sterile (contained no bacteria). Before a negative culture result is interpreted in this way it is important to consider the possibility that the result is falsely negative, i.e. the patient has bacteraemia but the test has failed to detect it. Causes of false negative results include

■ insufficient blood added to culture bottle
■ antibiotic therapy administered before blood sampled

'cont.'

'continued'

■ incubation period insufficient for growth of rare, slow-growing organisms.

Blood culture positive – pure growth. This means that a pure growth of a single identified species of bacteria (e.g. *E. coli, Strep. pneumoniae, Staph. aureus*, etc.) was isolated from the culture. This is the result which would be expected from a patient with septicaemia or bacteraemia. However, in around 10–20% of positive blood cultures, the bacterium isolated and identified is not derived from the patient's blood but is present as a result of bacterial contamination of the culture, due, most often, to poor aseptic technique at the time of sample collection. Since all species of bacteria have been implicated as a cause of septicaemia at one time or another, it is sometimes difficult to decide whether a positive blood culture is due to contamination (false positive) or reflects septicaemia or bacteraemia (true positive).

To illustrate this, suppose a blood culture yields a pure growth of the organism *Staph. epidermis.* This organism, which is normally present in abundance on the skin of us all, could quite easily be transferred from the skin of patient or staff to blood culture during the process of blood collection. In fact, it is one of the most common organisms to contaminate blood cultures. However, *Staph. epidermis* is also a quite common cause of septicaemia among patients whose focus of infection is an infected catheter. It is also the most significant cause of endocarditis among patients who have received heart surgery. The finding may reflect contamination, but in some circumstances can be of clinical significance.

It is bacteria such as *Staph. epidermis* which are part of the normal resident flora of skin that usually contaminate blood cultures. A pure growth of any organism in blood culture is more likely to be due to bacteraemia than contamination, if:

■ the same organism has been isolated from the same patient at some other infected site
■ the same organism is isolated from repeated blood cultures

Blood culture positive – mixed growth. This result indicates that more than one sort (species) of bacteria was isolated from the blood culture. It is rare for blood to be infected by more than one species of bacteria, although it may occur. A mixed growth of bacteria is strong evidence that the culture was contaminated, particularly if they are bacteria which normally inhabit the skin.

Case history 20

Until the evening prior to admission to hospital, 18-year-old Kevin Thomas was a fit and healthy student. On that evening he went to bed early complaining of a headache; he was also feverish. The next morning his mother, a nurse, went to check on him. He was clearly very ill, moaning quietly, with a very high temperature. He had vomited during the night. Mrs Thomas was so alarmed by Kevin's condition that she took him straight to the local A&E department where she worked, believing that he might be suffering from meningitis. On admission Kevin's temperature was 40°C, his heart rate was 126 and he was becoming increasingly drowsy. A rash was noted on Kevin's legs. Blood was sampled for among other tests, blood culture. In view of his rapidly deteriorating condition Kevin was given broad spectrum antibiotics intravenously and admitted to the intensive care unit. The next day the laboratory reported the presence of gram-negative bacteria in the culture of Kevin's blood which were later identified as *Neisseria meningitidis*.

(1) What was the diagnosis?
(2) What other serious infectious disease is caused by the same organism isolated from Kevin's blood?
(3) Is it possible to isolate the organism causing Kevin's illness from normally healthy individuals?

Discussion of case history

(1) Kevin was suffering from meningococcal septicaemia, a life-threatening infection of the bloodstream with the bacterium, *Neisseria meningitidis*.
(2) The same organism is one of the three main causes of bacterial meningitis; the other two organisms are *Haemophilus influenzae* and *Streptococcus pneumoniae*. When the causative organism is *N. meningitidis*, the condition is known as meningococcal meningitis. The majority of cases of meningococcal meningitis are accompanied by symptoms of meningococcal septicaemia, but in recent years there has been an increase in the number of patients whose infection is confined to blood and who have, like Kevin, no infection of the meninges.
(3) Yes. *Neisseria meningitidis* is present in the nose and throat of around 10–20% of the population.

References

(1) Eykyn S., Gransden W. & Phillips I. (1990) The causative organisms of septicaemia and their epidemiology. *J. Antimicrobial Chemotherapy* **25** (suppl. C): 41–58.

(2) Easmon C. (1990) Pathogenesis of septicaemia *J. Antimicrobial Chemotherapy* **25** (suppl. C): 9–16.

(3) Parillo J., Parker M., Natanson C., Suffredini A. *et al.* (1990) Septic shock in humans: advances in the understanding of pathogenesis, cardiovascular dysfunction, and therapy. *Ann. Intern. Med.* **113**: 227–42.

(4) Fagan E. & Singer M. (1995) Immunotherapy in the management of sepsis. *Postgrad. Med. J.* **71**: 71–8.

Further reading

Bihari D. (1990) Septicaemia – the clinical diagnosis. *J. Antimicrobial Chemother.* **25** (Suppl C): 1–7.

Edgeworth J., Treacher D. & Eykyn S. (1999) A 25-year study of nosocomial bacteraemia in an adult intensive care unit. *Crit. Care Med.* **27**: 1421–8.

Shanson D. (1989) Septicaemia. In: *Microbiology in Clinical Practice*, pp. 138–50. Butterworth, London.

Shifman R., Strand C., Meier F. & Howanitz P. (1998) Blood culture contamination. A College of American Pathologists Q-Probes study involving 640 institutions and 497 134 specimens from adult patients. *Arch. Pathol. Lab. Med.* **122**: 216–21.

Stucke V. (1993) *Microbiology for Nurses*, 7th edn. Baillière-Tindall, London.

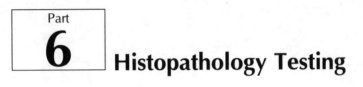

Part 6

Histopathology Testing

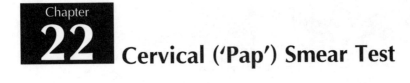

Cervical ('Pap') Smear Test

The purpose of most clinical laboratory tests is to aid clinical diagnosis and monitor the progress of disease or the effectiveness of therapy. By contrast, the purpose of the test which is the subject of this chapter is to prevent disease. The cervical smear test involves the microscopical examination of cells recovered by scraping the surface of the cervix. Abnormal changes in the appearance of these cells occurs up to 10–15 years before cancer of the cervix develops. Since early treatment of these changes prevents cervical cancer developing, all women are actively encouraged to have the test at regular intervals. In England and Wales around 4.5 million cervical smears are examined in laboratories every year.[1] This work accounts for a significant proportion of the total workload of cytopathology departments.

Normal physiology

The cervix

Anatomy

The cervix (from the Greek meaning 'neck' or 'neck-like') is part of the female genital tract. It is a tubular structure around 4 cm in length that forms the lower part or neck of the uterus, connecting the uterus to the vagina. There are four main anatomical features (Fig. 22.1) which comprise the cervix. The ectocervix is the lower part of the cervix which extends into the vaginal canal. At the centre of the ectocervix is the external os, the tiny opening to the endocervical canal. The endocervical canal is the tubular structure of the cervix which opens at the internal os to the body of the uterus.

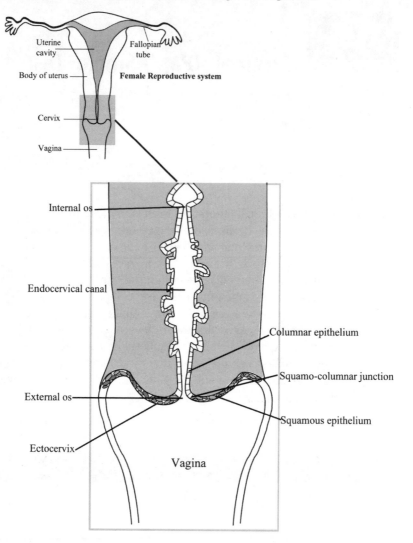

Fig. 22.1   The cervix.

As the connection between uterus and vagina, the endocervical canal is the first part of the birth canal. Late in pregnancy the normally tough and fibrous cervix softens or 'ripens', allowing it to dilate to several times its normal diameter for passage of the developed foetus from uterus to vagina during birth.

Cervical epithelium

The surface of the cervix is covered with a protective layer of epithelium. It is the epithelial cells, which make up this protective layer that are sampled in a cervical smear test. In the case of the cervix there are two sorts of epithelium: squamous epithelium covers the ectocervix, whilst columnar epithelium lines the endocervical canal. Four distinct layers of squamous epithelium can be distinguished on the surface of the ecto- cervix. The deepest of these is the basal layer, which comprises one row of immature squamous (basal) epithelial cells. Above this is the para- basal layer: two rows of immature squamous (parabasal) cells, which are constantly dividing to maintain the epithelium above. The intermediate layer comprises four to six rows of more mature cells, and the most mature squamous epithelial cells are those within the five to eight rows of the superficial layer. Cells in this superficial layer become increas- ingly less attached to each other and are cast off from the surface of the ectocervix by a process called desquamation or exfoliation. Constant regeneration of squamous epithelial cells in the basal layers is required to replace those that are lost from the surface of the ectocervix in exfoliation. Most of the squamous epithelial cells recovered in a cervical smear are from the superficial and intermediate layer. Cells from the parabasal layer constitute only around 5% of all squamous epithelial cells in a normal smear from a young woman. The cells in smears from older women contain slightly more parabasal cells, and disease of the cervix is associated with a significant increase in the number of parabasal cells in a cervical smear. Because of their relative depth, basal cells are rarely seen in a cervical smear.

The mucous-secreting columnar epithelium of the endocervical canal is composed simply of one row of columnar epithelial cells; some are mucus secreting and others have cilia on their surface. The mucus and cilia are thought to facilitate the passage of spermatozoa through the endocervical canal. When columnar epithelial cells are seen in a cervical smear, they are referred to as endocervical cells.

The squamo-columnar junction

The point where the squamous epithelium of the ectocervix meets the columnar epithelium of the endocervical canal is called the squamo- columnar junction (Fig. 22.1). This junction is of great pathological significance because it is here that most cases of cervical cancer origi- nate. Before puberty the junction lies at the external os (Fig. 22.2) but in response to the normal hormonal changes that occur at puberty, the

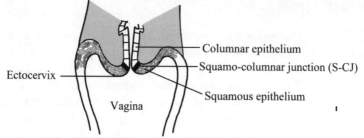

Ectocervix —

Columnar epithelium

Squamo-columnar junction (S-CJ)

Squamous epithelium

Vagina

Before puberty S-C junction at the external os

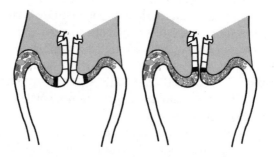

During reproductive age the S-J junction moves on to the ectocervix with formation of transformation zone (ectropion)

At the menopause S-C junction retreats into the endocervical canal

Fig. 22.2 Location of the squamo-columnar junction at different stages of a woman's life.

columnar epithelium of the endocervical canal grows outward so that the junction is on the ectocervix. The growth of columnar epithelial cells from the endocervical canal on to the ectocervix is called an ectropion. There is, then, a transformation as squamous epithelium grows over this columnar epithelium. The area of the ectocervix where this transformation of columnar epithelium to squamous epithelium occurs is called the transformation zone. Epithelial cells which are undergoing this transformation are called squamous metaplastic cells. At the menopause the squamo-columnar junction usually retreats into the endocervical canal.

Cancer of the cervix

Invasive cancer

Every year around 3000 women in England are told they have invasive cancer of the cervix. The annual death toll is close to 1100.[1] The disease is most often diagnosed after the age of 35 years, but younger women – as long as they are of reproductive age – are also at risk. The incidence of cervical cancer is increasing among younger women. The cause or causes of cervical cancer have not been established but there is much evidence to suggest that a sexually transmitted agent is involved. Early age of first sexual intercourse, a large number of sexual partners and sexual intercourse with a man who himself has had many sexual partners, all independently increase the risk of cervical cancer. Cervical cancer is rare among virgins. There is now convincing evidence that certain types of human papilloma virus (HPV), a sexually transmitted virus that can cause genital wart infections, is at least partly responsible in most cases. Oncogenic (cancer causing) DNA from HPV types 16 or 18 is present in the cells of over 80% of invasive cancers of the cervix,[2] suggesting that HPV infection is important for malignant transformation of normal cervical cells. Despite the emerging significance of HPV infection, it is important to remember that not all women who are infected with HPV go on to develop cervical cancer (it is only HPV types 16 and 18 which are significant), and not all women with cervical cancer have evidence of being infected with the virus.

Other significant risk factors include cigarette smoking, use of oral contraceptives and social class (incidence of and mortality from cancer of the cervix is highest in those of low socio-economic status).

There are no symptoms of early cervical cancer. The first sign of a problem is usually vaginal discharge or abnormal vaginal bleeding; some women experience discomfort during sexual intercourse. The prognosis for a woman with invasive cancer of the cervix depends, as with many other cancers, on the extent of cancer spread at the time of diagnosis. So long as the cancer is confined to the cervix, the prognosis is good. Treatment can effect a cure. Untreated, invasive, cervical cancer spreads from the cervix first to the upper part of the vagina, then to the ureters and lower part of the vagina. In the most advanced cases, invasion of the bladder wall and rectum may be evident at diagnosis. Such advanced disease is associated with a poor prognosis; only 10% of patients with advanced disease survive more than five years.

Natural history of cervical cancer

The importance of the cervical smear test is based on the knowledge that cervical cancer usually has a very long natural history. Identifiable pre-cancerous changes occur up to 10–15 years before invasive cancer develops. If these are identified and treated, cervical cancer can be prevented. As previously stated, most cases (around 90%) of cervical cancers originate at the squamo-epithelial junction. Such cancer is known technically as cervical squamous cell carcinoma. Many years before cervical cancer develops, microscopical changes to the squamous epithelial cells at the squamo-columnar junction occur. These changes are known as cervical intra-epithelial neoplasia (CIN). CIN is a potentially progressive lesion, usually associated with HPV infection, which may, if not treated, ultimately lead to cervical cancer. Three grades of severity of CIN have been identified. If the cellular changes which characterise CIN are confined to the lowest third of epithelium, a diagnosis of CIN I is made; if such changes are seen in the lower two-thirds, CIN II is diagnosed. The most severe form of CIN, CIN III, is diagnosed when atypical cells are seen throughout the full thickness of the epithelium; this is also called carcinoma *in situ*. The level of CIN determines the risk of invasive cervical cancer developing. For example patients with CIN I have a relatively low risk of cancer developing; in around 50% of cases the abnormality resolves spontaneously. However, CIN I may persist without any untoward effects, or, for an unpredictable small minority of patients, may progress through CIN II to CIN III. Around 30% of patients with CIN III if left untreated would progress to invasive cancer within ten years. At the present time there is no way of predicting with any certainty which patients with CIN will progress to invasive cancer, or how speedy that progression will be. All that can be said is that there is an increased risk of cervical cancer for women with CIN and that the risk is highest in those with CIN III. Treatment of CIN prevents cancer developing in nearly all cases.

The definitive diagnosis of CIN depends on microscopical examination of a piece of cervical tissue. However, the microscopical appearance of cells scraped from the surface of the cervix reflects the abnormalities which constitute CIN. This is the rationale for the cervical smear test as a screening test for prevention of cervical cancer.

Cervical screening

History

The cervical smear test is often referred to as the Pap smear test. This alternative name celebrates the research of George Papanicolaou, a Greek physician who worked in the United States. In the 1920s Papanicolaou first observed that cancerous cervical cells could be found in vaginal smears. To enhance the appearance of these cells he developed a staining technique using the Papanicolaou stain, which is used to this day to stain cervical smears. In the late 1940s Ayre demonstrated that scraping the surface of the cervix was a more reliable means of recovering cancerous cervical cells. He developed the Ayre's spatula for this purpose. At around this time, the concept of pre-cancerous disease of the cervix was introduced, allowing the rationale for the use of the cervical smear test to screen for early evidence of cervical cancer.

A screening programme using the cervical smear test was first introduced in the UK during 1964. However, the organisation of the scheme was not nationally co-ordinated and evolved in an *ad hoc* fashion. The result was that the scheme had much less impact in reducing the incidence of cervical cancer than expected. Experience of cervical screening in other European countries, particularly Denmark, Iceland, Sweden and Finland, demonstrated that a well organised scheme, in which all women at risk are regularly given a cervical smear test, can be successful. In these countries there has been a huge steady reduction in the incidence of cervical cancer from the time screening was introduced in the 1960s. In recognition of the relative failure of the *ad hoc* screening programme then in operation in the UK, a nationally co-ordinated cervical screening programme was introduced in 1988. With slight changes to the scheme in 1990, this is the scheme in operation today.

Organisation and success of cervical screening

The aim of the UK programme is to reduce the incidence of cervical cancer by performing a cervical smear on every woman between the age of 20 and 65 years at least every five years; in some areas women are screened every three years. The responsibility for cervical screening falls largely on the primary health care team. A computerised call and recall system organised by primary care workers (GPs, practice nurses and practice managers) ensures that every woman in the target population of each GP practice is offered a smear test. Full payment for smear testing is made to GPs if greater than 80% of their target population are screened. Before 1987 around 40% of women in the age range 20–65 years were being screened. With the introduction of the national screening programme in 1988 the coverage increased quickly. By 1994, 85% of the target population were being screened; this level of coverage has been maintained ever since. There is now evidence that this increased level of cervical smear testing is having the desired effect on the incidence of cervical cancer.[1] In England between 1971 and 1987 the annual incidence of invasive cervical cancer stayed fairly steady, fluctuating between 14 and 16 per 100 000 women (i.e. on average 3900 cases a year). Since 1990, however, the annual incidence has fallen steadily year on year; by 1995 the incidence was 10 per 100 000 women or 2900 new cases. The screening programme since 1987 has also had an effect on the number of deaths that are attributed to cervical cancer. From 1950 to 1987 mortality due to cervical cancer fell steadily at the rate of 1.5% every year. Since 1987 this rate of fall has trebled. In 1987, 1800 deaths in England were attributed to cervical cancer; in 1997 this number had fallen to 1150. An estimated 800 deaths in England were saved in 1997 by the cervical smear test.

THE CERVICAL SMEAR OR 'PAP' TEST

Around 80% of cervical smears are sampled in a primary care setting, most often by practice nurses.

PATIENT PREPARATION

The best time to take a cervical smear is mid-cycle to avoid contamination of the smear with menstrual blood. It is preferable to delay taking a smear for a few months following childbirth. The patient should be advised to avoid the use of vaginal creams and refrain from sexual intercourse for 24 hours before the test. Many women will be anxious, especially on the first occasion they attend for a smear, so that a calm reassuring manner is important. A brief explanation of the test will help to allay fears. Any effort made to reduce the tension or anxiety a woman might experience at the time of smear sampling will increase the chance of obtaining a suitable sample. Furthermore there is evidence to suggest that women who are dealt with in a sympathetic manner are more likely to reattend for future testing or further investigation if an abnormality is discovered.

'cont.'

'continued'

CERVICAL SAMPLING TECHNIQUE

The practical detail of collecting an adequate cervical smear is beyond the scope of this chapter but good technique is essential. A significant number of smears (up to 20% in some studies) are reported as inadequate in some way and have to be repeated. With expert technique acquired through training and experience, most inadequate or unsuitable smears are preventable.

The cervix must first be visualised by passing a vaginal speculum. The cervix must be well illuminated. The object is to sample cells from the squamo-columnar junction, so a smear should contain squamous epithelial cells as well as some endocervical cells and/or mucus derived from endocervical cells. Since the position of the squamo-columnar junction varies with age and parity, sampling technique must take account of these factors. Several sampling devices are routinely used. The endocervical brush and cotton-tipped swab are used to sample cells from the endocervical canal, whilst the Aylesbury spatula with its extended tip for insertion into the external os is used to sample cells from the transformation zone on the ectocervix. The full circumference of the transformation zone is sampled by rotating the spatula through 360°. The sample is transferred to a glass slide (pre-labelled with patient details), by spreading the material from both sides of the sampling device or devices evenly on to the glass slide. If more than one sampling device is used, sample material from both devices should be spread on to a single glass slide. It is vital that the cells in the sample be 'fixed' or preserved immediately. This is usually achieved by immersing the glass slide in 90% ethanol 'fixative' for 10–15 minutes. Spray fixative may be used. The slide is air dried and placed in a plastic slide box for transport to the laboratory. Alternatively slides can be transported in the fixative solution. If the smear is found to be inadequate or unsuitable in some way, the laboratory will request that the test be repeated. The most common reasons for having to repeat the test are

- inadequate number of epithelial cells due to
  - cervix not being scraped firmly enough
  - sample not completely transferred to glass slide
- no evidence that the squamo-columnar junction has been sampled (i.e. no endocervical cells, endocervical mucus or metaplastic cells seen)
- sample spread too thinly or too thickly on the glass slide

'cont.'

'continued'

- cells poorly preserved due to
  - ☐ sample being allowed to air dry before being 'fixed'
  - ☐ inadequate time in the fixative solution
- sample contaminated with, for example, blood, lubricant, spermicide, inflammatory exudate.

RESULTS OF SMEAR TEST

Around 90% of adequately collected smears are found on microscopical examination to be entirely normal and no further investigation, save recall in 3 or 5 years (depending on local policy), is necessary. The remaining 10% have some degree of abnormality ranging from the benign (the vast majority), through entirely curable pre-malignant disease (CIN) to invasive cancer. Only 1 in 1000 smears is found to show evidence of invasive cancer.

In the laboratory, cervical smears are stained with Papanicolaou stain and examined under the microscope. Having established that the smear is adequate, the main object of the examination is to search for the abnormal changes to epithelial cells associated with the pre-cancerous condition, CIN. These abnormal changes, which are known collectively as dyskaryosis (literally, abnormal nucleus), include an increase in the size of the nucleus compared with surrounding cytoplasm, along with irregularity in the shape and staining characteristics of the nucleus. There are three recognised grades of severity of dyskaryosis: mild, moderate and severe. In some cases only slight changes to the nucleus are present which may not be sufficient to warrant a report of even mild dyskaryosis; these are reported as 'borderline nuclear abnormalities'. The severity of dyskaryosis correlates to some degree with the level of CIN that might be expected if a tissue biopsy were examined. A report of a smear result from a patient with dyskaryosis would therefore usually include a prediction of the level of CIN. In broad terms CIN I would be predicted if mild dyskaryosis were present; CIN II or CIN III would be predicted if moderate dyskaryosis were present; and CIN III would be predicted if severe dyskaryosis were present. It is not possible to make a definitive diagnosis of CIN or invasive cervical cancer from examination of a cervical smear.

FOLLOW-UP OF ABNORMAL SMEARS

The cervical smear test is only a screening test; its value lies in its ability to exclude the 90% or so of women whose smear is negative. The severity of

'cont.'

'continued'

dyskaryosis found in an abnormal smear merely determines the next step in the diagnostic process. The majority of abnormal smears are either 'borderline nuclear abnormalities' or 'mild dyskaryosis'. There is a strong likelihood that these changes will regress to normal. However, there remains a slight risk that, over time, a pre-malignant lesion might develop. Such patients may require no treatment initially but, rather, more intensive monitoring. They might, for example, be advised to have a repeat smear test at three- or six-monthly intervals until the abnormality has resolved. For those whose smear shows signs of moderate or severe dyskaryosis, or mild dyskaryosis on two consecutive occasions, referral for colposcopy is indicated.

COLPOSCOPY

Colposcopy is usually a pain-free, outpatient diagnostic procedure in which the cervix is viewed directly through a specially modified microscope called a colposcope. A vaginal speculum is passed as for a cervical smear, and the cervix is 'painted' with acetic acid. Application of acetic acid turns CIN-affected tissue white. With a colposcope this area can be visualised and biopsied to determine the level of CIN or confirm the presence of micro-invasive cancer. The results of colposcopy and cervical tissue biopsy determine the treatment that may be offered. In the absence of invasive cancer, CIN can be treated in an outpatient setting by a variety of techniques which all involve the destruction (ablation) of abnormal tissue by extremes of heat (e.g. lasar vaporisation, cryotherapy, loop diathermy). Surgical excision (cone biopsy) may be necessary, and rarely, hysterectomy might be recommended in the absence of invasive disease. All patients who have been treated for CIN must be monitored for recurrence of disease. Instead of the normal 3- or 5-year interval between smears, such patients may be recalled every year for up to 10 years.

OTHER ABNORMALITIES IN A CERVICAL SMEAR

Microscopic examination of a cervical smear may reveal incidental genital tract infections. In such cases an inflammatory exudate (accumulation of dead and dying white cells recruited to fight the infection and other cellular debris) may be present in the cervical smear, obscuring normal epithelial cells. The epithelial cells themselves may show signs of very mild dyskaryosis during an inflammatory process. All these effects of infection may make it difficult to identify those changes in epithelial cells which are due to CIN, and a repeat sample may be requested.

'cont.'

'continued'

Specific infections that can be identified from microscopical examination of a cervical smear include

- Candida vaginitis (infection caused by the fungus (yeast) *candida albicans,* which results in a thick purulent vaginal discharge and severe itching). The organism itself can be seen in a cervical smear.
- Trichomoniasis (infection caused by the protozoon *Trichomonas vaginalis* which results in a thin watery discharge with an offensive smell. Symptoms include itchiness. The organism itself can be seen in cervical smears.
- Genital herpes (infection caused by the herpes simplex virus) gives rise to painful lesions (ulcers) on the genitalia. Recurrent infection (often asymptomatic) can result in chronic inflammatory disease of the cervix (cervicitis). The virus cannot be seen when examining a cervical smear, but virally infected cervical epithelial cells show characteristic changes which are evident on microscopical examination.
- Actinomycosis (infection caused by the bacterium, *Actinomyces israelii*). This organism is sometimes seen in cervical smears and is almost always associated with the use of a intrauterine contraceptive device (the coil). Infection can lead to pelvic inflammatory disease.
- Mention has already been made of the human papilloma virus (HPV) as a likely causative agent of cervical cancer. It is possible to see evidence of infection with this virus when examining a cervical smear. Epithelial cells infected with the virus have a particular appearance; such HPV-infected cells are called koilocytes.

Case history 21

Sally Turnbull is a 23-year-old mother of three who had her first cervical smear test five weeks ago. The report of the test arrived three weeks later and read 'borderline nuclear abnormalities'; it included the suggestion to repeat the test in six months' time. As soon as she received the appointment for the repeat test, Sally began to worry. She now telephones the surgery for a much earlier smear test booking, insisting, 'If I have cancer I want to know now, not wait for five months.'

(1) What do you understand the laboratory report to mean?
(2) What can you say to Sally to allay her fears?

Discussion of case history

(1) The principal objective of examining a cervical smear is to discover if the epithelial cells it contains show any signs of dyskaryosis (literally 'abnormal nucleus'). The nucleus of a dyskaryotic cell is typically larger than normal, occupying an increased volume of the cytoplasm. It is irregular in shape and staining characteristics. Dyskaryosis is a signal that the cervical epithelial tissue from which the cells have been sampled has CIN, a condition which may progress to cervical cancer. There are three grades of severity of dyskaryosis: mild, moderate and severe, which broadly correspond to the severity of CIN. If there are only very slight abnormal changes to the nucleus of epithelial cells, insufficient in magnitude to warrant them being labelled even mildly dyskaryotic, a report of 'borderline nuclear changes' is made.

(2) You can assure Sally that the smear showed no evidence that she has cancer. Whilst not normal, the changes seen in her smear are not uncommon; around 1 in 20 smears have such slight changes. You can say that in the majority of such cases the changes revert to normal over a period of months and that by the time of her next appointment it is quite likely that her smear will be entirely normal. However, she must know that there is a chance that the abnormality will persist and could, if ignored, progress slowly over many years to cancer. She should know that, if the abnormality does persist, cancer can be prevented and a 'cure' achieved by a simple outpatient procedure. It is important that women presenting for a routine cervical smear understand that the test is not a test for cancer but rather a test to detect a curable abnormality, CIN, which, if left untreated, might progress to cancer.

References

(1) Quinn M., Babb P., Jones J. & Allen E. (1999) Effect of screening on incidence and mortality from cancer of cervix in England: evaluation based on routinely collected statistics. *BMJ* **318**: 904–7.

(2) Austoker J. (1994) Screening for cervical cancer. *BMJ* **309**: 241–8.

Further reading

Bos A.B., van Ballegooijen M. & van Oortmarssen *et al.* (1997) Non-progression of cervical intraepithelial neoplasia from population-screening data. *Br. J. Cancer* **75**: 124–30.

Buntinx F. & Brouwers M. (1996) Relation between sampling device and detection of abnormality in cervical smears: a meta analysis of randomised and quasi-randomised trials. *BMJ* **313**: 1285–90.

Evans D., Hudson E., Brown C. *et al.* (1986) Terminology in gynaecological cytopathology: report of the Working Party of the British Society for Clinical Cytology. *J. Clin. Pathol.* **39**: 933–44.

Graham P. & Bromilow J. (1995) Cervical smear audit. *Practice Nurse* 7 June: 726–30.

Ibbotson T. & Wyke S. (1995) A review of cervical cancer and cervical screening: implications for nursing practice. *J. Adv. Nursing* **22**: 745–52.

McKie L. (1993) Women's views of the cervical smear test: implications for nursing practice – women who have not had a smear. *J. Adv. Nursing* **18**: 972–79.

McKie L. (1993) Women's views of the cervical smear test: implications for nursing practice – women who have had a smear. *J Adv. Nursing* **18**: 1228–34.

Mulvey V. (1997) The colposcopy clinic. *Practice Nurse* 4 April: 312–18.

Raffle A.E., Alden B. & Mackenzie E.F.D. (1995) Detection rates for abnormal cervical smears: what are we screening for? *Lancet* **345**: 1469–73.

Soutter W., deBarros Lopes A., Fletcher A. *et al.* (1997) Invasive cervical cancer after conservative therapy for cervical intraepithelial neoplasia. *Lancet* **349**: 978–80.

Index of tests

Index